MENTAL DISORDERS IN OLDER ADULTS

Mental Disorders in Older Adults

FUNDAMENTALS OF ASSESSMENT AND TREATMENT

Second Edition

Steven H. Zarit
Judy M. Zarit

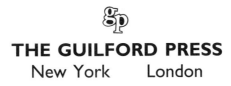

THE GUILFORD PRESS
New York   London

Library of Congress Cataloging-in-Publication Data
Zarit, Steven H.
  Mental disorders in older adults : fundamentals of assessment and treatment / by
Steven H. Zarit, Judy M. Zarit.—2nd ed.
     p. ; cm.
  Includes bibliographical references and index.
  ISBN 978-1-57230-946-3 (hardcover : alk. paper)
  ISBN 978-1-60918-232-8 (paperback : alk. paper)
    1. Older people—Mental health. 2. Older people—Psychology.   3. Mentally ill
people.   4. Geriatric psychology.   I. Zarit, Judy M.   II. Title.
    [DNLM: 1. Mental Disorders—diagnosis.   2. Aged.   3. Aging—
psychology.   4. Mental Disorders—therapy. WT 150 Z37m 2006]
    RC451.4.A5Z374 2006
    618.97′689—dc22   2006009239

For our parents—
Sara R. and Albert Zarit
Avis E. and Laurence A. Maes

About the Authors

Steven H. Zarit, PhD, is Professor and Head of the Department of Human Development and Family Studies at Pennsylvania State University, and is also Adjunct Professor at the Institute of Gerontology, Jönköping University, Jönköping, Sweden. He has conducted research on late-life issues, particularly family caregiving and adaptation for older adults.

Judy M. Zarit, PhD, has been in private practice in State College, Pennsylvania, since 1986. She specializes in neuropsychological assessment of dementia and clinical interventions with older adults. Dr. Zarit also provides consultation services to nursing homes and assisted-living facilities.

Acknowledgments

Many people have contributed to the development of this book. At The Guilford Press, Kitty Moore gave encouragement throughout and waited patiently when the project ran into delays, Sarah Lavender Smith provided insightful critiques of the manuscript, and Laura Specht Patchkofsky made the production process go smoothly. Donna Ballock provided valuable assistance with references and manuscript preparation.

Judy thanks her colleagues at Centre Psychology Group—Robert A. Franz, Leta F. Myers, and Lisa Young—who provided insights on difficult cases, and especially Michael M. Kiel, who helped us take a fresh look at geriatric neuropsychological assessment.

Steven thanks his colleagues in the Department of Human Development and Family Studies at Pennsylvania State University for sustaining a collaborative and intellectually stimulating environment. The many talented students with whom he has worked over the years have made valuable contributions to the ideas expressed here. Steven especially thanks Julie Bach, Adam Davey, Anne Edwards, Elizabeth Fauth, Elia Femia, Joseph Gaugler, Caryn Goodman, Shannon Jarrott, Sara Leitsch, Eileen Malone-Beach, Nancy Orr-Rainey, Suzanne Robertson, Victoria Steiner, and Carol Whitlatch. Steven's research has been enriched through collaborations with several people—Karen Fingerman, Rick Greene, Leonard Pearlin, Mary Ann Stephens, and Aloen Townsend. Through international collaborations, he has been able to develop new perspectives on aging, and would like particularly to acknowledge Yumiko Arai, Stig Berg, Murna Downs, Jamuna Duvuru, Boo Johansson, Yolande Kuin, Bo Malmberg, Anne Margriet Pot, and Gerdt Sundström.

Finally, we thank our children—Michael Weston, Thomas Weston, Jessica Sidman, Benjamin Zarit, Megan Manly, and Matthew Zarit—who continuously amaze and inspire us with their accomplishments.

Contents

CHAPTER 1

Introduction
CLINICAL PRACTICE WITH OLDER ADULTS

We have written this book for clinicians and clinical students interested in working with older people and their families, as well as for researchers seeking an overview of assessment and treatment of mental disorders in later life. The book provides a foundation for practice with older adults and addresses the most common problems clinicians are likely to encounter.

Colleagues of ours who do not see older adults in their practice often ask us if work with the elderly is boring. Quite the opposite! Clinical practice with older adults is intellectually challenging and rewarding. The rewards come in many ways. As with people of other ages, older adults can change and recover from problems such as depression or anxiety or can take control of their lives in ways that lead to greater personal fulfillment. In other cases, treatment can keep a bad situation from becoming worse. Assessment plays a prominent role in practice with older adults, because any particular symptom or problem may arise from several possible causes. We always feel a great sense of satisfaction when we can identify a treatable problem in someone who was considered "hopelessly senile," but even when we can only confirm bad news, we can provide the patient and family with knowledge about the problem and the opportunity to plan for future needs.

The book integrates clinical practice and research. A common complaint among practitioners is how frustrating it is to try to apply research findings that are based on standard protocols developed in university settings. In clinics and private practices, clients do not neatly conform to these standards, nor do they generally present with a single problem that meets the research requirements. At the same time, practice needs to be informed and guided by

1

research so that the best methods of assessment and treatment are used and so that insights into the aging process from basic research can be incorporated into our view of older people. We have backgrounds in both research and practice with older people and currently work in settings that emphasize these areas differently. One of us (SHZ) is in a primarily research and academic setting, and the other (JMZ) has 25 years of experience in private practice and as a consultant to nursing homes and retirement communities. We believe that the combination of these perspectives helps us integrate our discussions of research in a practical clinical context, while basing clinical approaches to the extent possible on a solid underpinning of empirical knowledge.

We draw heavily on our own professional training in clinical psychology, but we intend this book for all the mental health professions that work with older people. We emphasize psychosocial perspectives and expect the book to be most useful to psychologists, social workers, nurses, and gerontologists. Psychiatrists and geriatricians may also find the presentation of behavioral and neuropsychological perspectives a useful complement to their biomedical approaches.

An underlying assumption of our approach is that several professional groups can make valuable contributions to mental health care for the elderly. Clinical practice is best carried out in a context of multidisciplinary collaboration, with each field contributing its special expertise. The need for a multidisciplinary approach grows out of an understanding of mental health problems in later life. Medical, psychological, and social processes are frequently intertwined in later life, and an exclusive focus on one area to the neglect of the others can be detrimental. A major theme of this book is how to think about these interactions when conducting an assessment or treating an older person. As an example, a primarily medical approach to Alzheimer's disease (AD) can miss opportunities for behavioral or psychosocial treatment. These treatments can help patients with AD function optimally despite their disease: for example, by simplifying their environment and routines or by using behavioral management skills to control problems such as agitation or depressed mood. Conversely, an exclusively behavioral approach would overlook the potential benefits of medications in the management of disturbed behavior in dementia. Collaboration across disciplines makes it more likely that effective interventions will be identified, whether medical, psychological, social, or environmental.

One of our goals is to provide nonphysicians with information on illnesses and use of medications in later life. By understanding the effects of medical illnesses on psychological problems in later life and the uses and limits of psychoactive medications, the mental health professional can be a more effective collaborator with physicians. Nonphysicians should not, of course, give medical advice to their patients, but they can make assessments and observations that enable physicians to formulate better treatment choices. In the current health care climate, the physician's time is at a premium. By contrast, mental health professionals are often able to spend the time needed with patients to assess their symptoms and responses to medications, as well as to identify the best strategies for working with them. Development of collaborative relationships with physicians depends on establishing expertise in aging and mental health and in communicating findings in a succinct and jargon-free manner. Our experience shows that once physicians understand what information we can provide and how we can enhance treatment, barriers between professions fade away.

EMERGENCE OF AGING
IN MENTAL HEALTH PRACTICE

For many years, geriatric practice was a backwater, a minor field viewed condescendingly by clinicians who felt that little could be done for anyone over age 50. That viewpoint was a luxury of a society that had relatively few older people. The dramatic extension of life expectancy and growth in the proportion of people over age 65 in society, coupled with empirical findings of the effectiveness of treatment for many problems of later life, provides a solid foundation for geriatric mental health practice. The number of clinicians with geriatric expertise, however, falls far short of the need.

The aging of the population is one of the most profound and far-reaching changes affecting contemporary society. The number and proportion of older people in the population has grown dramatically in most developed countries and, more recently, in many developing nations. Among all the changes that occurred in the 20th century, one of the most profound and far-reaching was the dramatic increase in life expectancy. Throughout human history, only a very small part of the population enjoyed long life. Most people died young as a result of acute illness, injury, the effects of contaminated food or water, or, for women, from complications of childbirth. Improvements made at the beginning of the 20th century in public health and control of infectious diseases had a dramatic effect on the prospect of living to old age. Between 1900 and 2000, average life expectancy in the United States rose from 46 to 74 years for men and from 49 to 80 years for women (U.S. Census Bureau, 2003). The combined influence of greater life expectancy and smaller family size has led to growth in the proportion of people 65 and older in the population. As seen in Figure 1.1, only 4% of the population of the United States was 65 years of age or older in 1900. That figure rose to 12.3% in 2000 and is projected to increase to 20% by the year 2030 (Treas, 1995; U.S. Department of Health and Human Services, 2003). Canada and many of the European countries have experienced similar patterns of growth in their older populations (Kinsella & Velkoff, 2001). With so much of the population over age 65, mental health professionals with the expertise to assess and treat the problems of later life are sorely needed.

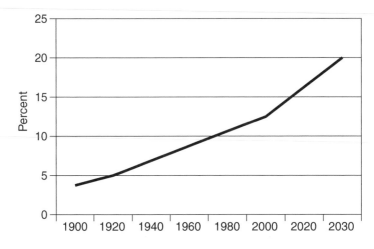

FIGURE 1.1. Proportion of the U.S. population ages 65 and older: 1900–2030. Data from U.S. Census Bureau (2003).

These demographic and social changes mean that an increasing number of older people are in need of psychological services. The mental health field, however, has been slow to respond with adequate numbers of trained professionals who have specialized training in geriatrics. Estimates from the United States indicate that in every mental health field—psychiatry, psychology, nursing, and social work—too few people currently have geriatrics training (Halpain, Harris, McClure, & Jeste, 1999; Shea, 2003). Shea (2003), for example, estimates the current need as an additional 2,400 psychiatrists, 2,800 psychologists, and 3,750 nurses with geriatrics training, as well as an indeterminate number of social workers. The failure to develop enough programs that provide specialized training in psychology, nursing, and social work will exacerbate the shortfall just as the baby-boom generation increases the number of older people dramatically.

The need for trained professionals comes at a time when steadily growing knowledge about the aging process and clinical problems of aging make research and practice with older people exciting and challenging. Studies of normal psychological and social processes of aging have challenged many negative stereotypes. In contrast to the image of older people as decrepit and depressed, studies repeatedly have demonstrated that older people are often competent and enjoy their lives (Carstensen, Pasupathi, Mayr, & Nesselroade, 2000; Rowe & Kahn, 1987, 1997). The aging process is characterized by the possibility of growth, as well as decline (e.g., Baltes, 1987, 1997). Many abilities once thought to undergo significant decline during the adult years, such as memory and intelligence, now appear to be stable on average or even to improve in some individuals until the 60s or 70s (Schaie, 1995). Dementia, depression, and other serious disorders typically identified with later life affect only a minority of the population and are not intrinsic or universal aspects of the aging process.

This optimistic picture of aging is reflected in the daily lives of older people. People are not just living longer; they are living *better* longer than ever before in human history. The prospect for successful aging, that is, for older people to lead healthy, active, and fulfilling lives, has become a real possibility (Rowe & Kahn, 1987, 1997). Improvements in disease prevention and health promotion, the widespread availability of public and private pensions and other financial benefits, and increased educational opportunities for each successive generation have dramatically improved the lives of today's older population. The next generation of older people will have had better education and have taken better care of their health across the lifespan, so their prospects for successful old age are even greater.

Successful aging is only part of the picture of later life. The increase in life expectancy means that people are more likely to live until their 70s, 80s, or even 90s, ages at which a variety of chronic illnesses and disabilities become common. Along with unprecedented numbers of vital and active old people, we have seen a dramatic increase in elders with significant mental and physical problems (e.g., Zarit, Johansson, & Malmberg, 1995). Their complex problems are costly for society and often overwhelming for their families. The dual existence of unprecedented numbers of successful agers and those with significant need is a key point for understanding old age.

Fortunately, timely and well-conceived clinical interventions can make a difference. Many older people retain resiliency and can respond positively to mental health interventions. A growing body of research documents the effectiveness of psychotherapy with older people and their families (Gatz et al., 1998). For disorders such as depression, response to treatment may be as good for older as for younger people (Scogin & McElreath, 1994). Even when confronted with the most devastating problems in later life, such as AD, clinicians can make interventions that dramatically improve the situation (e.g., Mittelman et al., 1995; Whitlatch, Zarit, & von Eye, 1991). Opportunities are emerging to design prevention programs for disorders such as depression and anxiety and to develop strategies for promoting health, as well as intellectual and functional competency, thus helping to make old age a productive and fulfilling period of life.

Older people themselves are increasingly turning to mental health professionals for help with their problems. In the past, clinicians often remarked that older people were not interested in psychotherapy. Indeed, when we first began our practices, we found that some older clients were reluctant or embarrassed to visit a psychologist. Increasingly, however, our older clients view psychotherapy positively. Some have been in treatment earlier in their lives and do not feel the stigma associated with seeing a therapist that typified previous generations. This trend is likely to increase with future generations.

The cohort of people currently in their 40s and 50s who are now consulting us about their parents will have even fewer inhibitions about seeking out appropriate mental health treatment for themselves when they are older.

One other major factor in the growth of clinical practice with older people in the United States is the inclusion of outpatient mental health treatment in Medicare. When Medicare was first implemented in 1965, it paid only for inpatient psychiatric treatment. Beginning in the late 1980s, however, coverage was extended to mental health services in outpatient settings and in nursing homes and other institutional settings. Although Medicare currently reimburses differently for outpatient mental health care than for other medical problems (50% of usual costs are covered, compared with 80% for most other treatments), a major financial obstacle to seeking treatment has been reduced. Increasingly, older people and their families are taking advantage of the options for mental health treatment available to them.

PURPOSE AND PLAN FOR THIS BOOK

We have written this book for the student who is exploring geriatric mental health for the first time, for the experienced professional who wants to learn the specialized knowledge and skills that are needed for meeting the growing needs of an aging population, and for the researcher wanting a broad foundation in clinical concepts and approaches. With knowledge in geriatric mental health rapidly expanding, we have chosen to emphasize some topics and not others.

Our decisions were guided by three considerations. First, we wanted to write a concise introduction that provides clinicians and students with the basic knowledge and framework necessary to begin practice with older adults. The book covers the topics recommended in guidelines for practice with older adults developed by the American Psychological Association (2004). We could have gone into greater depth on many topics, but instead we have chosen to present a foundation for each area while providing references for readers wishing to pursue an issue in greater depth. By organizing the book in this way, we believe we have created a practical introduction to clinical work with older adults. Second, we have been guided by the fact that clinical practice with older people is both similar to and different from practice with other adults. To be successful in assessing and treating older adults, clinicians need a combination of basic clinical skills that they might use with any adult client, combined with specialized knowledge about what is different about disorders in later life and when and how clinicians need to use different strategies in their clinical work with an older adult. In this book, we emphasize the issues and topics that are different in geriatric practice, topics that are usually not covered in clinical training. Third, we integrate research findings with our clinical experience. This will be most evident in discussions of treatment, in which we present findings about empirically validated treatment but also discuss approaches developed by JMZ through clinical experience. These examples illustrate different ways of implementing validated approaches, as well as treatment of problems on which there is as yet little empirical evidence. Each therapist will develop a unique style, and so these approaches are meant to be illustrative rather than a definitive blueprint for treatment.

Throughout, we use clinical examples to illustrate key points. These are drawn mainly from JMZ's clinical practice, with names and details changed to ensure confidentiality. As a stylistic note, because the clinical work was done by one person, we use the first-person pronouns "I" and "me" in all the examples.

What constitutes the basic knowledge needed for practice with older adults? We believe the starting point is being able to recognize when a client is suffering from one of the common disorders of aging. Assessment is important when working with people of any age, but it takes on an even more prominent role in practice with older adults. Given the negative stereotypes of and expectations for older people, the tendency exists to mislabel potentially treatable problems as irreversible aspects of age or disease. Geriatric mental health specialists must be able to make sophisticated assessments of symptoms, which, in conjunction with medical assessments, help differentiate between mild, everyday problems and the more pathological processes due to disorders such as AD.

Three main components contribute to assessment: (1) an understanding of the normal changes that occur with aging, (2) knowledge of the characteristics of the most common disorders in later life, and (3) familiarity with assessment approaches. In Chapter 2, we present an overview of the normal psychological processes of aging and summarize the usual and expected changes in intellectual functioning, memory, personality, and other areas. Knowing what is usual and expected is helpful for setting goals in treatment and for comparing findings from a clinical assessment to determine whether an individual has a problem that needs to be treated.

The next three chapters address the problems and disorders of later life. Chapter 3 focuses on disorders that impair cognition—dementia and delirium—and reviews their symptoms, prevalence, and etiology. Chapter 4 addresses the affective disorders—specifically, depression and anxiety. These are the most common psychiatric disorders in later life and also the ones for which the most treatment options exist. In Chapter 5, we look at the most disabling of the psychiatric diagnoses: personality and psychotic disorders. Although most cases of these disorders have their onset in earlier periods of life, they often continue to exert a major influence on older people and their support networks.

Building on this foundation, we move to methods for assessing older people, emphasizing approaches for differentiating dementia from other disorders. This is the most common assessment question that is raised and one that must be clearly answered before developing a treatment plan. Chapter 6 describes how to conduct a clinical interview, including the goals and process of the interview, topics to address, and brief testing. Chapter 7 focuses on psychological testing. We include examples of the tests used and how the results of testing contribute to determining diagnosis and competency.

Chapters 8 through 14 address treatment, with an emphasis on issues in treatment that are different or unique in practice with older people. Treatment of older people with mental health problems requires a multifaceted approach. Clinicians need to draw on basic skills of psychotherapy, to coordinate psychological with psychiatric and other medical treatment, and to intervene at different levels—that is, with patients, with patients' families, with community agencies that provide supportive services, and with nursing homes and other residential settings.

We begin the discussion of treatment in Chapter 8 by exploring basic concepts and approaches that underlie successful treatment of older people and by examining differences and similarities in treatment of older clients. Chapter 9 applies this framework to treatment of depressive disorders, and Chapter 10 takes a similar approach with anxiety disorders.

Chapter 11 turns to the problem of paranoid disorders in later life, when treatment is typically different from that for younger patients. Chapter 12 focuses on the treatment of people with dementia, including new medications and psychosocial interventions that help people function as well as possible despite their illness. In Chapter 13, we broaden the focus on treatment to include caregivers—the families of people with dementia and other serious disabilities. We examine the burden experienced by family caregivers and present treatments that alleviate stress.

Chapter 14 discusses the nursing home as a system and presents approaches for successful intervention. Nursing homes and other special housing are very important settings for mental health interventions. Many residents in nursing homes have mental health problems that often go undetected and untreated (e.g., Burns et al., 1993; German, Shapiro, & Kramer, 1986; Shea, Streit, & Smyer, 1994). Increasingly, mental health professionals are being called on to consult in nursing homes and other institutional settings. Clinicians working in these settings need to call on their knowledge of assessment and treatment approaches for older adults, as well as understand how to solve problems within a complex system.

We conclude in Chapter 15 with a discussion of ethical issues. Familiar ethical issues, such as maintaining confidentiality, take on a new twist when working with older adults, particularly when family members are involved or when the person lives in an institution. Some issues are more complicated in later life, such as how to assess consent for treatment when someone is cognitively impaired and making end-of-life decisions.

Working with older people is intellectually challenging and personally rewarding. Older clients often pose complex and varied assessment questions, which need to be addressed by integrating medical, psychological, social, and sometimes legal information. Treating an older person is sometimes like opening a window to the past. Our clients have lived through major historical events and have personally met many great figures of the past century. Unlike young adults, who often have limited experience and may lack basic practical skills for managing everyday life, our older clients can draw on a lifetime of adaptation, bringing it to bear on their current situation. In the end, we have always found that we can make a difference in the lives of older people and their families, and that is gratifying.

CHAPTER 2

Normal Processes of Aging

A familiarity with the characteristics of the older population and the changes that occur in functioning with normal aging can help clinicians differentiate the disorders that occur in later life. Knowing, for example, which patterns of intellectual performance are normal and expected and which suggest early changes associated with dementia is a basic component of practice.

HEALTHY AGING

I first met Margaret when she was living in a nursing home with her second husband, John. She came to the lobby to meet me, impeccably dressed in a silk blouse, skirt, and polished black pumps. Her hair was carefully arranged, and she appeared to be about 80 years old. She had asked to see a psychologist because she was having trouble controlling her temper when John's behavior disturbed her. He had a long history of cardiac problems, as well as Parkinson's disease, but he also was moderately demented. He was forgetful and at times incontinent. Margaret was very fastidious, and the incontinence incidents were quite upsetting to her, particularly when the staff did not respond to John's call in a timely way.

In the first interview I was astonished to learn that Margaret was, in fact, 94 years old. Nothing about her appearance, speech, or bearing gave the slightest indication that she was that old. She had only modest health problems and took minimal medications, an antihypertensive and multivitamins.

Margaret was the only child of older parents. She had studied nutrition at a small women's college and worked for several years as a dietician in a hospital. When she was in her late 20s, she met her first husband, Charles, and they lived together in a happy marriage for 40 years. They were not able to have children, but they spent much time with nieces and nephews. When Charles retired, they moved to Florida, where they spent about 10 good years until Charles became ill with cancer and ultimately died.

A few years later, Margaret met John, who was also recently widowed. They married and spent 22 years together. They traveled around the world and enjoyed a comfortable lifestyle, as both had good retirement incomes. When they reached the age of 90, they moved into a retirement community, anticipating that one or both might need assistance. When John first began requiring nursing care, he moved by himself into the nursing home. But he missed Margaret, so when a suite became available, they moved into it.

Margaret found herself in an unusual situation in the nursing home. She was perfectly well but living in a facility in which the only people she could relate to were the staff members. The staff became very attached to her, largely because of her gracious manners and ladylike appearance.

During the 6 months that she lived in the nursing home with John, Margaret used psychotherapy in sessions with me as a safe place to air her complaints about the staff, the food, and John's behavior. This served as a safety valve for her, so that her frustration would not build up and lead to aggressive behavior toward John, which she admitted fantasizing about. And it allowed her to meet an important goal: to be with John when he died. After his death, Margaret initially thought she would need only a few sessions to work through her grief. She moved into assisted living, because she no longer wanted to prepare meals for herself and she was comforted to know that staff members were around if she needed them.

Therapy became very important for Margaret. The sessions were the one situation in which she could be completely honest about how she felt and in which she could know that what she said was confidential. She was aware that life within the retirement community was much like living in a small town; everyone was curious about other people's business. At 94, Margaret had outlived all of the people she used to confide in. Now we meet weekly, and she looks forward to it as the high point of her week. She has had some small strokes (transient ischemic attacks) and is more aware than ever of how little time she has left. Margaret discusses the arrangements she wants to make for the changes she sees coming with clear eyes and a strong heart.

This example illustrates the possibility for healthy aging even at a very advanced age. Most older people report that they lead independent and satisfying lives and do not seem to experience as many stressful or distressing times as do younger people (Charles, Mather, & Carstensen, 2003; Mroczek & Kolarz, 1998). Older people today are healthier and wealthier than any previous generation has been. Through a lifetime of learning, they have developed strategies that help them manage the ups and downs of daily life.

Of course, there is another side to aging that appears in Margaret's story as well: the possibility of decline and deterioration. The aging process is characterized by this duality of successful aging and decline. Some people grow old gracefully, whereas others encounter setbacks and problems that lead to a deterioration in functioning. The tension between these positive and negative aspects of aging forms the foundation of mental health practice. For many older clients, clinical interventions can facilitate growth and overcome barriers to successful aging. When irreversible illnesses and other problems occur, clinicians can play an equally valuable role in containing the consequences of decline and in helping older people and their families cope effectively with illness and disability.

Using a lifespan perspective is important in understanding aging. People do not suddenly change when they reach a certain age, whether 65, 75, or older. Instead, the aging process is characterized largely by continuity. People remain recognizably similar over time. Changes tend to be gradual and, as is discussed, sometimes involve growth, as well as decline. People who have functioned well all their lives generally will continue to do so in old age. Conversely, someone who has always had emotional or personal problems will continue to struggle with those issues in old age. Aging, in other words, makes us neither wise nor foolish nor neurotic. Rather, people's personal histories, their life experiences and social circumstances, as well as broader generational and historical influences, affect the outcomes that we see in old age. When a sudden downward course occurs, often it is related to a specific cause. This lifespan perspective helps differentiate between long-standing patterns of adaptation and those more catastrophic events that disrupt the continuity of normal aging and lead to decline.

A lifespan perspective also allows the therapist to view an older person's current problems in the context of a lifetime of experiences and learning. These past experiences can provide information both about the origins of current problems and resources for their solution. In this chapter, we begin by reviewing the social characteristics of the older population. We then examine lifespan and life-course models of aging and conceptual issues that are critical for understanding how we age. We then consider psychological processes of aging in several domains, including intelligence, memory, personality, and emotions.

CHARACTERISTICS OF THE OLDER POPULATION

As a result of the improved life expectancy described in Chapter 1, old age has become for the first time in human history an expected rather than an exceptional part of the lifespan. What is this population of older people like? We describe the older population along several dimensions, including their social characteristics, health and functioning, and financial status. Each of these areas can play a role in assessment and treatment.

The majority of older people are women. Among people 65 and older, there are 70 men for every 100 women, and this discrepancy increases to 46 men for every 100 women by age 85 (U.S. Department of Health and Human Services, 2003). In the United States, life expectancy for women is currently a fraction short of 80 years, compared with 74 years for men (U.S. Census Bureau, 2003). Because of their greater longevity, women outlive their husbands, who, on average, are older than they are. About three-quarters of older men are married, compared with only 43% of older women (U.S. Census Bureau, 1998). Women who are widowed are also less likely than men to remarry (Treas, 1995).

These trends play out in important ways. When one person in a married couple becomes ill or disabled, the spouse is likely to take on caregiving responsibility. Being younger, on average, than their husbands, women more often take on this responsibility. Older women who outlive their husbands must depend on children or other relatives if they need assistance.

One of the most important social changes is that the racial and ethnic makeup of the older population is becoming more varied (Hobbs & Damon, 1996). In the United States, for example, the proportion of white non-Hispanic elders will drop from 85 to 67% by the year 2050. The biggest growth will occur among people of Hispanic origin. The proportion of Hispanics who are 65 and older will more than triple, to 16%. Other minority groups will show similar growth. African Americans will increase from 8 to 10% of the older population, and other groups (including Asian, Pacific Islanders, American Indians, Eskimos, and Aleuts) will increase from 2 to 8%. This growing diversity means that therapists need to understand a more varied range of cultural beliefs and practices and the roles that older people from different ethnic groups play in their families and communities.

Despite this projected growth, minorities continue to have a lower life expectancy than the non-Hispanic white population in the United States. As an example, life expectancies at birth for African Americans in the United States are 7 years less than whites for men and 5 years less for women (U.S. Census Bureau, 2003). The exception is Asian Americans, who have a slightly greater life expectancy than the white population (U.S. Census Bureau, 2003).

Another important trend is that the number of people at very advanced ages, 80 and older, is growing faster than any other age group in the population (Hetzel & Smith, 2001; Hobbs & Damon, 1996). Bernice Neugarten (1974), one of the pioneers in the study of aging, was one of the first people to notice the increase in very old people and how they differed from the rest of the elderly population. She proposed differentiating between the "young old" and "old old." According to Neugarten, the prevailing stereotype of older people as dependent, depressed, and possibly demented was incorrect. Rather, with improved health care and health promotion, older people were functioning better than ever before. She described the "young old," defined roughly as people between the ages of 55 and 75, as leading independent and active lives that differed little from those of middle-aged persons. In contrast, due to increasing rates of illness and disability with advancing age, people 75 and older were more likely to have chronic illnesses that limited their functioning. Neugarten characterized this group as the "old old." She also stressed that these categories were not tied rigidly to chronological age but represented normative patterns of functioning within the older population. It is possible that a person in his or her 60s might have disabilities typical of an 80-year-old, whereas an 80-year-old may be relatively free from impairment. As the number of people reaching very late life has increased, an additional category has been proposed—the oldest old—consisting of people 85 and older. These distinctions call attention to the fact that the large group of people we call "old" are quite diverse in their functioning. It is also possible that people living to advanced ages may develop new psychological perspectives and new patterns of adaptation even as they cope with disability and the nearness of death (Johnson & Barer, 1997).

Healthy Aging and the Compression of Morbidity

These population trends illustrate the two sides of aging. On the one hand, the number of healthy older people who are able to function at high levels is increasing; on the other hand, individuals living to advanced ages at which disease and disability are endemic are also becoming more common.

These trends have spawned a controversy about the significance of improved health and increased life expectancy in today's older population. Fries (1983) has proposed an optimistic theory, called "compression of morbidity." According to Fries, increased life expectancy is pushing up against a genetically determined maximum in the human lifespan. Improvements in health care and lifestyle changes in nutrition and exercise mean that people will be able to live healthier lives for a longer period of time, and then will have only a short period of decline at the end of life. Some evidence suggests that rates of disability are decreasing (e.g., Schoeni, Freedman & Wallace, 2001). Other researchers, however, have taken the position that both life expectancy and the length of morbidity at the end of life are increasing (e.g., Cassel, Rudberg, & Olshansky, 1992; Verbrugge, 1984). These investigators believe that people have longer, healthier lives *and* a protracted period of disability at the end of life. This debate has critical implications for the amount of health care and other supportive services that will be needed for the older population, particularly as the number of oldest old grows.

Regardless of how this debate turns out, we can draw some general conclusions about the individual lifespan. For most people, old age includes a period in which they are relatively healthy, active, and independent— Neugarten's "young old" period—followed by a period of decline prior to death. Whether or not the period of morbidity has been compressed at a population level, if we look at the individual level, we see that it can last for varying amounts of time, from a very brief decline prior to death to a span of 20 years or more. Put another way, most people will need help at some time during their old age.

Where Older People Live

Consistent with the portrait of the older population as predominantly healthy, the vast majority of older people live independently. Most live alone or with spouses (Treas, 1995). A relatively small proportion of older people—10%— live with adult children (Treas, 1995). Only 4.5% live in nursing homes (Hetzel & Smith, 2001). That figure, however, is a bit deceiving. It does not reflect the growing number of people in assisted living facilities, where they may receive similar amounts of assistance with activities of daily living as they would in nursing homes. It also indicates only how many people reside in nursing homes at any one time. For many people, nursing home stays are brief, resulting in discharge or death. As a result, the lifetime risk of spending some time in a nursing home is much higher—43% (Kemper & Murtaugh, 1991).

Education, Income, and Employment

Over the past 40 years, the successive cohorts of older people have been better educated and wealthier than prior generations. Most older people today have completed high school, and nearly 20% have completed college (Smith, 2003). Future generations of elders will have even more education.

The economic position of older people has also improved. Poverty among older people was once endemic in many countries, but passage of universal pension programs such as Social Security and the development of workplace pensions produced dramatic improvements in their financial situations. Indexing Social Security benefits to the cost of living, which was done in the early 1970s, brought about a steady decline in the number of older people living in poverty. As a result, only 10% of elderly people in the United States now live in poverty (Smith, 2003). This success has not been matched among the other vulnerable segment of the population, children, who are nearly twice as likely to live in poverty as older people (Lee & Haaga, 2002).

Although the overall financial picture for older people is positive, not everyone is well off. Many older people are considered "near poor," that is, with income levels between 100 and 125% of federal poverty levels. Those figures work out to $9,750 to $12,187 annually for households with one person and between $12,830 and $16,037 annually for two-person households (U.S. Department of Health and Human Services, 2003). These individuals barely get by on their income and can have considerable trouble meeting unexpected expenses, particularly health care costs not covered by insurance. Poverty rates also remain high in some segments of the minority elderly population and among women and people over age 80. Finally, although people may retire in a good financial situation, long life and, particularly, health care and long-term care costs can eat away their resources. It has been estimated that nearly one-half of the older population faces the risk of becoming poor or near poor before they die (Rank & Hirschl, 1999). In other words, although the overall situation for older people is positive, the threat of poverty lingers. Economic adversity can contribute to depression and other mental health problems, as well as limit people's ability to get the medical and mental health treatment that they need.

Employment is a potential source of income for older people, as well as an opportunity for meaningful engagement. A relatively small proportion of older people are in the workforce: 18% of men and 10% of women (Smith, 2003). Although this number has been decreasing since the 1950s (Treas, 1995), we may soon begin to see a reversal. One factor that may lead to increased labor force participation is the elimination of mandatory retirement for most occupations. As a result, people who want to work now have the opportunity to do so. There are also economic benefits of continued employment, both in terms of the income that older people receive and the broader social benefits. Many of the dire predictions about the current Social Security system are based on the assumption that most older people will retire completely from the workforce. The large baby-boom cohort, which will begin reaching age 65 in 2011, is followed by smaller birth cohorts. That means that there will potentially be fewer adults in the period traditionally considered working age (18–65) supporting a larger number of retirees. Increased workforce participation by older people, however, could reduce pressure on Social Security and also address projected shortfalls of workers in some occupations.

LIFESPAN DEVELOPMENTAL PERSPECTIVE ON AGING

We now examine psychological changes that occur with normal aging, beginning with basic concepts and research strategies for understanding the aging process. We then consider four central areas of psychological functioning: intelligence, memory, personality, and well-being.

Studying the Aging Process

Clinicians working with older people need to know how to evaluate new information presented about the aging process. The media and even scientific journals present a constant and often conflicting parade of new findings about old age. What should we tell our clients when they ask such questions as whether doing crossword puzzles will prevent AD? (Probably not, but keeping mentally active can help with everyday functioning.)

In many ways, late life is a more complicated developmental period to study than any other. In studying aging, we are typically trying to make comparisons over long periods of time. A developmental study of children might focus on the patterns of changes from ages 2 to 4. Following a sample of children over 2 years is a relatively manageable task. When studying aging, however, we often focus on much longer time periods. If we ask how aging might affect memory in a group of 70-year-olds, we are interested in comparing their current abilities with what they were like in the past, perhaps 30 or 40 years earlier. Conducting research that spans the whole of adulthood is beyond the capability of most researchers, though a few unique studies have done just that (e.g., Elder, Shanahan, & Clipp, 1994; Schaie, 2005; Vaillant & Vaillant, 1990).

The most common way of addressing this problem is to use a cross-sectional design. This design is illustrated in Figure 2.1. In a cross-sectional study, samples of younger and older individuals are tested at one point in time (e.g., the year 1990) and compared with each other.

A cross-sectional study provides practical information on "age differences," that is, how older and younger people differ from each other. An age difference may be due to the aging process, but two other factors might have also played a role: generational differences and historical influences. Consider this hypothetical example. A study compared the spending habits of college sophomores and people age 75 and older and found that the older people are more frugal and less willing to run up credit card debt. One possible explana-

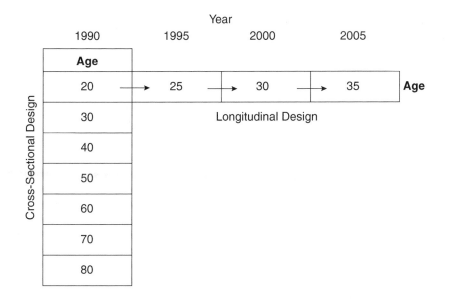

FIGURE 2.1. Cross-sectional and longitudinal research designs.

tion is that people become more careful with their money as they age. Indeed, there are many proverbs and sayings about frugal or stingy older people. But there are other explanations for this difference. Attitudes about money may be the result of generational influences, or what is referred to as "cohort" in the research literature. People today who are 75 and older came of age during the Great Depression. Their view of money was shaped during an era with unprecedented economic instability. Their frugality, then, might reflect these formative experiences and not the effects of aging. Another possibility is that current social and historical events, or what are called "period effects," influence their behavior differently than they do that of the 20-year-olds. Older people, for example, may be reluctant to spend money on discretionary items because they are concerned that growing threats to the viability of Social Security will lead to cutbacks in benefits. Cohort and period effects need to be considered in interpreting differences found in cross-sectional comparisons of young and old. In other words, older people and younger people differ in many ways, but not every difference is due to the aging process.

Other factors can account for differences in cross-sectional studies. The samples of young and old may not be comparable in some essential way, such as level of education or socioeconomic status. Some early research on aging compared college-age students with nursing home residents, a contrast likely to exaggerate differences. It is also possible that some artifact in the research may contribute to the differences—for example, the younger sample may be college students who are familiar with tests and testing procedures, whereas older participants experience more anxiety because of their lack of familiarity with the setting and procedures.

Findings from cross-sectional research can be useful despite their limitations. We often want to know whether old and young people differ, even if we do not know why they might differ. As an example, knowing that older people underreport negative feelings makes us aware that standard depression assessments may underestimate depression in an older client (Haynie, Berg, Johansson, Gatz, & Zarit, 2001). It does not matter whether this difference in reporting negative feelings is due to age, cohort, or some other factor. If we want to know, however, how aging affects emotional expression and depressive feelings, then we have to use a different research approach.

Longitudinal research follows the people from a single cohort over time. Figure 2.1 also illustrates a longitudinal design. Let's say we begin with a sample of 20-year-olds tested in 1990. This same group is then tested at 5-year intervals, when they are 25, 30, and 35 years old. This approach provides more direct evidence of an "age change"—that is, that the variability observed during the course of the study is due to aging (Schaie & Hofer, 2001). But longitudinal studies have their limitations as well. As noted, it is difficult to conduct studies that cover the full range of adulthood and old age. Another problem is that selective attrition can bias the findings; the people who subsequently drop out of a longitudinal study may have been less able to begin with or may have experienced declines in functioning since the preceding evaluation. Longitudinal studies can also be influenced by cohort and period effects. One cohort, for example, may score particularly high or low on a specific ability or may show a unique pattern of change over time. The same historical event could also affect cohorts in different ways, because the timing of that event occurs at different points in their lives. To illustrate this point, Jones and Meredith (1996) analyzed data from two longitudinal studies of men that were begun when both groups were children. The older cohort experienced increases in self-confidence in their 30s, whereas the younger cohort did not show an increase until they were in their 40s. The event that intervened was World War II, when the men in the younger cohort, in their late teens and early 20s, served in the military. Military service delayed their involvement in careers and developing families compared with the older cohort and probably also contributed to their gaining self-confidence at a later age.

Recognizing the limitations of longitudinal studies, Schaie (1967, 2005; Schaie & Willis, 2002) developed sequential research strategies as a way of separating the influences of aging, cohort, and period effects. The most common approach is called a "cohort sequential design," in which several cohorts are followed over time. A sequential design is shown in Figure 2.2. As with the cross-sectional design illustrated earlier, people could be enrolled in the study at ages 20–80. In this case, each cohort originally enrolled would then be

	Year		
1990	1995	2000	2005
Age			
20 →	25 →	30 →	35
30 →	35 →	40 →	45
40 →	45 →	50 →	55
50 →	55 →	60 →	65
60 →	65 →	70 →	75
70 →	75 →	80 →	85
80 →	85 →	90 →	95

FIGURE 2.2. Cohort sequential design.

tested at repeated intervals. In other words, we would be conducting a series of parallel longitudinal studies, one for each cohort.

The findings from a cohort sequential design can help sort out whether age differences are due to aging, cohort differences, or historical events. Let's say that we are conducting a study of sexual attitudes and behavior in adulthood, and we use the cohort sequential design shown in Figure 2.2. At our initial time of testing, let's say that we find differences in sexual attitudes, that younger people hold more liberal or permissive attitudes than older people. When we follow these cohorts over time, a number of different outcomes are possible. One possibility is that the younger cohorts become more conservative over time, becoming at age 30 similar to the older cohorts at that age. That would be evidence of an age change. Another possibility is that the initial differences between cohorts in 1990 might remain the same over time, that is, the younger cohorts could maintain more open or tolerant sexual attitudes as they age. The last possibility is that most or all of the cohorts might change in the same direction during a particular time interval, let's say between 1990 and 1995. When many people in the population are changing in the same way during the same time period, that is evidence of a historical effect. An example is the emergence of AIDS in the 1980s, which may have affected sexual attitudes in the population as a whole.

The problem of attrition can also be dealt with in a sequential design. At each new wave of testing, the investigators can add a new, independent sample from each cohort. By comparing this new sample with the longitudinal participants, it will be possible to determine whether attrition has biased the results (see Schaie & Willis, 2002, for a discussion of various design strategies for studying development).

Due to the cost and other logistical problems of longitudinal and sequential studies, most research on aging remains cross-sectional. But understanding what each type of research can say about aging is of critical importance. As will be shown, the changes with aging appear generally smaller and to occur later in life when viewed from a longitudinal than a cross-sectional perspective. Many of the differences we generally ascribe to aging are due to generational differences and to the effects of historical events.

Life-Course and Lifespan Approaches to Aging

Life-course and lifespan models of aging provide complementary frameworks for understanding the process and sources of change. A fundamental premise of both approaches is that aging is a lifelong process involving the interaction of biological, psychological, and social processes. Biological changes set the broad parameters for aging: people's reactions slow, they may lose some strength and flexibility, and their sensory functioning may diminish, but they can draw on psychological and social resources to compensate for these changes.

Life-course approaches (e.g., Elder, 1998; Neugarten, Moore, & Lowe, 1968; Settersten, 1999) emphasize the role of cohort and the timing of social and historical events in shaping development across adulthood. Recognizing the effects of cohort and the timing and influence of specific events is a fundamental part of clinical practice with older adults. Our older clients tell us about a world that we have only read about but that continues to influence their behavior and beliefs. Depression-era experiences, military service during wartime, or surviving a concentration camp may have obvious or subtle influences on current behavior. If we view the attitudes and beliefs of an older person as "old-fashioned" or out of step with the times, we miss the opportunity to engage him or her in a meaningful therapeutic process. By entering into an older person's world—for instance, understanding what it was like to grow up poor during the Great Depression—we can establish empathy and better identify strengths that we can build on.

The lifespan developmental perspective (e.g., Baltes, 1987, 1997) also presents concepts that help us understand the unfolding of the aging process. Changes with aging can be characterized as "interindividual" and "intraindividual" differences. Interindividual differences describe how people differ from one another on specific abilities. Some people score better on memory tests, for example, and others may do better on spatial ability. This comparison, however, does not tell us whether people who score poorly on some ability, such as memory, have always had a difficult time keeping track of names and appointments or whether they have declined in recent years. Intraindividual differences, by comparison, refer to the patterns among an individual's abilities. An individual may experience decline in some abilities and improve in others over time. This pattern of intraindividual difference can vary from one person to another. In other words, people do not necessarily experience psychological aging in the same way. Some people may show a decline in memory relatively early in life, and others may experience little or no decline. The clinical relevance of these concepts is that aging is not associated with a universal pattern of global decline. Some abilities are more likely to be affected than others, and the rate and timing of change in each ability can differ from one person to the next.

Another important concept is reserve capacity, the ability of a person to meet the challenges of a very stressful or demanding situation. According to Baltes (1987), aging has a greater effect on reducing reserve capacity than on functioning in everyday situations. To illustrate this point, Baltes uses the example of walking and running. Comparing a healthy older person with a younger person when they are walking will yield no meaningful differences. By contrast, most younger people can run faster and farther than most older people. This example shows that the effects of aging are not typically apparent in ordinary tasks but that they can be brought out under challenging and difficult circumstances that test the limits of an older person's capacity.

Of course, some older people remain fit and active and may be able to run farther and maybe even faster than a sedentary younger person. There is, in other words, the potential for plasticity in functioning (Baltes, 1987). Plasticity indicates that performance can improve with training or similar experiences. Whether we are considering physical or intellectual fitness, ample evidence exists that older people can improve their performance and that these improvements can be sustained over time (e.g., Ball et al., 2002; Willis, Blieszner, & Baltes, 1981; Willis & Nesselroade, 1990). As we show, these studies suggest that under certain conditions decline associated with aging can be minimized or reversed.

Older people can also compensate for decline. Baltes (1987) has described a process called selective optimization with compensation (SOC), by which older people are able to maintain a high level of functioning in valued domains despite declines in some of the underlying cognitive abilities that contribute to performance. One of the best examples of SOC comes from a study by Salthouse (1984). Salthouse observed that expert older typists were able to perform as quickly and accurately as younger typists, despite experiencing a decline in reaction time, which is one of the most notable changes with aging. They were able to compensate for slowing by anticipating upcoming words in the text better than younger typists. The high level of expert performance maintained by older people in activities such as music, chess, law, and business may be due to compensation processes. This ability to compensate, combined with continued potential for growth in later life, means that older people can sustain performance in valued activities and can respond to treatment to help them overcome losses.

Intelligence and Aging

When do older people need someone to take over complex situations, and when do they remain capable of making judgments themselves? Consider, for example, an older couple who have had a few minor problems managing their home and financial affairs. Although they want to stay in their home, their children are increasingly concerned about their decision-making capabilities. The adult children wonder whether they should take over managing the finances for their parents or encourage them to move to senior housing. Although it is clear that people suffering from AD and other dementing illnesses lose their ability to manage their affairs competently, what about older people not suffering from dementia?

Intelligence is an important marker of biological changes in the brain that occur with aging, as well as an indicator of continued capability to carry out complex everyday activities. Regular and expected changes in the brain occur as part of the normal aging process, though the amount of cell loss is less than early estimates suggested (Vinters, 2001). Imaging studies of the brain have generally found that the volume of the ventricles increases and the amount of brain tissue decreases with age (Kramer, Fabiani, & Colcombe, 2006). Losses are particularly evident in white matter and in the volume of the hippocampus and frontal lobes, although the extent and significance of these changes remains controversial. Nonetheless, it is logical to expect that brain aging will result in a decline in cognitive functioning. It appears, however, that decline occurs in some abilities and not others and at later ages than originally expected (Schaie, 2005).

The picture of how intelligence changes with aging is intrinsically tied to the type of research design used. Historically, studies of intelligence and aging used cross-sectional research designs and reported considerable differences between old and young. Using cross-sectional data from adults who took the original or the revised Wechsler Adult Intelligence Scale (WAIS and WAIS-R; Wechsler, 1987), researchers generally reported that verbal abilities, such as vocabulary and information, peak early in life and then show a moderate amount of decline, whereas scores on performance tests, such as block design, begin to decline quite early in life (late teens or early 20s) and then show a steeper decline than verbal skills throughout the adult years (e.g., Matarozzo, 1972; Wechsler, 1958).

Compared with cross-sectional results, longitudinal and sequential studies paint a somewhat different picture of changes in intelligence (e.g., Cunningham & Owens, 1983; Schaie, 2005; Schaie & Hofer, 2001; Siegler, 1983). The Seattle Longitudinal Study, conducted by Schaie and his associates (e.g., Schaie, 1983, 1996, 2005; Schaie & Hertzog, 1986), is the richest source of information about intelligence and aging. Initiated in 1957, this study uses a cohort-sequential design. The original sample of adults were ages 22–70. This sample has been retested at 7-year intervals, with new cohorts of people added at each wave of testing. As a result, it is possible to follow the same people over time, to compare performance among different birth cohorts, and to test for the effects of attrition.

The test used in the Seattle Longitudinal Study is Thurstone's Primary Mental Abilities Test (PMA; Schaie, 1985; Thurstone & Thurstone, 1949). The PMA has five components: verbal meaning, spatial orientation, inductive reasoning, number ability, and word fluency. Higher order factors correspond to fluid and crystallized intelligence (Schaie, 1996, 2005).

Compared with cross-sectional studies, which show that intellectual abilities peak early in adulthood and then decline, the Seattle Longitudinal Study found that intellectual ability on most components of intelligence increases into middle adulthood, is stable into the 50s or 60s, and then shows a gradual decline (Schaie, 1996, 2005). The difference in findings between cross-sectional and longitudinal analyses is illustrated in Figure 2.3. The dotted line indicates cross-sectional findings for one test from the PMA, verbal meaning. This cross-sectional analysis shows a peak around age 39, followed by a fairly steep pattern of decline. In contrast, the longitudinal analysis, illustrated with the solid line, shows that the peak for verbal meaning is reached at age 53 and

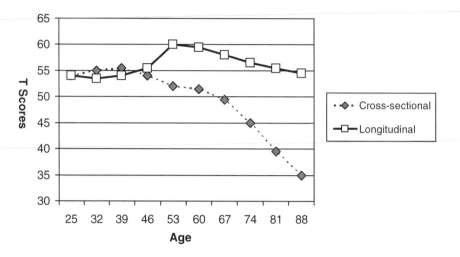

FIGURE 2.3. Cross-sectional and longitudinal gradients for verbal meaning. From Schaie, K. Warner, and Willis, Sherry, L., *Adult Development and Aging*, 5th Edition, © 2002, p. 365. Adapted by permission of Pearson Education, Inc. Upper Saddle River, NJ.

is followed by a more gradual decline. Word fluency and number ability show decrements between testing intervals beginning at age 53 and declines on other PMA tests appear after age 60 (Schaie, 1996, 2005).

Why do the cross-sectional and longitudinal findings differ so much? First, generational, or cohort, effects are pronounced (Schaie, 1996, 2005). The more recent cohorts have scored better from the start on tests of verbal meaning, spatial orientation, and inductive reasoning and have maintained this advantage over time. Number ability also was higher in successive cohorts born up to 1945 but has been lower in later-born cohorts. The fifth PMA test, word fluency, shows no generational differences. Following cohorts over time confirms that differences between old and young are in part generational. As they age, younger cohorts do not decline to the level of older cohorts; rather, they maintain their initial advantage. For example, a cohort born in 1945 might show better performance at age 20 than a cohort from 1931 at age 34 *and* will still perform better when they reach age 34 compared with the 1931 cohort's scores at age 34.

The other likely source of differences between cross-sectional and longitudinal findings is selective attrition. People who return for repeated testing in a longitudinal study are more likely to have better functioning initially and less likely to experience a decline over time. To test for the effects of attrition, new participants were added to the sample at each wave of testing and compared with ongoing participants. Even after adjusting for attrition, however, cohort differences remain a much more important factor than age until the decade of the 60s or later (Schaie, 1996, 2005).

Individual Differences in Intellectual Performance

Not everyone experiences a decline in later life at the same time or rate. Using data from the Seattle Longitudinal Study, Schaie (1996) reported that over 60% of participants over the age of 60 were stable or showed improved performance over the 7-year period between assessments. The proportion of people showing a decline between assessments increases with advancing age, but even after 80, a majority of participants had stable scores between testing intervals. Additionally, when decline occurs, it is most likely to be found for one or two abilities rather than across all tests.

There are several possible reasons that some people decline after age 60 whereas others remain stable in intellectual performance. Poor health contributes to decline (Schaie, 1996). It is also possible that many of the people who decline are exhibiting preclinical symptoms of AD or other dementias (Hofer et al., 2002; Sliwinski, Lipton, Buschke, & Stewart, 1996).

Several lifestyle factors may contribute to maintaining good intellectual functioning after age 60 (e.g., Gruber-Baldini, Schaie, & Willis, 1995; Schaie, 1996; Schooler, Mulatu, & Oates, 1999). People who seek out intellectually challenging experiences, who work in an intellectually challenging environment, who remain engaged, and who hold more flexible attitudes are less likely to decline in abilities after age 60. Having a spouse with high intellectual ability also contributes to stability in later life.

Disuse of intellectual abilities may also contribute to the rate and amount of decline. To test this hypothesis, Schaie and Willis (1986) selected participants from the Seattle Longitudinal Study who had previously declined in functioning on tests of either verbal meaning or spatial orientation. These participants were then given training either in skills related to the ability in which they had declined or in another area. The results indicated that training improved performance and that many people were able to function at or near their previous levels on these abilities. A multisite trial showed gains from several different types of cognitive training (e.g., Ball et al., 2002). It remains to be determined whether gains from cognitive training result from improved use of cognitive resources or whether cognitive stimulation produces new neural synapses (e.g., Diamond, Johnson, Protti, Ott, & Kajisa, 1985).

Finally, cognitive change in late life may be related to a process called terminal decline (see Berg, 1996, for a review). As people near death, cognitive functioning may suffer either due to physiological changes or to a psychological process of turning inward. From both these perspectives, the timing of decline and mortality are more critical for cognitive function than chronological age.

Wisdom

In many families, there is a grandparent or other older relative to whom people turn when they have a complicated life problem. They rely on that person's ability to identify what is important in the situation and to help them make a decision. Many cultures believe that some elders have special insight into major life problems.

Although cognitive aging studies usually focus on decline, it is also possible that new qualities, such as wisdom, might emerge (Baltes, 1997). Baltes and his colleagues (e.g., Baltes & Smith, 1990; Staudinger & Baltes, 1996; Staudinger, Lopez, & Baltes, 1997) have conducted a series of studies to explore wisdom in adulthood and old age. Wisdom was defined as expertise in the pragmatics of life, that is, in such things as planning, management, and decision making. Another quality of wisdom is virtue, which is defined as being able to focus on the well-being of others and not oneself. Other aspects of wisdom include knowledge of specific contexts, knowledge of strategies for reaching goals, and the ability to weigh the merits of conflicting goals and values. To assess wisdom, respondents are presented with scenarios involving life decisions and asked to respond. The scenarios involve dilemmas that are specific to particular stages of life. The responses are then rated with a multidimensional scoring system that reflects the definition of wisdom.

Wisdom was generally not related to age (e.g., Staudinger & Baltes, 1996), but there were two important caveats. First, there may be an age-matched effect in wisdom (Staudinger, 1999). People may be able to give the "wisest" responses when the scenario they are responding to involves life decisions at ages that are developmentally close to their own age. In other words, younger people tend to give the best responses involving situations specific to young adulthood, whereas older people give the best responses for dilemmas pertinent to later life. This finding suggests that wisdom is context specific and requires knowledge of the circumstances involved in a particular situation. Second, when given the opportunity to talk through their responses with a peer and then reflect on them, older people improved much more than younger people did (Staudinger & Baltes, 1996). Of course, not all older people were capable of providing high-quality responses, either before or after priming. These studies do not confirm the folk wisdom that all older people are wise but suggest that the experience gained with aging may play a role in the development of wisdom, especially in a supportive situation in which the older person has an opportunity to reflect about a life decision.

Several conclusions can be drawn from these studies of intelligence and wisdom. Changes in intellectual performance with aging have been demonstrated, but, except for speeded tests, average declines occur relatively late in the adult years (50s or 60s). Even at advanced ages, however, there are considerable individual differences in the timing and rate of decline. Differences in performance among generations have contributed to somewhat inflated estimates of intellectual decline in later life in results from cross-sectional studies. Tasks that cause more difficulties for older adults typically involve novel or unfamiliar procedures. At least part of this disadvantage can be offset by training. These findings, of course, reflect functioning of relatively healthy individuals and do not take into account the catastrophic changes in intelligence that occur with dementia.

The changes in these abilities associated with aging probably do not affect performance of familiar activities. Competency to perform many complicated intellectual activities in everyday life shows little decline with aging (Salthouse, 1990). Age effects will be more apparent, however, when people face new or overwhelming challenges, especially at older ages (75 and older). Finally, some individuals develop higher order conceptual skills as they age, or what is popularly termed "wisdom." Although wisdom is not a universal or normative outcome among the elderly, it represents one possible pattern of successful aging.

Memory and Aging

An older client reports having forgotten an appointment and worries, "Am I getting senile?" A colleague misplaces his glasses and says "I must be getting old." A woman juggling work and family stops at the grocery on the way home from work to pick up some items but forgets one thing she wanted to buy. She wonders whether the loss of memory that happened to her grandmother is beginning to show up in her. These examples of forgetting are common daily occurrences. The widely held expectation that memory declines with age makes older people more sensitive about these types of everyday forgetting. They forgot names and misplaced keys when they were younger but did not dwell on these incidents. Now that they are older, the same events take on much greater significance.

Memory impairment is the hallmark symptom in dementia, and so it is natural to worry that any instance of forgetting might herald the onset of decline. But the expectation of decline exceeds the reality. Most older people do not suffer from dementia or other disorders that impair cognitive functioning. Although they experience changes in memory, these changes are benign or, at worst, annoying (see Bäckman, Small, & Wahlin, 2001, for a review).

One of the most important tasks in geriatric mental health is to differentiate the mild changes typical of normal aging from more severe and persistent problems associated with dementing illnesses. An understanding of the normal and expected changes in memory with aging can be helpful both for differential diagnosis and for helping healthy older clients view their occasional lapses in memory as a minor irritant rather than a signal of impending deterioration.

Memory is not a unitary process but a set of interrelated systems that are involved in processing information (Smith, 1996). These systems can be

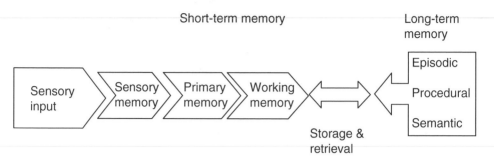

FIGURE 2.4. Memory processes.

broadly grouped into three levels: sensory memory, short-term memory, and long-term memory (Figure 2.4). "Sensory memory" refers to a brief holding system, which can be illustrated by the short-lived afterimage that forms after presentation of a visual image. Deficits in sensory memory increase with age (e.g., Parkinson & Perey, 1980; Walsh, Till, & Williams, 1978). The functional significance of these changes, however, is generally considered to be minimal. Sensory memory should be distinguished from sensory functioning, that is, the integrity of sensory systems, such as vision and hearing. Deficits in the senses can make it more difficult for people to learn and remember because information is not perceived easily or accurately at input.

"Short-term memory" comprises two related processes: primary memory and working memory. Primary memory refers to memory span, that is, the amount of information that can be actively attended to at any given time. Working memory involves the simultaneous processing and storage of information from primary memory (Baddeley, 1992). A digit-span task illustrates both these processes. Repeating digits forward (e.g., 1, 6, 4, 3 . . .) is an example of primary memory, whereas repeating those digits backward (e.g., 3, 4, 6, 1 . . .) is an example of working memory. In other words, information moves from primary to working memory, where it can be manipulated and moved into storage.

Age differences are generally not found for primary memory (Gregoire & Van der Linden, 1997). Older people, however, are at a disadvantage in working memory tasks in which they have to process some information while also remembering other material from a prior task (Salthouse, 1994a). One such task would be to have older people answer questions about sentences while trying to remember the last words of those sentences. This type of divided-attention test is similar to the demands we often face in everyday life. Age differences in working memory also become larger when a great deal of information is presented, when the material is complex, or when participants are required to manipulate the information in some way (Salthouse, 1994a; Salthouse & Babcock, 1991). Attentional processes are a central part of working memory, and their disruption in disorders such as AD may be a major source of patients' memory problems.

Information that is to be retained over a longer time must be converted from working memory into some type of permanent storage and then later retrieved. This process of storage and retrieval is called "long-term memory." Storage of information can be effortful or incidental; that is, the person may deliberately try to learn information for later retrieval, or the person may acquire information without any deliberate effort. Long-term memory can be divided into episodic, semantic, and procedural systems. *Episodic* memory describes what most people think of first as memory: the ability to remember a specific event. *Semantic* memory involves recall of words, meaning, and grammar. *Procedural* memory refers to recall of motor, perceptual, or cognitive skills involved in performing a series of actions; for example, how to ride a bicycle. These distinctions in types of long-term memory reflect differences in neural organization and storage of information.

Although there are some age differences in semantic and procedural memory, the greatest change with normal aging is seen in episodic memory (Bäckman et al., 2001). Changes in episodic memory begin in early adulthood but progress at a very slow rate (Zelinksi & Burnight, 1997). Several sources of these differences have been proposed. In a classic study, Schonfield and Robertson (1966) compared performances of old and young participants on a word list under conditions of both free recall and recognition (i.e., choosing the correct word from among alternatives). They found age differences in recall but not in recognition and argued that this pattern of performances suggested that older people have decrements in retrieval but not in acquisition of new information. Subsequent research, however, has provided inconsistent support for a retrieval deficit. McNulty and Caird (1966) suggested that this pattern of results is due to differences in how well the material is learned at acquisition. If material is learned less thoroughly in the first place, it will be more difficult to recall, but it may still be possible to recognize correct answers based on the partial memory traces that were formed. Whatever the reason for these differences, older people will perform better on tasks involving recognition than recall. The practical value of this finding comes when working with people with dementia, who also do better at recognition tasks. Caregivers can learn to ask questions that give choices, for example, "Would you like tuna or chicken for lunch?" rather than asking a more open-ended questions such as "What would you like for lunch?"

The differences in performance of older people on recognition and recall tasks may reflect a larger issue—that cognitive resources necessary for processing information decline with aging. According to Craik (1994), age differences are more pronounced on tasks that provide fewer cues during learning and retrieval, or what he calls "environmental support." As cognitive tasks provide more support, older people perform relatively better. When learning a list of words, for example, the learner receives more support when the words are grouped into categories. Older people are also less likely to provide their own supports, such as by placing words into categories or using other types of mnemonic devices (Hultsch, 1971; Witte, Freund, & Brown-Whistler, 1993).

Speed of processing is another important source of age differences. Older people do more poorly when stimuli are presented faster or when the period allowed for recall is shorter (Salthouse, 1994a, 1994b). When the speed of presentation of material is controlled and time pressure for responses is reduced, age differences in memory performance are greatly reduced. In our fast-paced world, however, even high-functioning older people can sometimes have difficulty when information comes at them too quickly. Add to that distractions and poor acoustics, and the performance decrement in that situation could be considerable. Whereas younger people are able to multitask at a rapid pace, both generational and age effects may make it more difficult for older people to do so.

Relatively few studies have been done of very old memories; that is, recall of events from the distant past. This is an interesting area because it corresponds to people's own conceptions of memory. Older people recall historical events as well as or better than younger people do (e.g., Botwinick & Storandt, 1974; Perlmutter, 1978), perhaps because they may have had greater exposure to the information in the first place. Lachman and Lachman (1980) explored recall for names of well-known political and entertainment figures. Older and younger participants were asked questions with identifying information about these famous people. If they could not recall a name, they were asked whether they had a tip-of-the-tongue response, that is, whether they felt they knew the answer but could not recall it right then. When they felt they knew the answer, both older and younger participants could pick out the correct name most of the time from a multiple-choice response format. Older people had more tip-of-the-tongue responses than younger individuals, but they also had a larger total amount of knowledge. Based on these findings, Lachman and Lachman suggest that older people's efficiency in recalling old information was probably as good as younger people's, taking into account the fact that the older group had a larger store of information to sort through.

Forgetting can occur at any point in the memory process. Information may fail to register on the senses, may not be processed in working memory, may not enter storage, or may decay in storage; or there may be a failure in retrieval. Clinical examination and testing can be used to pinpoint the source of forgetting (see Chapters 6 and 7), which can be useful for diagnostic purposes and for developing strategies for improving performance. As an example, an older woman may complain that she cannot remember the names of people that she meets. One possibility is that she cannot retain new information, a symptom of dementia. Testing in that case would show a low rate of initial learning and a drop-off with delayed recall. Other possibilities include that she is worried about what impression the other person has of her and does not pay attention to that person's name or that she is hard of hearing and does not hear the name clearly. That type of information would come out as part of the clinical examination, and patterns of learning and recall on standardized tests would be normal or near normal.

As with intelligence, considerable individual differences exist in memory (Bäckman et al., 2001). Health is a major source of those differences. Memory, of course, declines early in the course of dementia and may also be affected by other illnesses, such as diabetes (Zelinksi, Crimmins, Reynolds, & Seeman, 1998). As with intelligence, memory may also decline as a function of nearness to death (Berg, 1996).

What older people say about their memories is one of the most important pieces of information in clinical assessment. This aspect of memory has been called "metamemory" and comprises people's knowledge and appraisal of memory. Consistent with findings on age differences in memory, older people report more problems and concerns about their memories (Collins & Abeles, 1996). What people say about their memories, however, may not be a reliable indicator of deficits. In samples of healthy people not suffering from dementia, the degree of correspondence between subjective evaluations of memory and actual performance is modest. Some people who complain about failing memory actually perform at high levels, whereas others who report very few problems perform at low levels. One problem in these studies is that the information about subjective memory and memory performance is obtained at the same time. When older people complain about their memories, they are comparing their current performance with how they functioned in the past. In one of the few longitudinal studies of memory complaints (Johansson, Allen-Burge, & Zarit, 1997), a somewhat different picture emerged. People who said that their memories had declined in the preceding 2 years in fact showed slightly lower performance than they had 2 years earlier. They were also more likely to decline over the following 2 years. Even in this longitudinal study, however, subjective evaluations did not have a strong association with decline, and there was considerable overlap in objective test performance between people who complained of failing memory and those who did not.

Although subjective memory has only a modest association with objective memory performance, depression and dementia have a strong effect on what people say about their memories. Depression is generally associated with overly negative appraisals of oneself and one's abilities (Beck, Rush, Shaw & Emery, 1979). Among older people, as well as some younger clients we have worked with, these negative appraisals extend to memory. Complaints of failing memory have been found to correlate with depression and not with actual deficits in memory performance (Collins & Abeles, 1996; Johansson et al., 1997; Jungwirth et al., 2004; Kahn, Zarit, Hilbert, & Niederehe, 1975; Pearman & Storandt, 2004). In dementia, there is a paradoxical relation between memory complaints and performance. People suffering from mild dementia are more likely to be aware of and to complain about failing memory, whereas those with more severe deficits usually maintain that they have little or no trouble with memory (Johansson et al., 1997; Kahn et al., 1975; Kaszniak, 1996).

Memory complaints, then, are an important marker not for their relation to actual performance but for the other problems they might indicate. We return to this issue of subjective evaluations of memory when discussing clinical assessment (Chapter 6).

As with intelligence, researchers have attempted, through training, to improve participants' memory performance. These efforts have been based on the hypothesis that age-related deficits in memory are due to a lack of resources when processing information. Training has entailed teaching older people how to use cognitive strategies that enhance their resources. Strategies have included organizing a list of words into categories or employing a visual association strategy to link words in a list. These approaches have generally had positive results (Ball et al., 2002; Floyd & Scogin, 1996; Hill, Sheikh, & Yesavage, 1988; Meyer, Young, & Bartlett, 1989). Yesavage (1983) and his colleagues (Yesavage & Jacob, 1984) have conducted an interesting set of experiments that suggest that combining relaxation training with instruction in mnemonic strategies has a better outcome than using either approach separately.

The most intriguing training studies have been conducted by Paul Baltes and his colleagues (e.g., Baltes, 1987; Baltes & Kliegl, 1992; Kliegl, Smith, & Baltes, 1989; Staudinger, Marsiske, & Baltes, 1995). These studies used a testing-the-limits approach that makes it possible to examine the extent of plasticity or potential for improvement in memory among older people, as well as limits imposed by the aging process. Young and old participants learned a classic mnemonic device, the method of loci, in which information to be remembered is associated with a familiar place or location. Participants then were asked to apply this approach to learning lists of digits and nouns. Using this method, both young and old were able to learn very long lists, though younger participants consistently performed at a higher level. When the learning conditions were made more difficult, such as increasing the pace of presentation of new items, the advantage of younger individuals increased further. These studies suggest plasticity in memory ability for older people— that is, they can apply cognitive resources to improve performance—and that aging sets limits to performance under more stressful or demanding conditions.

The concern that older people have about their memories is likely to continue or even grow in response to the growing emphasis on early detection of AD and other dementias (see Chapter 3). Normal lapses in memory can readily trigger worries about a more serious decline. People are beginning to use nonprescription and natural substances that are potential memory enhancers (Jorm, Rodgers, & Christensen, 2004). Rather than promoting medications that people may not need nor benefit from, a public health strategy could combine ways of educating people that some forgetting is normal and expected with proven strategies for maintaining performance. These strategies might include practical steps to improve memory, such as better organization and the use of memory aids, as well as techniques such as visualization that enhance learning and memory.

Personality and Adaptation

As we age, do we change in the very core of who we are? Does our sense of self and the various traits, motives, behaviors, and emotions that make up the self change in a predictable way? Are there optimal ways of adapting to later life and preventing unwanted changes? Historically, aging has been associated with a variety of negative personality characteristics—irritability, rigidity, reactionary political and social attitudes, and self-centeredness. Competing theories and approaches to the study of personality have resulted in conflicting perspectives on the question of stability versus change with age, but most researchers agree on a central point: in the absence of catastrophic illness such as AD, personality deterioration is not an inevitable or even common consequence of aging.

Before turning to the research on personality, we want to comment on the reasons that negative stereotypes have dominated thinking about aging, especially in Western countries. One reason is the confusion of aging and disease. People have long attributed the catastrophic changes that occur in dementia to aging, not disease. A second factor is a failure to differentiate life-long characteristics from the effects of aging. People with unpleasant personality characteristics grow older and do not generally become more pleasant or easier to deal with. Because of negative expectations about aging, their irritating and abrasive behavior may be attributed to old age rather than to a life-long pattern. Finally, Western culture prizes innovation and change. In periods of rapid social and technological change, older people may be more disadvantaged and thus are perceived as old-fashioned or as blocking progress.

Early personality research usually focused on single traits that were expected to change with age, such as rigidity, cautiousness, and defensiveness. The results of these studies suggest that few of the stereotypes are borne out (e.g., Costa & McCrae, 1988; Haan, Millsap, & Hartka, 1986; Helson & Moane, 1987; Siegler, George, & Okun, 1979). Data from the Seattle Longitudinal Study (Schaie & Labouvie-Vief, 1974), for example, were used to examine three dimensions of behavioral rigidity: (1) motor–cognitive, (2) personality–perceptual, and (3) psychomotor speed. Cross-sectional analysis found large differences between young and old on these dimensions. In longitudinal analyses, however, only psychomotor speed showed a clear pattern of decline across the adult years. Both motor–cognitive and personality–perceptual rigidity were relatively stable, although with some evidence of decline (increased rigidity) in the oldest groups. Similar to the findings for intelligence, the differences found between cross-sectional and longitudinal analyses of rigidity appeared due to cohort. In other words, the amount of behavioral rigidity has been decreasing in successive generations, not increasing with age. Another cohort difference is that extroversion has been increasing in generations born since World War II (Schaie, 1996; Schaie & Labouvie-Vief, 1974).

One of the dominant ideas in modern psychology is the primacy of early childhood experiences in shaping later development. To what extent can development in adulthood be understood as shaped by early experiences? The theory most often applied to the adult years is attachment. There is, undoubtedly, some continuity in the type of relationships formed early and those made later in life, but on the whole, correlations from measures of attachment from one part of childhood to another show only moderate degrees of association (Kagan, 1996; Rubin, Bukowski, & Parker, 1998), and so it is likely that the contribution to personality later in life is even more modest. Another consideration is the role of early social and psychological deprivation. Life-course sociologists have drawn attention to the cumulative effects of social adversity on health and other outcomes (e.g., Alwin & Wray, 2005). Positive experiences, however, such as when children from a chaotic and impoverished family develop a good relationship with an adult or gain attention for a skill or ability, can help them overcome early deprivation (Werner, 2001). Experiences in adolescence and young adulthood, such as military service and marriage, have also been found to help people from impoverished backgrounds make a successful transition to adulthood. Not everyone, however, is fortunate enough to overcome early hardship. For many of our clients, traumatic or other conflicted experiences early in life remain vivid or real and appear to have an enduring influence, even in very old age. And those people who appear successful sometimes are still struggling with issues from an earlier, harsher time of life.

Although some theories suggest little change after childhood, other approaches have proposed that adulthood is characterized by a series of qualitatively distinct stages (Erikson, 1950; Erikson, Erikson, & Kivnick, 1986; Jung, 1933; Levinson, 1986; Loevinger, 1976). The possibility of a midlife crisis has received considerable attention in scientific journals and the popular media. Erikson's (1950) notion that later life involves the dichotomy of integrity–despair has probably received more attention than any other theoretical proposition. According to Erikson, the central psychological process in later life revolves around either gaining a sense of integrity—that is, that one's life has been lived well—or feeling despair over missed opportunities and unfulfilled dreams.

In contrast to these expectations for change, Costa and McCrae (e.g., Costa & McCrae, 1988; McCrae & Costa, 1990) have proposed that there is considerable stability in personality in adulthood after age 30. Their studies have used an empirically derived model of personality, the NEO+2, that has five dimensions: neuroticism, extraversion, openness to experience, agreeableness, and conscientiousness. Using findings from a longitudinal study, they have shown that scores earlier in adulthood generally have high correlations with personality later in life. Other studies have supported these findings (e.g., Plomin, Pedersen, McClearn, Nesselroade, & Bergeman, 1988).

Even in very old age, there may be continuity. Troll and Skaff (1997) examined responses of community-dwelling people ages 85 and older to questions about perceived changes in their core selves (*I*) and in self-concepts (*me*). Respondents reported a high degree of continuity in their core selves, but acknowledged some changes in specific characteristics. Changes were both positive and negative. In a similar analysis done by Costa and McCrae (1989), most people reported that they changed only a little or not at all over time.

New methods for studying change longitudinally—particularly, the use of growth curve modeling—have presented a somewhat different picture of stability and change in personality. Rather than correlating scores between early and later times of measurement, which has the effect of masking individual differences, growth curve modeling makes it possible to look at individual patterns of change over time. Mroczek and Spiro (2003) used two dimensions of the NEO+2, neuroticism (the tendency to overreact emotionally and experience distress) and extraversion (the tendency to be outgoing and enjoy social activity), to examine longitudinal changes in personality. The sample consisted of men who were between 43 and 91 years of age at the start of the study. The sample as a whole showed a mean decline in neuroticism over time and no change in extraversion. Many people, however, deviated from these average patterns of change. For extraversion, although no mean change occurred with age, some people increased over time and some decreased. Likewise, for neuroticism, the average score for the whole sample decreased over time, but many individuals differed from the mean pattern of change. Some decreased in neuroticism more than the average, some showed a smaller decrease than average, *and* some increased in neuroticism as they aged (see also Jones & Meredith, 2000; Small, Hertzog, Hultsch, & Dixon, 2003). In other words, people age in different ways.

In addition, Mroczek and Spiro (2003) found significant cohort differences for both personality dimensions. Younger cohorts showed higher extraversion, which increased over time, whereas the oldest cohort showed lower initial levels, which decreased over time. For neuroticism, the oldest cohort showed the highest level, and this declined more slowly than it did for the youngest cohort. Life events, such as death of a spouse and marriage or remarriage, were significantly associated with changes in neuroticism. As noted earlier, historical events can also affect the timing of changes in personality (Jones & Meredith, 1996).

What can we conclude, then, about stability or change in personality, particularly in later adulthood? On average, there is probably greater continuity than change. Undoubtedly, some people have life-transforming experiences during the adult years, but that is not the norm. One does not become a completely different person at midlife or on reaching age 65. Changes are gradual, and there are individual differences in the direction and amount of those changes. Some people change a little over time, and others change a lot. The timing and amount of change varies with cohorts and in response to historical and life events. Broad psychological principles such as integrity versus despair are inherently appealing, but they are probably too simplistic to capture the developmental issues of later life, given the diversity of the older population and the large span of years involved (e.g., 65–95 or older). Clinicians should not become overly enamored with these types of poetic descriptions of the life course. A sense of integrity is important in later life, and issues related to integrity or despair that arise in therapy should not be ignored, but we also should not force the full variety of aging to fit into that narrow framework.

One point on which there is agreement is that people do not usually experience significant deterioration in personality over time. Commonplace beliefs, such as that aging involves a "hardening of the attitudes," are prejudices with little basis in fact.

Emotions and Aging

At the heart of this trend of improved psychological functioning with aging is that people generally feel good and in control of their emotions and their lives. Reports of negative emotions decrease across the adult years, at least until age 60 (e.g., Carstensen et al., 2000; Charles, Reynolds, & Gatz, 2001; Filipp, 1996; Gross et al., 1997; Lawton, Kleban, Rajagopal, & Dean, 1992; Mroczek & Kolarz, 1998). Positive emotions, in contrast, have been found to be stable during adulthood or to decline only slightly after age 60.

Why do many older people present themselves as happy and having few negative emotions? One possible explanation is that they use better strategies for managing negative experiences and emotions. Using in-depth interviews to study emotional expression and control, Labouvie-Vief and colleagues (Labouvie-Vief, Hakim-Larson, DeVoe, & Schoeberlein, 1989) found that older people used more sophisticated ways of modulating their emotional experiences. This finding that older people have better control over their emotions than younger people has been reported in many other studies (e.g., Gross et al., 1997; Lawton et al., 1992).

Carstensen (1992; Carstensen, Isaacowitz, & Charles, 1999) has proposed that older people maximize their well-being not just through control of emotional expression but by regulating their social interactions. In her theory of socioemotional selectivity, she proposes that older people view the time that they have left in their lives as limited. As a result, they structure their social interactions to maximize positive experiences, actively seeking out people with whom they have positive relationships and avoiding those people who generate negative feelings. Findings from studies of daily irritants and hassles also support this idea. Older people are less likely to report negative interactions in their daily lives than are younger people (Mroczek & Almeida, 2004).

Part of the selection process may be choosing to emphasize positive experiences in important relationships and minimizing or not admitting negative ones. In a study of mother–daughter relationships, Fingerman (2000) found that daughters frequently reported complaints about their mothers but that mothers mainly emphasized positive features of their relationships with daughters. Fingerman posited that older women could not acknowledge to an interviewer, and perhaps to themselves, that their relationships with their daughters had negative qualities. Daughters, however, were quite willing to bring up negative experiences they had had with their mothers.

Not all older people, however, experience this emotional mellowing. Some remain locked in intense conflicts with a spouse, child, or even a parent. Others experience high levels of distress and depression. One source of this difference may be long-standing personality characteristics. Mroczek and Almeida (2004), for example, found that whereas older people, on average, showed less distress than younger individuals in reaction to daily stressors, those older people who were high in neuroticism had high negative reactions to daily stressors. These findings illustrate that aging does not mold everyone in the same way. Personality differences, as well as health and social resources, have strong influences on behavior and emotion.

Control and Adaptation

As we have seen, older people may be able to exercise greater control over emotional expression and perhaps also over the situations that are likely to evoke negative feelings. The control that people apply in shaping their daily lives may be a pivotal element in adaptation in later life. According to Schulz and Heckhausen (1999), these processes can be differentiated into primary and secondary control. Primary control refers to active efforts to modify the external world, whereas secondary control strategies are directed at changing one's own beliefs, motivation, and emotions—for example, making the best of a bad situation. These types of control have different age trajectories. Use of primary control strategies is believed to increase through childhood and adolescence, peak in adulthood, and then gradually decline in old age. Secondary control also increases from childhood on but continues to increase into old age. Older people are less likely to try to exert primary control over the events in their lives and more likely to alter their expectations or judgments to take into account losses or disappointments. As an example, an older man who once had the goal of becoming a millionaire may deal with the failure to achieve that goal by changing his goals, stating that he would rather be happy than rich. This may be the process by which older people maintain positive and minimize negative emotions, or it may be wisdom.

Feeling in control of their lives may help people function better, even when faced with mounting threats to their independence. In their study of the oldest old, Johnson and Barer (1997) describe how very frail persons structured their days into a series of manageable steps that allowed them to get through daily tasks, such as cleaning and meal preparation. They were able to exercise control over only these very mundane activities within their apartments, yet they reported feeling in control of their lives and positive about what they were able to accomplish. The perception of being in control may contribute to independence. Focusing on a type of control belief, mastery, Femia, Zarit, and Johansson (1997) found that people with higher levels of mastery at an initial assessment were more likely to remain independent 2 years later. People with low mastery, however, were more likely to develop disabilities. These effects were found even after controlling for initial levels of health (see also Kempen, van Sonderen, & Ormel, 1999). A sense of control may also be critical in institutional settings. In their classic study, Langer and Rodin (1976) found that nursing home residents who were given the responsibility of caring for a plant in their rooms improved in functioning and well-being compared with residents whose plants were cared for by staff members. Believing oneself to be in control and being able to assert control, even over a very small domain, may be beneficial for maintaining independence and well-being.

Successful Aging

We began the chapter with an example of a person who had had a long, full, and "successful" life. Rowe and Kahn (1987, 1997) first introduced the distinction between usual and successful aging. They argued that much of the geriatrics literature had focused primarily on average levels of functioning but that research on individual differences in later life demonstrates that it is possible to maintain high levels both in health and in psychosocial functioning. According to Rowe and Kahn, processes that have been found to contribute to successful aging are maintaining a sense of control over one's life, good health habits, social relationships that provide emotional support and assistance, and having a meaningful commitment. They believe that the goal for geriatrics practitioners should be to promote the processes that underlie successful aging.

Other researchers have highlighted similar processes that lead to optimal outcomes in later life. Ryff (1989), for example, stressed the importance of having a positive and caring relationship, maintaining a sense of humor, enjoying life, and being able to accept change. Blazer (2002) proposed that self-efficacy plays a pivotal role in successful aging. Older people who believe that they can have an impact in such important areas of their lives as their health or finding meaningful activities are less likely to suffer from depressive symptoms or to have other problems. Blazer also suggests that interventions that build self-efficacy in areas such as managing one's health and social relationships might prevent depression in later life. As baby boomers grow older, interventions designed to promote successful aging and prevent mental health problems are likely to become increasingly popular.

CONCLUSIONS

In contrast to the commonplace negative views of aging that are grounded more in prejudice than in fact, we have presented an optimistic perspective that has emerged from research on the normal aging process. Today's older people are healthier and better educated than ever before, and this trend will continue as future generations reach old age. Research on psychological functioning suggests both stability and change, but in the absence of dementia, decline in intelligence, memory, and other abilities is relatively mild and does not interfere with the ability to carry out everyday activities. Older and younger people differ in many ways. Some of those differences are due to the experiences that come with aging. Many differences, however, have been shaped by generational experiences, as well as historical and cultural influences.

These findings on the normal processes of aging form a foundation for psychological assessment and treatment. Decline and disability are important aspects of later life, but aging is not just a process of unremitting decline. Rather, older people have resources and abilities that can be utilized in dealing with difficult life transitions, such as retirement, illness, or widowhood, or with other problems they encounter. They have the capacity to regain lost functioning and make a successful adaptation to the challenges facing them. Older clients also bring a unique resource to treatment: a lifetime of learning and experience. Age is a barrier neither to leading a meaningful and satisfying life nor to treatment of psychological problems.

CHAPTER 3

Disorders of Aging

DEMENTIA, DELIRIUM, AND OTHER COGNITIVE PROBLEMS

Our discussion of disorders of aging starts with dementia because it is the most devastating problem in late life and the one that mental health professionals are least likely to have encountered in their prior training. We describe the general pattern of symptoms of the dementia syndrome and studies of its prevalence and then discuss the more common types of dementia, such as Alzheimer's disease (AD), frontotemporal dementia (FTD), and vascular dementia (VaD). Also included in the chapter are two syndromes, reversible dementia and delirium—which present with cognitive symptoms and so are often mistaken for dementia—and mild cognitive impairment, which is believed to be an early or preclinical manifestation of dementia. We have provided abundant detail on these disorders for two main reasons. First, the most important and most frequent assessment question that the geriatric specialist must address is whether or not someone is suffering from dementia. The description of dementia and delirium in this chapter, in combination with our discussion of assessment in Chapters 6 and 7, prepares clinicians to tackle that question. Second, opportunities for meaningful interventions, especially with families of people with dementia and also with patients themselves, are increasing, especially regarding efforts to diagnose dementia as early as possible in the course of the illness.

This is a rapidly changing field, with significant new research appearing regularly. We find ourselves frequently sorting through new findings to identify advances in our understanding of these disorders. Several useful websites provide new and reliable information; these are provided in Table 3.1. The

TABLE 3.1. Useful Websites for Information on Dementia

- Alzheimer's Disease Education and Referral Center (ADEAR) of the National Institute on Aging
  www.niapublications.org/adear/
- Alzheimer's Association
  www.alz.org
- Association for Frontotemporal Dementia
  www.ftd-picks.org
- Family Caregiver Alliance
  www.caregiver.org
- Lewy Body Dementia Association
  www.lewybodydementia.org
- National Institute of Neurological Disorders and Stroke
  www.ninds.nih.gov/disorders/multi_infarct_dementia/multi_infarct_dementia.htm

best single source for in-depth information is the book *Dementia: A Clinical Approach* by Mendez and Cummings (2003).

DEMENTIA

ONSET OF DEMENTIA

Al and Donna entered old age relatively healthy, had good friends, and took part in many satisfying activities. At age 73, Al was taking only an antihypertensive and a baby aspirin.

Donna wasn't sure when the changes in Al had first started. He had always been independent, and he had always had a temper. Al was jealous of Donna's close relationship with their children. On more than one occasion, he had stormed out of one of their son's homes and had gone home alone. But now Al was unpredictable. Sometimes he actually seemed sweeter and more affectionate than he had ever been. Then, with no apparent provocation, he would slam books to the floor, yelling angrily and grabbing his car keys as he raced out the door.

Donna tried to get Al to go for counseling, thinking that it was a problem between the two of them. He refused to consider it. Finally, without telling him, she sought help for herself, at the urging of her children. She described to me the changes in his personality and how she no longer knew how to soothe him. When I asked Donna about Al's memory, initially she said he had no problems that she had noticed. However, she had begun finding rolls of cash hidden in odd places in the house. This was especially surprising to her because he usually carried very little cash. She had asked him about it once, and he became very angry. So she just tried to keep track of the money and said nothing further about it to him. She also found projects he had started and not completed, which was also unusual.

Over the next few years, Donna came to therapy one or two times a month. During this period, Al's behavior problems gradually increased. She began to realize that his memory was unreliable. He was a very proud man and quite intelligent, so his ability to hide these lapses continued for some time. When he could not recall a name, he would cover with a friendly greeting. When he wasn't able to find the word he wanted, he would substitute another. Eventually, as Al's language started to become more problematic, he withdrew angrily and spoke less and less.

One day, Donna came in with a very troubling story. Earlier in the week, Al had disappeared, and several hours later, Donna got a call from a police department in a town 2 hours away. They had stopped Al because he was driving erratically. He had told them he was on his way home, but, when asked where home was, he gave the name of the town he was born in, which did not match his driver's license. Donna and her children could no longer deny the fact that something was seriously wrong.

They decided to take Al to a university medical center for an evaluation. A complete neurological workup was done, including blood work, a magnetic resonance imaging test (MRI), an electroencephalogram (EEG), and neuropsychological screening tests. The only findings were scattered white-matter hyperintensities (abnormalities associated with vascular problems) and mild enlargement of the ventricles, which suggests the possible loss of neurons. These findings alone would not be indicative of dementia. But the neuropsychological screening tests showed moderate disorientation and moderate anomic aphasia. The neurologist made a diagnosis of possible mixed dementia, AD, and VaD. Al was given a trial of a cholinesterase inhibitor (a medication for AD), and for a few months, things seemed a little better.

Then one evening Al got in his car to drive around town, something he had done every night for nearly 40 years. Instead of being gone for 30 minutes, he was gone for more than 2 hours, returning home with a dent in the left front fender. Donna was never able to determine what he might have collided with, but she realized that he was no longer safe driving. Unfortunately, Al disagreed. First, Donna hid his keys and pretended to have lost them. But Al called the dealer and had a new set made. Next, she had her son disconnect the battery and told Al the car wouldn't start. After a few days, she moved the car to her son's house and told Al it was in the shop. He pestered her constantly, asking when it would be fixed, and she hoped that eventually his poor memory would work to her advantage in this. Curiously, he never attempted to drive her car, and he allowed her to do the driving from that time on.

The Dementia Syndrome

The symptoms Al experienced—progressive memory impairment and deterioration of habits and personality—are hallmarks of dementia. Though it is not a universal feature of aging, dementia occurs with sufficient frequency to be the most costly disorder in later life, both in its human toll and in the expense of caring for patients. Nancy Reagan poignantly characterized the decline of her husband, former President Ronald Reagan, who suffered from AD, as "the long goodbye" (Barrett, 1997). This phrase captures the slow, painful process of decline associated with this disease.

The term "dementia" refers to a syndrome of progressive decline in memory and other intellectual abilities. Dementia is a syndrome, not a disease, and it can, in fact, be caused by many different illnesses. The dementia syndrome is characterized by three key features: it is acquired, it is persistent, and it involves impairment in multiple domains of intellectual functioning (Cummings & Mega, 2003). Dementia differs from mental retardation in that it is an acquired disability. Symptoms of dementia persist and worsen over time. In contrast, cognitive symptoms in other psychiatric disorders, such as depression, tend to be transitory. Finally, dementia involves deficits in multiple cognitive functions—language, memory, visual–spatial skills, and general intellectual abilities. By comparison, head trauma or stroke often result in deficits in specific functions controlled by the areas of the brain affected by the trauma.

The dementia syndrome can develop from many different disorders, including some that are currently potentially reversible. Common causes of dementia are shown in Table 3.2.

According to the fourth edition of the *Diagnostic and Statistical Manual of Mental Disorders* (DSM-IV) of the American Psychiatric Association (1994), three main criteria for diagnosis of dementia are (1) memory impairment, (2) cognitive disturbances in at least one other area of functioning (e.g., aphasia, apraxia, agnosia, or a disturbance in executive functions) that are (3) severe enough to interfere with social or occupational functioning. The pattern of symptoms, however, varies depending on the site of brain damage. Mendez and Cummings (2003) make a distinction between cortical and frontal–subcortical dementia. Cortical dementias are characterized by prominent deficits in language, memory, and visual processing. Patients are also typically unable to carry out complex functional tasks, such as dressing. AD and FTD are the most common types of cortical dementia. In contrast, frontal–subcortical dementias have a greater impact on the frontal cortex and subcortical areas, such as the basal ganglia and thalamus and the pathways between them. The typical changes associated with these disorders involve movement disorders, a slowing of mental functioning, and lack of motivation. Patients have difficulty with learning and retrieval, but in contrast to the cortical dementias, they can improve performance when provided with cues and prompting. Vascular dementia, dementia due to Parkinson's or Lewy body disease, and HIV dementia all have prominent frontal–subcortical involvement. As Mendez and Cummings point out, disorders do not always follow this pattern. In AD, for example, some subcortical regions are affected. Rather, this scheme represents a heuristic approach that can guide clinicians in

TABLE 3.2. Common Types of Dementia

Primary dementia—Dementia such as Alzheimer's disease that does not result from any other disease.
- Alzheimer's disease
- Vascular dementias
- Lewy body dementia
- Frontotemporal dementia
- HIV-associated dementia
- Huntington's disease
- Dementia pugilistica
- Corticobasal degeneration
- Creutzfeldt–Jakob disease

Secondary dementia—Dementia that may occur in conjunction with another illness or injury.
- Parkinson's disease
- Multiple sclerosis
- Presenile dementia with motor neuron disease, also called ALS dementia Olivopontocerebellar atrophy (OPCA)
- Wilson's disease
- Normal pressure hydrocephalus

Other conditions—Conditions that can cause dementia or dementia-like symptoms, including reversible causes.

Reactions to medications

Metabolic problems and endocrine abnormalities, including:
- Thyroid problems
- Hypoglycemia
- Too little or too much sodium or calcium
- Impaired absorption of Vitamin B_{12} (pernicious anemia)

Nutritional deficiencies, including:
- Deficiencies of thiamine (Vitamin B_1)
- Severe deficiency of Vitamin B_6
- Deficiencies of Vitamin B_{12}
- Dehydration

Infections, including:
- Meningitis and encephalitis
- Untreated syphilis
- Lyme disease
- Progressive multifocal leukoencephalopathy (PML)

Subdural hematomas

Poisoning
- Exposure to lead, other heavy metals, or other poisonous substances

Brain tumors

Anoxia

Heart and lung problems

Note. From National Institute of Neurological Disorders and Stroke. (2006). *The dementias: Hope through research*. Retrieved from www.ninds.nih.gov/disorders/alzheimersdisease/detail_alzheimers-disease.htm#58683045 what systems to assess for possible impairment. Although in some cases the pattern of symptoms is not clear, most people present with predominantly cortical or frontal–subcortical symptoms.

Prevalence of Dementia

The incidence and prevalence of dementia rise with age. Dementia is virtually unknown before age 35, but it may affect 30% of the population age 85 and older. Estimating the exact number of people who suffer from dementia is complicated, mainly because there are as yet no definitive biomedical or psychological markers for diagnosis of the illnesses that cause it, such as AD. A state-of-the-art diagnostic evaluation draws on behavioral, neuropsychological, and medical data (see Chapters 5 and 6) and can be very accurate in identifying people with dementia. By contrast, epidemiological studies that estimate the prevalence in the population necessarily rely on brief mental status or cognitive screening evaluations that are not as reliable as a thorough assessment. Identification is most difficult for early and mild cases. Factors such as low education, health problems, and medications and psychiatric symptoms such as depression and anxiety affect cognitive functioning and may lead to overdiagnosis of dementia (Crum, Anthony, Bassett, & Folstein, 1993; Johansson & Zarit, 1997). Conversely, screening tests do not necessarily identify mild dementia in well-educated people, who can score in normal ranges on these tests despite developing obvious deficits in other areas of functioning.

It is not surprising, then, that there is generally a consensus on the prevalence of moderate and severe dementia but not on mild cases. Most studies from North America, Europe, and East Asia report rates of moderate and severe dementia as ranging between 3 and 7% for the population over age 65 (Anthony & Aboraya, 1992; Canadian Study of Health and Aging Working Group, 1994; Kay, 1995; Kim, Jeong, Chun, & Lee, 2003; Liu et al., 1995; Wimo, Winblad, Aguero-Torres, & von Strauss, 2003). Similar estimates of prevalence have been found for Latino, African American, and non-Latino white groups in the United States (Gurland et al., 1995). These estimates are lower than the 10% prevalence typically cited in the United States. That rate, however, was based on a single study (Evans et al., 1989), which used an unusual method of computing prevalence that inflated the estimate (Johansson & Zarit, 1995).

There is much more variability in rates of mild cases of dementia, with estimates varying from 3 to 64% (Busse, Bischkopf, Riedel-Heller, & Angermeyer, 2003; Mowry & Burvill, 1988). Recently, attention has turned to identifying people with preclinical symptoms of dementia. The term "mild cognitive impairment" (MCI) describes people with cognitive problems that do not yet meet diagnostic criteria. As with mild impairment, rates of MCI show considerable variability, with estimates ranging between 3 and 20% of the older population. There is undoubtedly some overlap between cases identified as early and as mild dementia in previous studies and those regarded as MCI now. Estimates of early-stage dementia and MCI are likely to remain problematic until more reliable ways of determining early signs and symptoms of dementia are developed.

Whatever the true prevalence turns out to be, it is clear that rates of dementia increase with age (Figure 3.1). Prevalence of dementia among people in their 60s is around 1%. It increases to 7% by the mid-70s and then rises dramatically in the 80s, to between 20 and 30% of the population (e.g., Canadian Study of Health and Aging Working Group, 1994; Johansson & Zarit, 1995; Kay, 1995; Skoog, Nilsson, Palmertz, Andreassen, & Svanborg, 1993). The cumulative risk of developing dementia at some point in one's life is even higher. Among people in their 80s, slightly more than 50% developed dementia before they died (Johansson & Zarit, 1995, 1997).

The prevalence of dementia is higher among women than men, though the reasons for this difference are still controversial. It has been speculated that hormonal changes with menopause may place women at increased risk, although new studies raise questions about that hypothesis (Shumaker et al., 2003). An obvious factor contributing to the sex difference is that, in general, women live longer than men and thus are more likely to survive to ages at which the risk of dementia is greatest (Kay, 1995). Another reason for differences in prevalence is that women live longer than men do after the onset of the disorder (Heyman, Peterson, Fillenbaum, & Pieper, 1996). When studies have focused just on the incidence of new cases of dementia, rather than its prevalence, no sex differences were found (Edland, Rocca, Petersen, Cha, & Kokmen, 2002; Gatz et al., 2003).

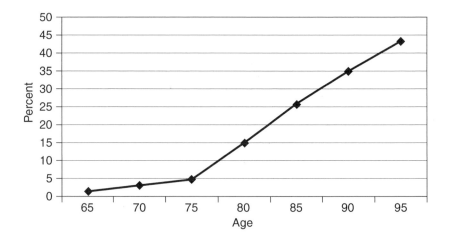

FIGURE 3.1. Prevalence of dementia with advancing age. Data from Canadian Study of Health and Aging Working Group (1994) and Johansson and Zarit (1995, 1997).

Alzheimer's Disease

AD is the most frequent cause of dementia. It is characterized by an insidious onset and gradual, steady deterioration. Impairment in memory and new learning is typically noticed first, but visual–spatial and language problems may also be present early in the disease. The person gradually loses the ability to perform everyday tasks. Early on, the ability to carry out complex activities, such as work-related tasks or managing finances, is impaired. Later in the disease, people can no longer perform basic activities of daily living, such as dressing and bathing. Personality changes may occur, including increased apathy, dependency, anger, aggressiveness, and inappropriate sexual behavior. Patients' awareness of their condition varies. In the early stages of the disease, people sometimes recognize that something is wrong, although denial and covering up of problems is common. As the disease progresses, some people continue to have at least occasional awareness of their disorder, but it is more typical for patients to deny having any difficulties or problems and to be unaware of their limitations. Depression occurs with some frequency in the early and middle stages of AD (Reifler, Larson, & Hanley, 1982; Teri & Wagner, 1992).

This disorder was first described by Alois Alzheimer in 1907 in a 51-year-old patient. Using new staining techniques for tissue samples prepared for the microscope, Alzheimer identified the types of pathology in brain tissue that have come to be regarded as the hallmarks of the disease: amyloid plaques and neurofibrillary tangles. Because the disorder was identified initially in patients in their 40s and 50s, it was originally considered a "presenile dementia." In contrast, dementia after 65 was regarded as an inevitable deterioration associated with the aging process or as the result of restricted blood flow, or hardening of the arteries. Beginning in the 1960s, studies reported that many older people with dementia had similar or identical brain pathology to that of "presenile" cases (Terry & Katzman, 1983), leading to a reconceptualization of AD as occurring both early and late in life.

The major significance of age of onset is that early cases (before age 55) are likely to be related to a strong inherited pattern (Harvey & Rossor, 1995). In late-onset cases, genetics contributes to the etiology but is not sufficient by itself to account for the cause. There have been reports that symptoms differ in early- and late-onset cases. Greater difficulties in spatial orientation (Raskind, Carta, & Bravi, 1995) and language (Imamura et al., 1998) have been reported in early-onset cases. Cases with early onset have also been reported to progress more rapidly (Jacobs et al., 1994). Other studies, however, have not confirmed these differences in symptoms or progression (Lehtovirta et al., 1996; Swearer, O'Donnell, Drachman, & Woodward, 1992; Swearer, O'Donnell, Ingram, & Drachman, 1996).

AD accounts for the majority of cases of dementia in the United States and Europe (Kokmen, Beard, Offord, & Kurland, 1989; Ott et al., 1995; Skoog et al., 1993). Based on postmortem examinations, about three-quarters of cases of dementia involve Alzheimer-type pathologies—amyloid plaques and neurofibrillary tangles (Barker et al., 2002; Knopman et al., 2003; Mendez, Mastri, Sung, & Frey, 1992). Many of these patients also show evidence of other types of pathology, particularly vascular changes and Lewy bodies (Knopman et al., 2003; Snowdon et al., 1997).

Clinical characteristics remain the main way of identifying AD in the absence of an autopsy. Although there have been frequent reports of new biomedical tests that improve diagnosis of AD, including various types of brain scans, as well as laboratory findings, none has yet proven more reliable than assessment of cognitive and functional impairment. Clinical criteria for diagnosis are found in the DSM-IV (American Psychiatric Association, 1994). A diagnosis of AD can be made when there is impairment in memory and at least one other area of cognitive functioning and when these cognitive deficits cause significant impairment in social activities and work. Other possible causes of cognitive symptoms must be ruled out, particularly reversible illnesses and delirium and other types of dementia.

AD has often been described as having distinct stages. Among the more widely used stage models are the Global Deterioration Scale (Reisberg, Ferris, de Leon, & Crook, 1982), and the Clinical Dementia Rating (Hughes, Berg, Danziger, Coben, & Martin, 1982). Distinct and unique stages probably do not occur, but these models are useful for illustrating the pattern of decline. Cognitive symptoms progress from mild memory and other cognitive problems to pronounced difficulties that make it difficult to carry out even simple activities to a final stage in which patients may be largely unresponsive. Parallel to these cognitive changes, the ability to perform everyday activities declines, beginning first with complex activities that demand considerable cognitive resources, such as work, and then proceeding to basic activities of daily living such as dressing or bathing.

The rate of progression of symptoms in AD can vary (Teri, Hughes, & Larson, 1990). In some cases, the patient progresses to severe disability and death in a few years. More typically, deterioration is gradual and prolonged. Aneshensel, Pearlin, Mullan, Zarit, and Whitlatch (1995) found that the median life expectancy of a sample of persons with various types of dementia was 11 years after onset of symptoms. Many patients survive as long as 20 years after diagnosis. Progression is more rapid among patients who are agitated, who have other neurological diseases, and who abuse alcohol (Teri et al., 1990). Death is brought about by other illnesses or by complications of AD, such as loss of the ability to swallow or greater susceptibility to infections.

Neuropathology of AD

The classic pathological features described originally by Alzheimer are amyloid plaques, neurofibrillary tangles, and brain atrophy. Amyloid plaques (which are sometimes called neuritic or senile plaques) are accumulations of degenerative nerve endings and other material, with a core of the peptide beta amyloid. Located near synapses, plaques probably interfere with communication between neurons and may also be toxic to healthy cells. Neurofibrillary tangles are twisted strands of protein found within the bodies of nerve cells. Tangles probably interfere with the cells' energy metabolism and the movement of chemicals to cell endings, and they eventually lead to cell death.

Atrophy is due to a loss of neurons. Damage is selective, affecting some parts of the brain and types of neurons more than others. Cell loss is most pronounced in the temporolimbic region, particularly the hippocampus, entorhinal cortex, and amygdala, as well as in frontal and temporoparietal areas of the brain (Mendez & Cummings, 2003). Sensorimotor areas are relatively spared. These patterns of cell loss correspond to typical neuropsychological performance found in patients (Chapter 7).

Accompanying the loss of cells is a decrease of certain neurotransmitters, the chemicals that permit communication across the synapses between neurons. Among the affected neurotransmitters are acetylcholine, serotonin, and norepinephrine (Mendez & Cummings, 2003).

The Search for Causes of AD

The main search for a cause for AD has centered on the role of amyloid. Amyloid is produced normally by cells, released into the bloodstream, and broken down by an enzyme called alpha-secretase. In AD, other enzymes, called beta- and gamma-secretase, produce a variant form that is called beta-amyloid. Beta-amyloid is sticky and begins clumping together to form plaques. These amyloid plaques, in turn, are believed to contribute to further degeneration (Hardy, 1993; Lansbury et al., 1995).

Neurofibrillary tangles may also make an important contribution to the development of AD, either in combination with beta-amyloid or independent of it. The protein that makes up the tangles, A68, is an abnormal variation of the tau protein (Lee, Balin, Otvos, & Trojanowski, 1991). The tau protein is found throughout the central nervous system and helps stabilize microtubules, which form a skeleton to support normal cell structure. This structure serves as a pathway for nutrients and other molecules from the cell nucleus to the axon. Abnormal variants appear to be the result of errors in the phosphorylation process in which phosphates are added to tau. These errors cause tau to aggregate into tangled strands, which weakens cell structure. Tau pathologies play a role in other neurodegenerative diseases, particularly some of the FTDs.

Genetic factors may set off the processes that lead to production of beta-amyloid and neurofibrillary tangles. Genetic risk factors have been found for the formation of tau protein tangles (Bird et al., 1999). Most of the focus, however, has been on genetic abnormalities, which may be related to overproduction of beta-amyloid. Mutations have been identified on chromosome 21, chromosome 14 (called presenilin-1), and chromosome 1 (called presenilin-2). Each of these mutations leads to early-onset AD (Schellenberg et al., 1992; St. George-Hyslop et al., 1987, 1990). Inheritance follows an autosomal dominant pattern; that is, the children of a parent with one of these mutations have a 50% chance of carrying the mutant gene and developing the disease (St. George-Hyslop et al., 1990).

In addition to these three mutations, susceptibility genes have been identified for late-onset AD. In contrast to autosomal dominant genes, susceptibility genes contribute to the etiology of disease, in combination with environmental and/or other genetic risk factors. They do not appear sufficient in and of themselves to cause the disease, and the inherited risk is lower than for the autosomal dominant Alzheimer's genes (e.g., Gatz et al., 1997).

Four or five susceptibility genes associated with late-onset cases have been identified. The best characterized site is on chromosome 19. This genetic site codes apolipoprotein (Apo E), which is involved in cholesterol transport and also appears to have a role in binding amyloid. Three variants of Apo E have been identified: Apo E2, Apo E3, and Apo E4. Increased risk of AD is associated with Apo E4. About 15% of the population carry one or two copies of the E4 allele. People with one copy of Apo E4 have 2 or 3 times the risk of developing AD by age 75 than people with other types of Apo E, whereas people with two copies of the Apo E4 gene have between 5 and 10 times the risk (Corder et al., 1993; Kuller et al., 2003). The presence of E4 has also been found to be associated with milder forms of cognitive decline in later life, indicating possible early changes due to AD (Haan, Shemanski, Jagust, Manolio, & Kuller, 1999; Hofer et al., 2002; Lopez, Jagust, Dulberg, et al., 2003). In some population groups, however, such as Finns and possibly African Americans, high rates of Apo E4 are not associated with greater prevalence of AD (Mayeux, 2003).

Other possible risk genes have been identified on chromosomes 9, 10, 12, and 14 (Kamboh, Sanghera, Ferrell, & DeKosky, 1995; Myers & Goate, 2001; Stephenson, 1997; Wang, DeKosky, Ikonomovic, & Kamboh, 2002). These diverse findings about genetic markers of AD indicate that more than one cause and different genetic sites or combinations of genetic and environmental influences are related to its cause (St. George-Hyslop et al., 1990). Given this heterogeneity, AD may be best thought of as a spectrum of diseases rather than a single disorder (Gatz, Lowe, Berg, Mortimer, & Pedersen, 1994).

The role of genetic influences naturally raises concern among children and grandchildren of people with AD. Genetic testing, which has proven to be helpful to families with other genetic disorders such as Huntington's disease, is available for the known variants of early-onset AD and for the Apo E4 allele. Counseling children of people with early-onset AD can address the implications of genetic risk to themselves and their children and the advisability of genetic testing. Given the lower risk of inheritance in late-onset cases, even for people with two copies of Apo E4, genetic testing is not recommended at this time (Post et al., 1997).

Amyloid plaques and neurofibrillary tangles appear to be the core of the pathology in AD, but they set off a cascade of other events in the brain that may increase the damage and dysfunction. The areas around plaques become inflamed, and there may be oxidative stress due to an excess of free radicals. As noted, there are also decreases in the availability of certain neurotransmitters, as well as excessive amounts of other substances, such as glutamate.

One of the most intriguing hypotheses is that factors such as hypertension, high cholesterol, and coronary artery disease that have long been regarded as risk factors for VaD may also increase risk for AD (Mendez & Cummings, 2003; Newman et al., 2005). Cerebrovascular disease may increase the risk of AD in a couple of ways. Cognitive impairment may occur when a critical threshold of the amount of cortical damage is passed. The source of brain damage may be less critical than the amount. In this scenario, small amounts of damage due to early AD and vascular changes have an additive effect that results in dementia, whereas the amount of either pathology by itself would not be sufficient to produce symptoms (Newman et al., 2005). Another possibility is that vascular disease could have a potentiating or triggering effect on AD through added stress to the brain (Mendez & Cummings, 2003).

Insulin resistance and type-2 diabetes have also been hypothesized to play a role (e.g., de la Monte & Wands, 2005; Fishel et al., 2005). In addition to contributing to vascular disease (see later in this chapter), insulin resistance may potentiate the release of beta-amyloid.

The toxic effects of metals, especially aluminum, have been considered as a possible trigger for the pathologies found in AD. The accumulation of aluminum as a result of kidney dialysis has been found to produce dementia (Davison, Walker, Oli, & Lewins, 1982). It remains unclear, however, whether people with AD have been exposed to excessive amounts of aluminum or have greater brain levels of aluminum than age-matched controls (Graves et al., 1990).

Head injury early in life, particularly involving loss of consciousness for 5 minutes or more, may increase risk of AD (Schofield et al., 1997). Boxers frequently develop dementia symptoms later in life and have been found on autopsy to display some characteristic brain pathologies similar but not identical to AD (see Corsellis, Bruton, & Freeman-Browne, 1973; McKenzie, Roberts, & Royston, 1996).

Anesthesia is another possible stressor to the brain. Onset of dementia symptoms is sometimes reported after surgery in which a general anesthetic has been used. Studies that have examined the possible association of exposure to anesthesia and AD have not been able to establish a clear relationship

(Bohnen, Warner, Kokmen, Beard, & Kurland, 1994). An alternative explanation is that anesthesia and the other stresses of a hospital stay may uncover a preexisting dementing illness. Symptoms that were minimal and went unnoticed by the family before surgery become more pronounced afterward. For people who already show definite symptoms of dementia, anesthesia and other stressors can lead to a major decline in functioning.

Promising Leads in the Treatment and Prevention of AD

The search for a treatment for AD has increasingly focused on amyloid plaques and neurofibrillary tangles as possible primary factors in the disease. Drug trials are under way of substances that might alter the formation of the abnormal variant of tau that makes up neurofibrillary tangles. Researchers are also attempting to prevent the accumulation of beta-amyloid either by mobilizing the immune system to break it down, by blocking the enzymes, beta- and gamma-secretase, that are associated with its formation, or by increasing the availability of alpha-secretase.

Some medications, the cholinesterase inhibitors and memantine, a glutamate inhibitor, have been approved for treatment of AD. These medications have been found to provide mild short-term benefits (Areosa Sastre, Sherriff, & McShane, 2005; Birks & Harvey, 2006; Knapp et al., 1994; Reisberg et al., 2003), and are discussed in more detail in Chapter 12.

A number of medications used for other purposes have been explored for their effect on AD. For many years, estrogen has been reported to decrease the risk of AD. Unfortunately, in a trial involving estrogen replacement in women 65 and older, the experimental group showed an increase in the incidence of AD (Shumaker et al., 2003). Treatment of women who already have AD with estrogen has also not been effective (Thal et al., 2003). Despite these negative findings, some hope is held that unopposed estrogen (administered without progesterone) could have a protective effect.

Statins, which lower cholesterol, have also been reported to lead to lower risk of AD, perhaps because they lower the risk of small strokes and VaD. A definitive test of the role of statins remains to be made.

One of the consequences of AD is an increased amount of oxidative damage in the brain due to an excess of free radicals. Vitamin E and other antioxidants (carotene, vitamin C) could reduce the amount of free radicals in the brain, thereby reducing some of the damage that is occurring. Studies that have examined intake of antioxidants and subsequent risk of developing AD have had mixed results. Some studies have reported reduced risk (e.g., Englehart et al., 2002; Maxwell, Hicks, Hogan, Basran & Ebly, 2005), but other studies have found no protective effect (Luchsinger, Tang, Shea, & Mayeux, 2003; Petersen et al., 2005). Benefits to patients with AD have not been established, and there is a risk of significant side effects with high doses (Mendez & Cummings, 2003). The antioxidant selegiline also has been found to have no therapeutic benefits in AD, though it may have a role in treatment of patients with Parkinson's disease (Birks & Flicker, 2003).

Another focus of treatment has been the use of nonsteroidal anti-inflammatory medications (NSAIDs). These common medications are thought to reduce the inflammation that occurs when plaques form. As with antioxidants, there is some evidence that people who take NSAIDs may have reduced risk of developing AD (see e.g., t'Veld et al., 2001). A trial of common anti-inflammatories, however, found no benefit for patients with the disease (Aisen et al., 2003). Recently, one class of NSAIDs, the cox-2 inhibitors, was found to increase the risk of cardiovascular problems and mortality (Juni et al., 2004). Other NSAIDs can lead to gastrointenstinal problems, including stomach bleeding, particularly for older patients. As a result, any potential benefits need to be weighed against potential adverse effects.

As evidence has accumulated that genetic risk alone cannot account for most cases of AD, an extensive search has been undertaken for other factors that might contribute to the disease or potentially protect against it. A long list of possible protective factors has emerged, including some noted earlier— estrogen replacement and use of antioxidants and anti-inflammatory medications, as well as cognitive stimulation and education (Fritsch, McClendon, Smyth, & Ogrocki, 2002; Gatz et al., 2001; Liu et al., 1995; Stern et al., 1994), low cholesterol (Miller, 2004), low intake of dietary fats (Morris, Evans, Bienias, Tangney, Bennett, Aggarwell, et al., 2003), moderate consumption of alcohol (Mukamal et al., 2003), foods high in antioxidants (Ortiz & Shea, 2004), normal blood sugar and weight (Fishel et al., 2005; Whitmer, Gunderson, Barrett-Connor, Quesenberry, & Yaffe, 2005), and normal blood pressure (Qiu, von Strauss, Fasborn, Winblad, & Fratiglioni, 2003). Depression and other psychiatric symptoms have emerged as possible risk factors (Copeland et al., 2003; Green et al., 2003).

Understanding Contradictory and Improbable Findings about Treatment for AD

The number of potential risk and protective factors that have been reported for AD has grown exponentially in recent years, and it is likely that by the time you read this chapter, more additions have been made to this list. Some findings have not been confirmed, and others seem to have no plausible basis. As each new potential treatment hits the media, families of patients with AD will want to know its value for their relative and also for themselves.

In evaluating these various studies, the primary question is whether the evidence is based on an experimental or a correlational design. A study that has used an experimental design with random assignment and double-blind evaluation of the outcomes provides the most definitive results. Most of the evidence on risk and protective factors for AD has come instead from large population studies that conduct correlational analyses. These studies are very useful for the initial testing of hypotheses, but the results cannot be viewed with as much confidence as those from an experimental trial.

Correlational studies are prone to three types of error that may lead to incorrect or misleading results. First, as every student learns in introductory statistics, correlation is not causation. The association may not be due to the effects of variable A on variable B. Instead, some third variable may influence both A and B. In the case of estrogen replacement, for example, the third variable might be education: Women with more education may be more likely to receive estrogen replacement therapy; thus education level may account for the findings of a lower risk of AD. The relation of education and cognitive stimulation to lower risk may be an artifact of how we detect cases. People with less education will reach the threshold at which the diagnosis is made sooner because they start out with lower cognitive functioning or have fewer compensatory processes for the early changes in dementia. In a well-designed study, every effort will be made to control statistically for these types of alternative explanations that might account for the findings, but those controls will not necessarily eliminate the problem.

Second, because many of the studies of risk and protective factors have used large samples, a finding could be significant yet account for only a trivial amount of variance. It may be that eating more green vegetables, for example, protects against AD, but the benefit could be small.

Finally, a correlational design does not necessarily take into account possible adverse effects of the protective factor. When subjected to more rigorous investigation, both estrogen replacement and anti-inflammatory medications were found to increase the risk of adverse health events.

Families will often ask clinicians about new findings, and so it is important for clinicians to review reports in light of how the studies were conducted. We generally advise families to be cautious about new findings, especially when the treatment might involve some risk. Some potential protective factors, however—such as mental and physical exercise and maintaining a healthy diet—carry very little risk of negative consequences and may do some good for overall health, if not for AD.

AD is the most frequent cause of dementia and the one about which the most is known. The other main types of dementia are discussed next.

Frontotemporal Dementia

Several degenerative disorders primarily affect the frontal and temporal lobes. These disorders, which have come to be called frontotemporal dementia (FTD), involve neural degeneration primarily in the frontal and temporal lobes of the brain, although some variants also include deterioration in motor areas. Types of FTD are shown in Table 3.3. The disorders are distinguished from one another by their underlying pathologies (McKhann et al., 2001).

TABLE 3.3. Types of Frontotemporal Dementia

Pick's disease

Frontotemporal dementia with parkinsonism linked to chromosome 17

Primary progressive aphasia

Semantic dementia

Corticobasal degeneration

Progressive supranuclear palsy

Note. From the National Institute of Neurological Disorders and Stroke (2006).

Pick's disease is characterized by the presence of Pick bodies, large, dense structures found in the cytoplasm of brain neurons, and by swollen, ballooned cells called Pick cells. Most cases of FTD, however, do not have the typical Pick pathology (Mann, 1997). Some of these disorders, including Pick's disease, are marked by abnormal variants of the tau protein, whereas other disorders have another protein that appears to be involved in degeneration, ubiquitin (McKhann et al., 2001; Murman, 2003). In contrast to AD, there is no evidence of amyloid plaques. Criteria for a neuropathology diagnosis include atrophy in the frontal and temporal lobes, without evidence of pathologies specific to AD or Lewy body disease (McKhann et al., 2001).

Estimates of the prevalence of FTD vary between 3 and 10% of dementia patients (Bird et al., 2003; Gustafson, Brun, & Passant, 1992; Massoud et al., 1999). Onset typically occurs at relatively young ages, between 35 and 75 (McKhann et al., 2001), although some cases with frontal symptoms have been reported among 85-year-olds (Gislason, Sjogren, Larsson, & Skoog, 2003). Among early-onset dementias (before age 65), cases of FTD may be as prevalent or nearly so as AD (Ratnavalli, Brayne, Dawson, & Hodges, 2002). It has been estimated that between 20 and 40% of cases have a positive family history (Mann, 1997; McKhann et al., 2001; Neary, 1990). One variant, frontotemporal dementia with parkinsonism linked to chromosome 17, is named specifically for its link to a genetic site, as well as for its combination of behavioral, cognitive, and motor symptoms. Other genetic abnormalities have been identified on chromosomes 3 and 9. FTD is also more common among men than women. There are no current treatments, though compounds that address the formation of abnormal variants of tau are under development.

Clinicians familiar with the symptoms of people with frontal head injuries will recognize the behavioral and cognitive symptoms of FTD. Behavioral symptoms typically involve impairment of executive functions, including personality changes, disinhibition of behavior, impaired social behavior and judgment, and lack of insight, as well as impairment in language, speech, and movement. Patients may act in impulsive ways, for example, with outbursts of profanities, or may exercise poor judgment in managing their finances.

Patients may lack initiative, have poor hygiene, and neglect their responsibilities. Mood is either blunted or slightly euphoric. Some stereotyped and repetitive behaviors may also occur.

Language problems are often prominent, particularly difficulties in naming and expressing oneself. Patients have trouble with word finding and naming familiar objects, and they may use circumlocutions when they cannot recall a name. A characteristic speech pattern in Pick's disease is echolalia, that is, excessively repeating certain words or syllables. A patient who is asked, "How are you today?" might reply, "Today, today, today. . . . " In some patients, understanding of the meaning of words is preserved, but that is not the case for others. The terms "primary progressive aphasia" and "semantic dementia" are sometimes used to describe these patterns (McKhann et al., 2001). Memory can also be impaired, though deficits are less prominent early in the disease than in AD. As FTDs progress, however, a more generalized pattern of intellectual deficits develops.

McKhann and colleagues (2001) suggest that there are two patterns of presentation of FTD. The first and most common involves primarily behavioral symptoms, with little cognitive impairment. In the second, language problems are noted first, and behavioral problems develop only later in the illness. Differences in the clinical presentation of symptoms have not been found to differentiate reliably among the types of underlying pathologies in FTD (McKhann et al., 2001).

Clinical characteristics are central for identifying FTD. Typical behavioral and cognitive symptoms that distinguish FTD from AD are shown in Table 3.4. Clinical criteria for diagnosis have been proposed by Neary and colleagues (1998) and by McKhann and colleagues (2001). In empirical tests of these criteria, patients with FTD had higher rates of behavioral problems than patients with AD, particularly a decline in social and personal conduct and emotional blunting. Language differences were found only in a small group of FTD patients (Rosen et al., 2002). These findings, as well as other tests of the criteria (e.g., Mendez & Perryman, 2002), suggest the need for further refinement.

Patients with FTD provide a challenge for families and other caregivers because of their impulsivity and other behavioral changes. A starting point in management of these patients is correct recognition, yet FTD is frequently misdiagnosed. Patients are often mistakenly diagnosed as having a psychiatric problem or as having AD. As a result, their special needs for care are not identified, and both patients and their families may be subjected to frustrating experiences and incorrect treatment. The cholinesterase inhibitors, for example, do not have any benefit in FTD, and patients may also be very sensitive to neuroleptics (Mendez & Cummings, 2003). Typical institutional environments may not have staff with sufficient training or appropriate environmental features to accommodate patients with FTD.

TABLE 3.4. Frontotemporal Dementia and Alzheimer's Disease: Similarities and Differences

Features	Frontotemporal dementia	Alzheimer's disease
Age at which disease generally occurs	• Usually after age 40 and before 65	• Usually after 65
Brain areas affected	• Frontal and temporal lobes (and motor areas in some frontotemporal dementias)	• Starts in the medial temporal area, usually in the hippocampus; spreads to other areas of the brain
Pathological features	• Loss of nerve cells • No amyloid plaques • Tau tangles seen in certain frontotemporal dementias	• Loss of nerve cells • Amyloid plaques • Tau tangles
History and progression	• Insidious onset and gradual progression	• Insidious onset and gradual progression

Symptoms	• Early symptoms characterized by behavioral and/or language deficits
	• Personality and behavior changes may include:
	  • Hyperactive or apathetic behavior
	  • Impairment in regulation of personal conduct (impulsiveness)
	  • Loss of empathy toward others
	  • Decline in social interpersonal conduct
	  • Emotional blunting
	• Language difficulties may include:
	  • Problems with expression and naming
	  • Problems with word meaning
	  • Memory is preserved early on
	  • Compulsive eating and oral fixations
	  • Repetitive actions
	  • Later in the disease, loss of motor skills, speech, and muscle movement
		• Begins with memory loss

Note. Data from Alzheimer's Disease Education and Referral Center (2002), Hodges et al. (1999), McKhann et al (2001), and Neary et al. (1998).

Vascular Dementias

VaD is a heterogeneous category of disorders in which the common feature is vascular pathology (O'Brien et al., 2003). Like FTD, VaD does not refer to a specific disease but rather to the outcome of several disease processes that differ in type of pathology, areas of the brain that are affected, and symptoms. The most widely known type of VaD, multi-infarct dementia, involves the occurrence of multiple strokes or "infarcts" in the cerebral cortex. The most common forms, however, are characterized by small-vessel ischemic changes, or lacunes, and extensive white-matter lesions (Mendez & Cummings, 2003). Other types of VaD are described in Table 3.5. Cerebrovascular disease, including strokes and other changes, may also cause cognitive impairment that does not meet criteria for dementia (O'Brien et al., 2003).

The term "vascular dementia" has replaced the older concept of arteriosclerotic dementia. At one time, the predominant belief was that dementia was caused by blockages in arteries that reduced blood flow to the brain. Arteriosclerosis per se does not result in generalized intellectual decline and dementia. Rather, it is one of the risk factors for small strokes and other pathological changes that lead to decline (Funkenstein, 1988).

The prevalence of VaD has been estimated at between 8 and 30% of cases of dementia (Mendez & Cummings, 2003; O'Brien et al., 2003; Peisah, Sachdev, & Brodaty, 1993). A recent population-based study found rates of VaD at age 80 to be nearly as high as those of AD (Fitzpatrick et al., 2004). As was noted, VaD and AD often coincide and appear to have additive effects. Between 8 and 30% of cases of dementia have been found to have mixed vascular and Alzheimer's pathologies (Gearing et al., 1995; Knopman et al., 2003). In fact, as many as one-half of cases with vascular changes may also show AD pathology. Some evidence of racial and/or cultural differences has been found, with higher rates of VaD in Japan and among Japanese American men in Hawaii, among Latinos in the United States (Fitten, Ortiz & Ponton, 2001), and in some European populations (Skoog et al., 1993), although the latter may be due to the use of different diagnostic criteria. There have been conflicting reports about rates among African Americans, with some research supporting increased risk (e.g., Froehlich, Bogardus, & Inouye, 2001; Heyman et al., 1991), and other studies showing no differences compared with European Americans (Fitzpatrick et al., 2004). It is also generally thought that men have a higher risk of VaD than women (Barclay, Zemcov, Blass, & Sansone, 1985; Kay, 1995), but some studies have not confirmed this association (Fitzpatrick et al., 2004). These conflicting results are probably due, in part, to the difficulties in identifying VaD and differences in the diagnostic criteria used in various studies.

Similar to AD, onset of VaD can occur as early as the fourth decade of life, though it is rare until the 50s and 60s. Prevalence increases with age,

TABLE 3.5. Classification of Vascular Dementia

Subtype	Mechanism	Structures involved
1. Macrovascular thromboembolic (multi-infarct dementia)	Thrombosis or emboli involving large or medium arteries	Cerebral cortex in distribution of anterior, middle, or posterior cerebral arteries or in border zones between them
2. Single strategic strokes	Single ischemic lesion in behaviorally critical areas	Thalamic, caudate nuclei, left angular gyrus, anterior cingulate/basal forebrain or genu of internal capsule
3. Multiple subcortical lacunar strokes (lacunar state)	Arteriolosclerosis of deep penetrating end-arterioles	Basal ganglia and thalamus with involvement of frontal–subcortical circuits/symptoms
4. Extensive white-matter lesions or Binswanger's disease	Arteriolosclerosis of deep penetrating end-arterioles	Periventricular and deep white matter with involvement of frontal–subcortical circuits/symptoms
5. Mixtures of types 1, 2, 3, and 4, especially lacunar–Binswanger's		
6. Postischemic dementia	Decreased blood pressure and cerebral perfusion below critical threshold	Frontal and other cortical laminar necrosis, loss of cells in striatum and hippocampus (possible sclerosis), pyramidal cell loss in cerebellum
7. Hemorrhagic dementia	Malignant hypertension, amyloid angiopathy, and vascular defects	Varies with location of hemorrhages
8. Genetic cerebrovascular disorders	Cerebral autosomal dominant arteriopathy with subcortical infarcts and leukoencephalopathy, Fabry's disease, etc.	Tend to involve deep white matter and subcortical gray nuclei
9. Vascular–Alzheimer's dementia	Combination of cerebrovascular disease and neuropathological features of developing Alzheimer's disease	Involvement of frontal–subcortical circuits/symptoms plus hippocampal memory loss and other features suggesting Alzheimer's disease
10. Vasculitides and other miscellaneous causes	Variable mechanisms and locations	

Note. From Mendez and Cummings (2003), p. 122. Copyright 2003 by Elsevier. Reprinted with permission from Elsevier.

though with some decline after age 85. Life expectancy of patients with VaD is lower than that of patients with AD or age-matched controls, probably due to the association of VaD with stroke and other symptoms of vascular disease (Knopman et al., 2003). Within 5 years of diagnosis, 64% of patients have died, compared with 32% of patients with AD (Peisah et al., 1993).

Multi-infarct dementia, which accounts for about 20% of cases of VaD, involves multiple strokes or infarcts that occur when blood vessels in the brain are blocked. Infarcts result in the death of surrounding tissue due to insufficient blood supply. The strokes are usually bilateral, that is, affecting both hemispheres. Blockages can be caused by thrombosis or embolism. Thrombosis refers to formation of a blood clot within the blood vessel and occlusion of the vessel at that point. In contrast, an embolism is a blood clot that forms at a different site and migrates to a vessel in which it causes an occlusion. Some patients experience short-lived events, called transient ischemic attacks (TIAs), which are brought about by brief blockages of vessels. Loss of consciousness and temporary motor, language, and sensory changes can occur. Single strokes that occur in strategic areas of the brain can also lead to dementia (Mendez & Cummings, 2003; Peisah et al., 1993).

The distinction between multi-infarct dementia and stroke is a matter of the magnitude and site of damage and resulting cognitive impairment. People who experience a single stroke are at a higher risk of developing dementia. About one-quarter of stroke patients with no prior evidence of cognitive impairment subsequently develop dementia, with the risk higher among people who have evidence of brain atrophy (Cordoliani-Mackowiak, Hénon, Pruvo, Pasquier, & Leys, 2003; Hénon et al., 2001). Some patients with multi-infarct dementia have typical symptoms of stroke (unilateral motor weakness, aphasia), but others do not.

Lacunar states are caused by occlusion in small vessels in the frontal lobes, basal ganglia, and other areas. White-matter lesions are found among both healthy older people and those with dementia. They are associated with stroke and other vascular risk factors such as hypertension, heart disease, and diabetes. Rates of white-matter lesions increase with advancing age (Piguet et al., 2003; Skoog, Berg, Johansson, Palmertz, & Andreasson, 1996). Findings of white-matter lesions on MRIs are diagnostic only in the presence of cognitive impairment or behavioral disturbances. Dementia is found when white-matter lesions are more extensive (Pantoni et al., 1999) and when they occur in combination with other vascular and nonvascular pathology, including AD and Lewy body dementia (Peisah, et al., 1993). People with white-matter lesions but no dementia may show mild cognitive deficits (Schmidt et al., 1993; Skoog et al., 1996). A finding of extensive white-matter lesions is sometimes called Binswanger's disease.

Symptoms of VaD

The symptoms of VaD are variable because the type of pathology and sites and extent of damage can differ. Typically, both cortical and subcortical damage is involved (Cummings & Benson, 1992). Impairment usually occurs in memory, abstract thinking, and language, though deficits in other neuropsychological functions, such as visual–spatial ability, can also be found. Depression, anxiety, emotional lability, and psychotic symptoms such as paranoid delusions are common in VaD, perhaps occurring with greater frequency than in AD (Cummings, Miller, Hill, & Neshkes, 1987; Sultzer, Levin, Mahler, High, & Cummings, 1993). Neurological symptoms such as rigidity, altered gait, dysarthria, and dysphagia are also frequently found.

It is difficult to differentiate among types of VaD because of overlap in types of symptoms and because many cases have multiple types of VaD pathology and perhaps also AD pathology. The symptoms of multi-infarct dementia depend on the site of the lesions. Mendez and Cummings (2003) characterize neuropsychological functioning as "patchy"; that is, some functions are impaired, but others are relatively preserved. Some cases will show greater language disturbances, for example, and others will show more visual–spatial problems. Symptoms of lacunar states often involve attentional deficits, decreased inhibition, lack of insight, and decreased memory and verbal fluency. Motor and sensory symptoms are also common. Dementia due to white-matter lesions has similar cognitive and motor symptoms. Changes in mood and behavior, including a trend toward apathy and urinary incontinence, are also common.

One of the more reliable indicators of multi-infarct dementia and other stroke-related syndromes is the history of onset and progression. Onset is usually sudden, and decline often occurs in a stepwise fashion. Patients are stable for periods of time and then experience a sudden drop in functioning. Onset with lacunar states and white-matter lesions is more insidious.

Several diagnostic criteria have been proposed for VaD (Chui et al., 1992; Hachinski et al., 1975; Román et al., 1993). One of the more widely used, the National Institute of Neurological Disorders and Stroke–Association Internationale pour la Recherche et L'Enseignement en Neurosciences criterion, is shown in Table 3.6. All of the criteria, however, have been found to have limitations and should not be the sole basis for diagnosis (see Norris, MacNeill, & Haines, 2003, for a review). The differentiation of VaD from AD is mostly based on history of onset and evidence of cerebrovascular disease and focal neurological symptoms. Many studies have compared symptoms of VaD and AD. Some commonly reported differences are shown in Table 3.7. The overlap in pathology, as well as problems in equating patients with VaD and AD in the severity of dementia (Mast, MacNeill & Lichtenberg, 2002), suggest that differentiating these syndromes solely on the basis of symptoms is problematic.

TABLE 3.6. Criteria for Diagnosis of Vascular Dementia

I. Criteria for the clinical diagnosis of *probable* vascular dementia include *all* of the following:

   A. Dementia (i.e., cognitive decline in memory and two or more other intellectual domains)
   B. Cerebrovascular disease (focal neurological signs; evidence from brain imaging of large vessel infarcts or a strategically placed single infarct, white-matter lacunes or extensive periventricular white-matter lesions, or combinations of these features)
   C. Onset of dementia within 3 months following a recognized stroke, an abrupt deterioration in cognitive functions, or fluctuating, stepwise progression of cognitive deficits

II. Clinical features consistent with the diagnosis of *probable* vascular dementia include the following:

   A. Early presence of a gait disturbance (small-step gait or march à petit pas, or magnetic, apraxic–ataxic, or parkinsonian gait)
   B. History of unsteadiness and frequent, unprovoked falls
   C. Early urinary frequency, urgency, and other urinary symptoms not explained by urological disease
   D. Pseudobulbar palsy
   E. Personality and mood changes, abulia, depression, emotional incontinence, or other subcortical deficits including psychomotor retardation and abnormal executive function.

Note. From Román et al. (1993). Copyright 1993 by Lippincott-Raven Publishers. Adapted by permission.

Risk Factors for VaD

Several risk factors have been identified for VaD. These include hypertension, cardiac disease, atherosclerosis, diabetes, inflammatory diseases (e.g., systemic lupus erythematosus), and conditions that can produce embolisms, such as a heart attack and plaques in the aorta and carotid arteries (Cummings, 1985; de la Monte & Wands, 2005; Hassing et al., 2002; Mendez & Cummings, 2003; O'Brien et al., 2003; Skoog, 1994). Cigarette smoking, high alcohol use, and obesity are also risk factors.

   The role of hypertension may be especially important for cognitive impairment and dementia. Hypertension is a risk factor for stroke and white-matter lesions (Skoog, 2003). Chronic hypertension has been linked to cell loss in the brain, particularly in the temporal and occipital lobes (Strassburger et al., 1997). Complicating this situation is the fact that some of the antihypertensive medications can affect cognition, producing symptoms that mimic dementia. These changes may be reversed by switching to another type of medication that is less likely to affect cognition.

   There is increasing interest in treatment of these risk factors as a way of preventing VaD or slowing its progression. Treatments include lowering blood pressure, preventing or improving control in type 2 diabetes, lowering cholesterol, and using antiplatelet (e.g., aspirin) and anticoagulant medica-

TABLE 3.7. Vascular Dementia and Alzheimer's Disease: Similarities and Differences

Features	Vascular dementia	Alzheimer's disease
History	• Sudden onset and stepwise progression • More variable decline than in Alzheimer's disease	• Insidious onset and gradual progression

Symptoms	• The sites of damage and associated symptoms can vary more than in Alzheimer's disease
	• Compared with Alzheimer's disease, patients with vascular dementia have more impairment in:
	  • Psychomotor functions
	  • Attention
	  • Frontal executive abilities (self-regulation, planning, and perseveration)
	  • Depression, emotional lability, apathy, anxiety
	  • Working memory, retrieval, and procedural memory
	  • Verbal fluency for letters
		• Compared with vascular dementia, patients with Alzheimer's disease have more impairment in:
		  • Episodic memory
		  • Recognition and cued recall
		  • Orientation
		  • Naming and comprehension
		  • Verbal fluency for categories
		  • Visual–spatial functioning
		  • Insight

Note. Data from Mendez and Cummings (2003); Norris, MacNeill, & Haines (2003); and O'Brien et al. (2003).

tions (Gorelick et al., 1999; Mendez & Cummings, 2003). Medications used in the treatment of AD have shown some benefits for VaD, including the cholinesterase inhibitors and memantine (O'Brien et al., 2003; Román, 2003).

Dementia with Lewy Bodies and Other Parkinsonian Syndromes

People with dementia often suffer from parkinsonian symptoms such as rigidity, tremor, difficulty initiating movement, and problems with posture and equilibrium. Three common syndromes of dementia and parkinsonian symptoms have been identified: (1) dementia with lewy bodies (DLB), (2) Parkinson's disease with dementia (PDD), and (3) AD with parkinsonian symptoms. All three syndromes involve both cognitive and parkinsonian motor symptoms. They differ, however, in the timing of these symptoms and in the type and location of underlying brain pathology. These syndromes are frequently misdiagnosed (Lopez et al., 1999), sometimes leading to treatments that make symptoms worse. Other, rarer syndromes can also cause parkinsonian and dementia symptoms, including progressive supranuclear palsy (see Mendez & Cummings, 2003).

Dementia with Lewy Bodies

DLB is characterized by progressive impairment in cognitive and motor symptoms. Onset of the disease comes typically after age 65, though some cases of younger patients have been reported. In contrast to both PDD and AD with parkinsonian symptoms, motor and cognitive symptoms appear at about the same time, or within a year of one another (Mendez & Cummings, 2003). Attention and visuospatial abilities are the cognitive functions most likely to be affected. Memory impairment may not be present early in the disorder, but it becomes prominent over time. Psychiatric symptoms such as hallucinations and delusions are common (Klatka, Louis, & Schiffer, 1996).

The pattern of symptoms and pathology that characterizes DLB was first described in the 1960s (Masterman & Swanberg, 2003). Several other names are used in the literature for this syndrome—"diffuse Lewy body disease," "senile dementia of the Lewy body type," and "Lewy body variant of Alzheimer's disease" (Cercy & Bylsma, 1997; Kosaka, Tsuchiya, & Yoshimura, 1988; McKeith, 1997). The name "dementia with Lewy bodies" was selected as part of a consensus conference on diagnosis (McKeith et al., 1996). Lewy bodies are insoluble filaments of protein that have a dense core and that are found within neurons or adjacent to them in affected parts of the brain. Alpha-synuclein, a protein found at the ends of neurons and at neural synapses, is a major component of Lewy bodies (Lee, Giasson, & Trojanowski, 2004). Lewy bodies are usually found throughout cortical and subcortical areas of the brain. Lewy bodies are also the main pathology in Parkinson's disease (PD), but in PD they are primarily located in the substantia nigra and other subcortical areas. Most DLB patients also have the characteristic pathologies found in AD, amyloid plaques and neurofibrillary tangles, although with fewer tangles (Heyman et al., 1999). Pure cases of Lewy body disease are relatively rare.

There has been increasing interest in DLB because of its high prevalence and possible connections to AD. A study of people ages 75 and over in Finland found that DLB affected 5% of the population and accounted for 23% of all cases of dementia. Other estimates are that DLB accounts for between 10 and 36% of cases of dementia (Masterman & Swanberg, 2003; McKeith et al., 1996).

Compared with patients with AD, people suffering from DLB display more impaired attention, slower cognitive reaction times, poorer working memory, more difficulty shifting mental set, poorer search strategies, poorer verbal fluency, more perseveration, confabulatory responses, and intrusions, and more visual–spatial deficits (Doubleday, Snowden, Varma, & Neary, 2002; Mendez & Cummings, 2003). They are also more likely to have motor symptoms and to have somewhat better memory recall (Heyman et al., 1999). Using family members' reports, Ferman and colleagues (2004) found four features that distinguished DLB from AD and normal aging: daytime drowsiness and lethargy, sleeping 2 or more hours during the day, staring into space for long periods of time, and periods of disorganized speech.

Consensus guidelines have been developed for the diagnosis of DLB (McKeith et al., 1996, 2005). The consensus criteria include:

- Progressive cognitive decline, especially in attention, visuospatial abilities, and frontal–temporal skills (e.g., mental slowness, inertia, lack of initiative, poor executive functioning.
- Fluctuations in cognition, particularly for attention and alertness.
- Parkinsonian symptoms, including rigidity, difficulty initiating movement, and problems with posture and equilibrium.
- Recurrent visual hallucinations.
- No evidence of brain damage due to cerebrovascular disease or other illnesses that could account for the symptoms.

Of particular importance is the temporal sequence of symptoms. A diagnosis of DLB can be made when cognitive and parkinsonian symptoms develop within 1 year of one another (McKeith et al., 2005). When parkinsonian symptoms develop more than 1 year before cognitive symptoms, a diagnosis of PDD should be considered. If parkinsonian symptoms appear after the development of severe cognitive impairment, then AD with parkinsonian symptoms should be considered.

These guidelines are effective in identifying pure cases of DLB, but they are less effective when both DLB and AD pathologies are present in substantial amounts, leading to a more mixed pattern of symptoms (Lopez et al., 2002; see McKeith et al., 2004, for a review).

There are practical reasons for differentiating DLB from AD. Patients with Lewy body disease may be more likely than patients with AD to respond positively to cholinesterase inhibitors (McKeith, 1997). They are also more likely to have adverse reactions to neuroleptics than AD patients, including a worsening of their parkinsonian symptoms (Ballard, Grace, McKeith, & Holmes, 1998).

Parkinson's Disease with Dementia

In contrast to DLB, PD is characterized at its onset mainly by motor symptoms. Cognitive symptoms in the early years of PD are mild and may include decreased attention, psychomotor slowing, poor cognitive flexibility, and poor visuospatial skills (Mendez & Cummings, 2003). Dementia may develop, however, as the disease progresses. Typical estimates of dementia in PD have ranged widely, between 10 and 80% (Brown & Marsden, 1984). Summarizing results from several ongoing studies, Kay (1995) estimates the cumulative incidence of new cases of dementia in patients with PD as ranging between 19 and 65% over a 5-year period. Using a population-based sample of patients with PD, Aarsland and colleagues (2003) found that 78% developed dementia within 8 years.

The primary site of brain damage in PD is the substantia nigra, a small region in the brain stem, which is involved in the synthesis of the neurotransmitter dopamine. A loss of neurons occurs in the substantia nigra, resulting in significant dopamine deficits. In addition, Lewy bodies are found in other subcortical areas.

The characteristic features of PD are difficulty initiating movements, rigidity, and tremors in the arms and/or legs. Because of rigidity of facial muscles, patients appear expressionless. They can no longer swallow spontaneously, and so saliva accumulates in their mouths and they may drool. Speech is usually abnormal as a result of these motor problems. Patients with PD are prone to depression, anxiety, and sleep difficulties. They also may have psychotic symptoms, particularly visual hallucinations, often as a result of the treatment for their dopamine deficiency (Masterman & Swanberg, 2003).

Because of the deficits that patients with PD have in motor functions and speech, it can be difficult to evaluate cognitive functioning. Impairment is pronounced on tests that are timed or that involve motor performance. In most cases, at least some cognitive impairment is found that appears independent of motor deficits and response speed, including deficits in memory and visuospatial performance (Pirozzolo, Hansch, Mortimer, Webster, & Kuskowski, 1982). The distinction between PD with and without dementia is based primarily on functional grounds. More extensive memory, intellectual, and behavioral impairment results in patients needing greater amounts of assistance and more stress on family caregivers. The clinician assessing a patient with PD should be less concerned with whether testing meets the criteria for a diagnosis of dementia than with the problems that the patient's motor and cognitive deficits cause for everyday activities. We return to these issues in assessment in Chapters 6 and 7.

Patients with PD can benefit from treatment with levodopa and other medications that increase the synthesis of dopamine in the brain. The benefits of levodopa diminish over time, however, and symptoms worsen again in 1–4 years, although occasionally patients may maintain gains for longer periods. New medications are becoming available that prolong the effectiveness of treatment. Side effects of levodopa and other dopaminergic medications can be considerable. These side effects include nausea, postural hypotension, cardiac dysrhythmias, psychotic symptoms, delirium, and anxiety. Patients with PD with dementia are especially prone to these adverse reactions (Mendez & Cummings, 2003). Treatment for depression can also improve functioning.

AD with Parkinsonian Symptoms

The third pattern is AD with parkinsonian symptoms. The main distinction between AD with parkinsonian symptoms and DLB or PD with dementia is the timing of symptoms (Mendez & Cummings, 2003). In AD, parkinsonian symptoms develop several years after the first onset of cognitive symptoms. In PD with dementia, cognitive symptoms worsen after several years of motor symptoms. In DLB, motor and cognitive symptoms develop concurrently, or nearly so. It is estimated that between 10 and 45% of patients with AD develop parkinsonian symptoms and have parkinsonian types of pathology (e.g., Lewy bodies, cell loss in the substantia nigra) prior to death (Ditter & Mirra, 1987; Gearing et al., 1995; Liu et al., 1997; Schmidt, Martin, Lee, & Trojanowski, 1996). There are two practical reasons for identifying these parkinsonian changes. First, as noted, neuroleptics may worsen patients' motor symptoms. Second, patients with parkinsonian motor symptoms become more prone to falls and other accidents.

Other Dementing Illnesses

As stated at the beginning of the chapter, a variety of disorders can result in dementia. We discuss a few of those disorders—dementias due to viral or bacterial infections and prion diseases. Although these disorders do not primarily affect older people, they are very important from a public health perspective. Another reason to note these problems is that they frequently present with a puzzling array of cognitive and behavioral symptoms that can be mislabeled as psychiatric.

In HIV-associated dementia (HAD), the HIV virus affects the white matter of the brain and subcortical areas, including the basal ganglia. Dementia can also be caused by disorders that are secondary to HIV infection, such as opportunistic brain infections. Although estimates vary, symptoms of dementia affect between 6 and 20% of patients with AIDS (Bacellar et al., 1994; McArthur et al., 1993; McArthur, Sacktor, & Selnes, 1999), with rates somewhat higher among those over age 50 (Becker, Lopez, Dew, & Aizenstein, 2004). Antiretroviral therapy has reduced one source of HAD, the occurrence of opportunistic infections. Even with treatment, however, the HIV virus still can cause cognitive problems and dementia (Sperber & Shao, 2003).

Symptoms are more common when the full AIDS syndrome has developed, but some people with HIV infection, though not AIDS, experience mild cognitive changes, especially in executive functions (Mendez & Cummings, 2003). The onset of dementia symptoms is generally gradual, but progression can vary. Some patients may stabilize or decline slowly, whereas others deteriorate rapidly (Mendez & Cummings, 2003). Symptoms of HAD include psychomotor slowing, forgetfulness, and poor attention and concentration (Holland & Tross, 1985; Mendez & Cummings, 2003). Memory impairment and other cognitive problems increase over time. Behavioral changes may occur, including apathy, withdrawal, inertia, agitation, mania, or obsessive–compulsive behavior.

Differential diagnosis of mental-status changes in patients with HIV is important. Early symptoms of HAD dementia can resemble depression. In turn, depressive and other psychiatric symptoms are common in individuals infected with HIV and should be treated (Holland & Tross, 1985). An increase in cognitive and behavioral symptoms may also indicate a complication of HIV infection, such as an opportunistic infection. Thus mental-status changes in individuals infected with HIV should be evaluated carefully to differentiate among psychiatric symptoms, secondary brain disorders, and primary infections of the central nervous system.

Other infectious causes of dementia include syphilis, Whipple's disease, viral encephalitis, meningitis, malaria, and certain amebas (Mendez & Cummings, 2003). Another infection, Lyme disease, has increased in prevalence considerably in recent years. Lyme disease often presents with a confusing array of symptoms, including attention problems, emotional lability, fatigue, chills and fever, and muscle and joint pain. These changes emerge weeks to months after infection, and so the infection may be overlooked as a possible cause of the symptoms.

Dementia may also be caused by prions, which are abnormally folded proteins that act as infectious agents (DeArmond & Prusiner, 1995). Prions are implicated in the disease scrapie, which affects sheep, and in bovine spongiform encephalopathy (BSE), which is better known as "mad cow disease." It seems likely that some people who ingested meat from infected cows have developed a form of dementia that is considered a new variant of a disorder called Creutzfeldt–Jakob disease (CJD). There are also sporadic and genetically linked forms of CJD (Mendez & Cummings, 2003). CJD can be distinguished from AD by a more rapid progression and the presence of focal neurological signs, particularly myoclonus (Van Everbroeck et al., 2003). Other diseases caused by prions include *kuru*, which is prevalent in New Guinea, and Gerstmann–Sträussler–Scheinker disease.

Mild Cognitive Impairment

As noted, the term "mild cognitive impairment" (MCI) denotes subtle cognitive changes that may be the first symptoms of dementia. The impetus to make the diagnosis of dementia as early in the disease process as possible comes from the belief that once primary treatments are developed for the underlying pathology, it will be necessary to intervene before too much damage has occurred. The development of the MCI category represents an attempt to identify the first noticeable changes from normal functioning.

Several criteria for MCI are available that emphasize measurable memory deficits that are greater than those expected with age (e.g., Morris et al. 2001; Petersen et al., 1999; Ritchie, Artero, & Touchon, 2001). The usefulness of the criteria for MCI depends on how accurately cases of early dementia are identified. Although some studies claim high rates of conversion from MCI to dementia, a review of the available evidence suggests that the average rate of conversion is approximately 25% in the first year and 50% after 5 years (Busse et al., 2003; Tuokko & Frerichs, 2000). In one study (Larrieu et al., 2002), almost half of the people originally diagnosed with MCI returned to normal levels of functioning over time. The problem with early diagnosis is that considerable individual variability exists in cognition independent of dementia. Some people score lower on cognitive tests because they have always had poorer functioning or because they are experiencing transitory health or psychological events that have temporarily impaired performance. When only one assessment is available, it is difficult to determine whether a person has, in fact, declined in performance. As a result, the MCI category mixes together people with early dementia and those with poor performance for other reasons, such as low formal education or nonprogressive brain damage from a stroke or head injury (Lopez, Jagust, DeKosky, et al., 2003). Thus a finding of MCI indicates an increased risk of dementia, but it cannot be viewed as definitive evidence of diagnosis.

Reversible or Secondary Dementia Syndromes

An important yet poorly described phenomenon is dementia due to reversible causes. Dementia symptoms have been associated with a variety of diseases, toxins, and medications (Clarfield, 2003; Mendez & Cummings, 2003; National Institute of Aging Task Force, 1980). These various problems do not necessarily cause diffuse damage to the brain, except when left untreated. Timely treatment results in considerable improvements in cognitive functioning. Among the most frequent causes are nutritional deficits, such as vitamin B_{12} deficiencies, chronic hypothyroidism and other endocrine disorders, exposure to heavy metals, and normal-pressure hydrocephalus. Medications, acting singly or in combination, can result in dementia symptoms. Chronic alcoholism can also produce dementia, which may partly reverse with treatment.

Reversible dementia is also associated with psychiatric disorders, particularly depression. This pattern of symptoms is frequently referred to as "pseudodementia" or "depressive pseudodementia." According to Caine (1981), pseudodementia involves intellectual impairment that resembles dementia but is reversible. Examination of the patient reveals other psychiatric symptoms but no evidence of a primary neurological disorder.

Maletta (1990) proposes using the term "secondary dementia" rather than "reversible" or "treatable" dementia. He points out that the distinction between reversible and irreversible dementia is inaccurate. Secondary dementia from causes such as excessive exposure to heavy metals may not be completely reversible, whereas primary dementias such as AD may have treatable components. Although the term "secondary dementia" has not been widely adopted, Maletta's point that the search for reversible aspects must be part of the evaluation of anyone with dementia has become a fundamental though sometimes overlooked principle in geriatric practice.

Estimates of the prevalence of reversible dementias have varied widely, depending on the definition and population studied. In perhaps the most systematic study to date, Hejl, Høgh, and Waldemar (2002) examined 1,000 consecutive cases seen in an outpatient memory clinic. They found that 4% of patients who met the diagnostic criteria for dementia had reversible conditions. A somewhat larger group that did not meet the criteria for diagnosis of dementia had reversible cognitive symptoms. These low rates are consistent with other studies (see Clarfeld, 2003). Additionally, 23% of patients had what was termed a "concomitant" condition, that is, a treatable disorder that made dementia symptoms worse but that was not the primary cause. The most common causes of all these reversible conditions were depression, hydrocephalus, and alcoholism.

Among patients with pseudodementia—that is, in whom cognitive symptoms are primarily psychiatric in origin—depression is the most common cause (e.g., Caine, 1981; Kiloh, 1961; Roth & Myers, 1975; Wells, 1979). In a sample of 10 patients who met criteria for pseudodementia, Wells (1979) reported extensive depressive symptoms among 7. He also found evidence of personality disorders, particularly dependency, among the entire group. Caine (1981) identified 11 patients with cognitive deficits resembling dementia that were subsequently found to be treatable. Of the 11 cases, 6 met criteria for a diagnosis of major depression, and the rest of the sample had other psychiatric diagnoses. Both Caine (1981) and Wells (1979) reported that some patients showed subtle signs of neurological abnormalities, which may have contributed to their cognitive impairment.

These findings indicate clearly the need to investigate patients for reversible causes at the time the dementia diagnosis is first made, as well as during the course of the disease, as reversible factors may make symptoms worse than they need to be. People with a primary dementia can also have illnesses or take medications that worsen their cognitive symptoms. As an example, a patient with AD who is depressed or has a nutritional deficit will function more poorly than he or she would with AD alone. Treatment of these secondary problems often improves functioning. The overlap of psychiatric disorders such as depression and primary dementia is a central diagnostic issue to which we return in subsequent chapters.

DELIRIUM

Probably no clinical skill is more important for a geriatric specialist than being able to recognize a delirium. Delirium is frequently misdiagnosed as dementia or a psychiatric disorder (e.g., Farrell & Ganzini, 1995), and older people with a delirium are often mislabeled as having dementia or AD. In a systematic review of hospital patients on a geriatric ward, Laurila and colleagues (Laurila, Pitkala, Strandberg, & Tilvis, 2004) found that only 40% of cases of delirium had been identified correctly in medical records. These diagnostic errors are critical because, if left untreated, the factors that have caused the delirium can result in permanent brain damage or death.

ACUTE ONSET OF DELIRIUM

Donald, an 80-year-old man, returned home from the hospital following minor surgery. He had been prescribed an anti-inflammatory medication to aid the healing process. Waking up in the middle of the night, he telephoned his grown children. His children quickly realized that Donald did not know what time it was, that his thoughts were disorganized, and that he reported the events of a dream as having actually happened. Donald seemed fearful and agitated. Prior to hospitalization, he had been functioning well, although with occasional memory lapses, especially in unfamiliar surroundings; but he had never had symptoms like these. His children were concerned that he was becoming senile and consulted with me. I encouraged Donald's children to involve their father's physician and to review the medication that had been prescribed following the surgery. The physician agreed that the medication was a possible cause of the patient's difficulties and discontinued it. In a few days the symptoms subsided, and Donald was able to function independently again.

This sequence of events is very common. An older person who has been functioning adequately suddenly develops global impairment in intellectual functioning. The onset of symptoms can occur in a few hours or a few days. Changes may include impaired perceptions, delusions or hallucinations, altered mood that can range from euphoria to fear, impaired ability to attend to or focus on events, very high or very low levels of activity, and other disruptions of thinking and behavior.

Although delirium can occur at any age, it is most frequent among older people. It results from a disruption of brain metabolism or an alteration in levels of certain neurotransmitters (Lipowski, 1990). Delirium can be brought about by several factors acting singly or in combination. Various illnesses, medications, and stressors have been associated with delirium. Often the causes are treatable and the outcome positive, as in the example. In that instance, the likely cause of delirium was the medication acting in conjunction with stress associated with surgery. The mental symptoms usually remit when the precipitating causes are identified and treated.

Terminology contributes to the problem of identifying delirium. Many different terms are used to refer to delirium, such as "acute brain syndrome," "acute confusional state," and, as we saw earlier, "reversible dementia." The confusion over terminology has been compounded by vague and inconsistent definitions.

In the effort to develop more precise operational criteria for delirium, the DSM definition eliminated two terms that were long associated with delirium: "clouding of consciousness" and "confusion." Lipowski (1990) points out that the term "clouding of consciousness" was used to refer to many different features of delirium, including drowsiness, a reduced awareness of self and surroundings, deficits in short-term memory, disorganized thinking, deficits in perception and misperceptions, and impairment in new learning. "Confusion" is one of the most overused terms in geriatrics, referring variously to behaviors of people with delirium, dementia, schizophrenia, and other disorders. Some of the different meanings ascribed to the word "confusion" have been disorientation, inability to think clearly or coherently, poor contact with reality, and reduced awareness of the environment (Lipowski, 1990). These global terms have been replaced with more specific descriptions of behavior.

Delirium is most likely to be encountered in an acute-care hospital, where the patient's illness and medications and the stressors associated with hospital routines can combine to produce the syndrome. Most estimates of the prevalence of delirium range between 10 and 26% of older inpatients (Inouye & Charpentier, 1996; Levkoff, Cleary, Liptzin, & Evans, 1991; Lindesay, Rockwood, & Rolfson, 2002; Pompei et al., 1994). The prevalence of delirium among older patients seen in the emergency room has been found to be 14% (Hustey & Meldon, 2002). In intensive care units, prevalence rates have been found to range between 31 and 80% (McNicoll et al., 2003; Pisani, McNicoll, & Inouye, 2003). Estimates of delirium after surgery range widely, between 5 and 52% (Lindesay et al., 2002). The risk associated with certain kinds of surgery seems especially high; delirium has been reported in between 28 and 52% of people having orthopedic surgery for hip fractures and in approximately 30% following heart surgery (Levkoff et al., 1991; Santos, Velasco, & Fráguas, 2004; Tune, 1991). Even minor surgery, such as cataract removal, is followed by delirium in a small proportion of cases (Milstein, Pollack, Kleinman, & Barak, 2002).

Patients who develop delirium in the hospital stay longer and have higher mortality rates (Pompei et al., 1994). Those who survive are more likely to go to nursing homes (Inouye et al., 1999). Surprisingly, many acute-care hospitals are unprepared to deal with delirium and may even adopt a punitive attitude toward the patient and his or her family.

Relatively few studies have been done of the incidence and prevalence of delirium in nursing homes. In one recent study, it was found that nearly one-quarter of admissions to a post–acute-care facility (which treats people who need transitional care between hospital and home) met diagnostic criteria for delirium. Of these patients, most were still symptomatic 1 week later, and nearly half were symptomatic 1 month later, suggesting that the causes of their delirium had not been adequately addressed (Kiely et al., 2004; Marcantonio et al. 2003). Among long-stay residents, an estimated 6–12% develop a delirium during a 1-year period (Katz, Parmalee, & Brubaker, 1991).

The prevalence of delirium among community populations is low, given that the symptoms often result in hospitalization. Nonetheless, one epidemiological survey estimated the rate of delirium at approximately 1% among community-living people over the age of 55 (Folstein, Bassett, Romanoski, & Nestadt, 1991).

Onset is typically rapid, occurring over a period of a few hours or days, and represents a dramatic change in a person's level of functioning. Delirium often develops at night. Thinking is often characterized by a dreamlike quality, with some merging of dream content with reality. Delusions, hallucinations, and illusions are very common. Patients also have difficulty focusing and sustaining or shifting attention. Symptoms fluctuate over the course of the day, often with a worsening toward evening.

Three patterns of delirium have long been recognized (Lipowski, 1990; Ross, Peyser, Shapiro, & Folstein, 1991). The first type is characterized by hyperalertness and hyperactivity; patients are restless, agitated, and vigilant. In contrast, the second type involves hypoalertness and hypoactivity. Patients are quiet and subdued and may be drowsy and difficult to arouse. The third pattern involves fluctuations between the other two types. The mixed type may be the most common variant, accounting for almost twice as many cases as the other two types (Sandberg, Gustafson, Brannstrom, & Buch, 1999).

Many different conditions can produce a delirium (Table 3.8). A classic report by the National Institute on Aging (NIA) Task Force (1980) stressed that any disruption of the internal environment of an older person can bring about a delirium. The more risk factors to which someone is exposed, the greater the likelihood of a delirium.

The most frequent cause of a delirium is a medication reaction, either to a single medication or to the interaction among drugs (Inouye, 1994; Marcantonio, 2002). Common over-the-counter (OTC) medications such as antacids can on rare occasions cause cognitive impairment and other delirium symptoms. The risk is greater, however, when OTC drugs are used in combination with prescription medications that add to or potentiate their effects.

This vulnerability to delirium and other types of adverse medication reactions is due to physiological changes in the aging body that affect how drugs are processed. Older people absorb, distribute, metabolize, and eliminate medications more slowly (Jacobson, Pies, & Greenblatt, 2002). As a result, medications reach a therapeutic level more slowly and remain in the body longer, increasing the risk that drugs will build up to toxic levels. Compounding this problem are changes in how medications affect the target tissue or organ, or what is called "pharmacodynamics." Changes with aging can decrease the effectiveness of a medication at its target site or can increase sensitivity (Jacobson et al., 2002). Multiple medications increase the potential for adverse reactions. Adverse effects are especially pronounced in some patients; for example, people with reduced kidney function eliminate most medications very slowly.

Infections, metabolic and endocrine disorders, and fractures can also trigger a delirium in an older person. Sometimes the first symptoms that are noticed are mental changes associated with the delirium syndrome rather than

TABLE 3.8. Precipitating Causes of Delirium

- Medications
    - Substance withdrawal
        - Alcohol
        - Sedative–hypnotics
    - Substance intoxication
        - Sedative hypnotics
        - Narcotics
        - Anticholinergics
        - Antipsychotics
        - Antiparkinsonians
        - Antidepressants
- Severe acute illness
- Infections
    - Urinary tract infection
    - Pneumonia
- Metabolic abnormalities
    - Hyperglycemia/hypoglycemia
    - Hypercalcemia/hypocalcemia
    - Thyrotoxicosis/myxedema
    - Adrenal insufficiency
    - Hepatic failure
    - Renal failure
    - Hypernatremia/hyponatremia
    - Hyperkalemia/hypokalemia
- Hypoperfusion states and pulmonary compromise
    - Hypoxemia
    - Shock
    - Anemia
    - Congestive heart failure
    - Chronic obstructive pulmonary disease
- Urinary and fecal retention
- Environmental/psychological contributors
    - Sensory deprivation
    - Sensory overload
    - Psychological stress
    - Sleep deprivation
    - Pain
    - Physical restraint use
    - Bladder catheter use
    - Any iatrogenic event
    - Intensive care unit treatment
- Surgery, anesthesia, and other procedures
    - Orthopedic surgery
    - Cardiac surgery
        - Duration of cardiopulmonary bypass
    - Noncardiac surgery
    - High number of procedures in hospital
- Neurological illness
    - Subdural hematoma
    - Stroke
    - Malignancy
    - Cerebral infection
    - Seizures

Note. From Rolfson (2002). Copyright 2002 by Oxford University Press. Reprinted by permission.

physical symptoms or complaints. A patient who has fallen, for example, may not complain about pain but may instead develop hallucinations, delusions, or other symptoms of delirium. Delirium can also indicate the presence of a brain disease. Focal events such as a stroke or TIA or more pervasive disorders, such as a rapidly growing tumor or infection, can produce symptoms of delirium. A delirium can also follow a head injury.

Alcoholism has been found to be a common cause of delirium (Pompei et al., 1994). Alcoholic intoxication is itself a form of delirium, and alcohol can also interact with medications an older person is taking. Older people who abuse illegal drugs or psychoactive medications are also at greater risk of suffering delirium or cognitive impairment.

Lipowski (1990) proposes a useful distinction of predisposing, facilitating, and precipitating factors for delirium. *Predisposing factors* increase susceptibility to delirium. These factors include increasing age and brain damage, either focal damage or that due to a progressive disease such as AD. Patients with dementia are at highest risk of delirium (Fick, Agostini, & Inouye, 2002). *Facilitating factors* such as psychological stress, sleep deprivation, sensory deprivation or overload, and immobilization can contribute to the development of a delirium or can worsen or prolong its course. In some instances, death of a spouse or a move to a new location appear to facilitate a delirium. *Precipitating factors* are the immediate medical conditions involved—the medications, illnesses, and other physiological problems that lead to the delirium.

Many of the conditions that produce delirium can also lead to a reversible dementia, the difference being in the types of presenting symptoms. With a reversible dementia, memory impairment is a prominent symptom, whereas in delirium, fluctuations in attention and alertness and a greater likelihood of delusions and hallucinations are characteristic. How the underlying physiology differs is not known.

The outcomes of delirium are variable, depending on the course and treatment of precipitating factors. Complete recovery is the most common outcome (Lipowski, 1990). It occurs when the factors that precipitated the delirium are treated or run their course. Recovery may be relatively rapid, for instance, in about a week, or it may be more gradual. Conversely, delirium can progress to coma and death or to irreversible brain damage. Some cases may persist, even after all possible precipitating causes have been removed. In our experience, however, it is more common for symptoms to persist when possible causes have been inadequately investigated.

The following case contains many elements typical of delirium, including sudden onset, the interaction of several risk factors, and the possibility of full recovery.

ONSET AND COURSE OF DELIRIUM

Sarah, age 74, had surgery for breast cancer and went to a rehabilitation hospital. While there, she fell and broke her hip. After the fracture was repaired, Sarah was moved to a nursing home, and soon after this, her husband died.

During the funeral, Sarah showed no grief, and afterward she talked about her husband as though he were still alive. An assessment uncovered evidence of delirium; she did not know where she was, nor the time or date. Three factors probably contributed to Sarah's delirium. The first was the trauma of having suffered a hip fracture; the second, the shock of learning that her husband had died; and the third, the pain medication that Sarah was receiving. As the fracture healed and she required less pain medication, the delirium gradually cleared. Follow-up evaluation indicated no lingering cognitive deficits, and Sarah was fully aware that her husband had died.

People often have amnesia for the events and experiences they had during delirium (Roth, 1991). Sometimes, however, a patient remembers a hallucination or delusion and is convinced that it actually happened. Even long after the delirium has cleared, some people persist in the belief that the imagined events actually took place.

The main approach to treatment of a delirium is a vigorous search for the cause, combined with a calming and reassuring environment. A thorough medical evaluation, including a review of medications, is essential (Inouye, 1994; Marcantonio, 2002). Neuroleptics are often prescribed for managing the more disruptive symptoms in a delirium, but they can worsen the situation. We have observed many patients who have paradoxical reactions to the neuroleptics, becoming more rather than less agitated. A calming, supportive environment, including using family members rather than hospital staff, may decrease behavioral agitation (Marcantonio, 2002).

It may be possible to prevent delirium in patients in high-risk situations. Inouye and colleagues (1999) used a protocol to identify and manage risk factors associated with delirium in an inpatient hospital setting. The risk factors included cognitive impairment, sleep deprivation, immobility, visual impairment, hearing impairment, and dehydration. For each risk, hospital staff implemented specific procedures to reduce the potential impact. For example, patients with hearing impairment had their ears cleaned. Staff members would use portable amplifiers, if needed, and speak clearly, with little background noise. This preventive approach lowered the rate and duration of delirium episodes compared with a control group that received usual hospital care.

Unfortunately, cutbacks in nursing staff in many hospitals and the trend toward shorter hospital stays make it more difficult to identify, treat, and care for patients with delirium. There is an increasing tendency just to throw medications at the problem rather than to identify the cause or provide the type of supportive environment that can calm patients down. Families are an invaluable resource for providing information that helps differentiate between delirium and dementia, but they are often overlooked in the hospital setting. An important role for the geriatric mental health specialist is to identify delirium and to advocate for its proper treatment.

OTHER COGNITIVE DISORDERS: NONPROGRESSIVE BRAIN INJURIES

With the attention given to dementia and, to a lesser extent, delirium in older populations, other sources of brain damage are sometimes overlooked. Accidents that involve head trauma can lead to both transitory and permanent cognitive deficits. Surgery is another important source of cognitive disorders. In addition to the risk of delirium in the period immediately following surgery, some people experience permanent cognitive deficits. Loss of oxygen to the brain, the occurrence of a stroke, or other adverse events during the surgery can lead to significant cognitive changes. Most reports of cognitive change following surgery rely on histories obtained from patients or their families, but a few prospective studies have confirmed this pattern. In a study that conducted cognitive testing prior to coronary bypass surgery, 53% of patients showed cognitive declines at discharge, as indicated by a change of 1 standard deviation on one or more of four tests (Newman et al., 2001). By 6 months, the rate had fallen to 24%, though that still represents a considerable risk.

It is important to differentiate these causes of brain damage from dementia because they have very different consequences and prognoses. Often, the deficits caused by the damage are focal, not global. As a result, more opportunities exist for compensation and rehabilitation. These conditions are also not progressive and do not result in the type of catastrophic decline found in dementia.

CONCLUSIONS

The syndromes of dementia and delirium are, in many ways, the most important mental health problems of the elderly. Dementia is a devastating condition that involves the gradual loss of the person. Delirium is usually of short duration but is frequently misidentified and mistreated. We return to these disorders in Chapters 6 and 7, in which we examine assessment approaches and criteria for making a diagnosis, and again in Chapters 12, 13, and 14, which focus on their treatment in community and institutional settings.

CHAPTER 4

Mood and Anxiety Disorders

This chapter reviews some of the most common problems in later life: depression, anxiety, and adjustment disorders. We have included suicide, because anxiety and particularly depression are frequently risk factors. We consider the prevalence of each of these problems in the older population, presenting characteristics and theories about their etiology. We also focus on what might be different about these disorders when they occur in later life compared with at younger ages. Is the presentation of depression different, for example, in an older person than in a younger person, and are different risk or causal factors involved? Chapters 6 and 7 expand on assessment issues, and Chapters 9 and 10 address the treatment of these disorders in older adults.

We begin with an example that illustrates the common pattern of comorbidity of depression and anxiety with each other, as well as with illness and medication. The case also shows links to events earlier in life that contributed to the depression and anxiety.

THE INTERPLAY OF DEPRESSION, ANXIETY, ILLNESS, AND MEDICATIONS

Henry, age 79, was referred by a family friend for treatment. In the initial interview, a complex medical and psychosocial history emerged. Henry had been born in France. At age 12, he suffered a closed head injury while playing soccer. He was unconscious for 2 days, then seemed to recover without incident. Several years later, after the Nazi invasion, Henry joined the underground. Because of his activities, he was arrested by the SS and placed in a concentration camp. While in the camp, he suffered his first grand mal seizure.

After the war, Henry emigrated to the United States, and he subsequently had a successful career. He continued, however, to be plagued with seizures, although a combination of medications reduced their frequency. Henry would have a major seizure about every other year, which would require him to sleep for several hours. Between major seizures, he would have minor seizures characterized by aphasia and light-headedness.

Henry was a widower. He had grown children from his first marriage. After his wife died, he married again. This marriage was intense and romantic. Sadly, after 8 years of marriage, his second wife died from pancreatic cancer. Henry reported being depressed for years after her death.

He then started communicating with an old school friend from France, Madeleine, who was also widowed. They discovered that they had much in common and began spending their time together, alternating between France and the United States so that they could be near their children and grandchildren.

Then the terrorist attacks of September 11, 2001, occurred, and it became difficult for Madeleine to obtain a long-stay visa. Shortly before I first met Henry, he and Madeleine had been in Paris, where he had had to be hospitalized with anxiety. Eventually, the doctors treated him for a urinary tract infection (UTI). Feeling better, Henry returned to the United States with Madeleine, but his anxiety symptoms worsened. He presented in the office as depressed and anxious. He had early-morning anxiety that improved as the day progressed, but his cognitions were pessimistic and hopeless. To further complicate the situation, Madeleine had only 3 weeks left on her visa, and Henry was worried that he would not be able to return to Paris with her. He was also afraid to travel because he was experiencing an increase in the frequency of his seizures.

We spent several sessions understanding and then challenging Henry's complex web of negative cognitions. In time, it became clear that he was a highly anxious individual and a worrier. Some of Henry's worries may have been an understandable reaction to his seizure disorder and to other circumstances in his life. Clearly, as he found himself nearing 80 in a complicated life situation, he had fears of what the future might hold.

Henry responded well to cognitive-behavioral therapy (see Chapters 8 and 9) and appreciated better the sources of his anxiety. But the anxiety did not abate. One day he came to a session with a fever, and I sent him immediately to his internist, who discovered that the UTI had not been effectively treated. The doctor started Henry on another and longer course of antibiotics. Henry became more depressed on the antibiotics, which occasionally happens, but he was able to attribute his mood correctly to the treatment.

This episode provided valuable lessons that would come in handy 3 years later when Henry returned for treatment. Henry learned that he has a depressive reaction to certain antibiotics and that he needs follow-up urinalysis to be certain that his UTIs have cleared. And I learned that an undertreated UTI can present anxious depression, with very few other somatic indicators. Consequently, when Henry returned to treatment, we were able to separate his recurrent anxiety from his medical problems much more quickly and efficaciously.

DEPRESSIVE DISORDERS

Depression has long been regarded as a defining characteristic of later life. The belief that the elderly are more prone to depression dates back at least to the 2nd-century Roman physician Galen, who described a link between melancholia and aging (Jackson, 1969). In contemporary society, older people are frequently portrayed in the media as sad, lonely, and isolated. They are seen as buffeted by losses and declining health and as increasingly irrelevant in a youth-oriented culture. Like most popular stereotypes, these images contain elements of truth and also distortions. It turns out that older people are generally satisfied with their lives and somewhat less likely than people at younger ages to suffer from depression. Nonetheless, the number of older people who do suffer from depression remains substantial, and it is the most likely reason for their seeking mental health treatment.

Rather than being an intractable problem embedded in the aging process, depression often improves with treatment. The field of geriatric mental health has its origins in a classic 1955 paper by the British psychiatrist Sir Martin Roth, "The Natural History of Mental Disorder in Old Age" (Roth, 1955). In that paper, Roth examined the outcomes of geriatric patients who were seen as inpatients in an English mental hospital. He described the prevailing pessimism about treating older patients and the belief that any mental disorder that occurred in later life was a manifestation of brain disease. Not much was expected of older patients except further decline. What Roth observed, however, was quite different. Recovery depended on the type of presenting problem, not on the patient's age. People who were hospitalized with affective disorders were much more likely to be discharged as recovered and to have higher survival rates at 6 months and at 2 years than were people with symptoms of dementia. This positive finding, during an era when few effective treatments were available for severe depression, spurred interest in mental health and aging.

The term "depression" refers, of course, to both symptoms and disorders. This duality introduces some confusion into discussions of depression and into estimates of the prevalence of depression. The primary diagnostic categories in DSM-IV (American Psychiatric Association, 1994)are major depressive disorder (MDD), dysthymic disorder, and adjustment disorder with depressed mood. Depression is also a defining feature of bipolar mood disorders. Depressive symptoms can occur with some degree of severity and regularity among people who do not meet criteria for any of these diagnoses.

Rates of Depression in Community Populations

Studies in the United States and Europe show that the prevalence of MDD among older people ranges between 1 and 5% (Blazer, 2002; Kessler et al., 2003; Ritchie et al., 2004; Weissman et al., 1988; Weissman & Myers, 1978).

These rates are lower than those in early or middle adulthood. The prevalence for women is about twice as high as for men at every age.

MDD usually does not first appear in late life. Rather, most people who suffer from MDD in later life have histories of prior episodes of depression. The most frequent age of onset is late teens through about age 30. In a multinational study of the lifetime prevalence of major depression, Andrade and colleagues (2003) reported that the median age of onset was between 20 and 25. In a large population survey in the United States, the peak ages of onset were found to be 15–19, and 25–29 (Burke, Burke, Regier, & Rae, 1990). Rates of first onset of MDD dropped steadily after age 29 and then rose slightly after age 75. Women had higher risks of MDD than men during the adult years, but in later life, rates were similar.

Why are the rates of MDD lower among the elderly than at earlier ages? Certainly, one factor may be that at least some of the people who have episodes of MDD earlier in life recover fully and do not experience recurrent episodes in old age. This explanation is consistent with findings on emotional well-being in representative populations of older people (see Chapter 2). Selective survival may also occur: People with severe depression earlier in life may be less likely to survive to old age, either because of a greater risk of suicide or because depression has an adverse effect on health (see later in this chapter). It is also possible that the diagnostic criteria for MDD may be too restrictive to apply to older people. These criteria have largely been established based on younger and middle-aged persons, with little consideration of whether the presentation of severe depression might change as people age. Younger people may find it more acceptable to express their emotional state as "depressed." In turn, older cohorts may be more likely to express distress indirectly or in the form of physical symptoms. In some other cultures, people who are depressed do not complain about dysphoric mood but instead report cognitive and somatic symptoms (Caine, Lyness, King, & Connors, 1994).

In contrast to the low rates of MDD, depressive symptoms are quite common among older people. The proportion of older people with "clinically significant" depressive symptoms has been found to range between 10 and 25% (Gurland et al., 1983; Kay et al., 1985; Lindesay, Briggs, & Murphy, 1989; Livingston, Hawkins, Graham, Blizard, & Mann, 1990; see Blazer, 2002, for a comprehensive review). Although not defined in a consistent way across studies, clinically significant depression usually involves symptoms that are severe enough to interfere with functioning and that warrant treatment but that do not meet the criteria for MDD. Blazer (1994) proposes adoption of the term "minor depression" for this pattern.

The prevalence of depressive symptoms also appears to decline with age. Rates of symptoms are highest in young adulthood, decrease until about age 75, and then increase somewhat among the oldest old (Heikkinen & Kauppinen, 2004; Zarit, Femia, Johansson, & Gatz, 1999). There may also be cohort differences in depression and other mental health symptoms, with younger generations more likely to report depressive symptoms than older ones (Blazer, 2002; Kessler et al., 2003).

Comorbidity of depression with other psychiatric disorders is quite common. Anxiety disorders are often a precursor of a major depression (Kessler et al., 1996; Wetherell, Gatz, & Pedersen, 2001), and depressive symptoms are frequently found in people with anxiety diagnoses (e.g., Judd et al., 1998; Kessler et al., 1998). Depressive symptoms are often prominent in many other disorders, including dementia, personality disorders, and schizophrenia.

PREVALENCE OF DEPRESSION AMONG MEDICALLY ILL OLDER ADULTS

People who have serious medical problems, as well as those living in nursing homes or other institutional settings, often suffer from depressive symptoms. Rates of MDD among older hospital patients have been found to range between 6 and 44%, depending on the population studied, with an average of about 12% (Koenig & Blazer, 1992). Rates are higher among patients with more severe illnesses, such as cancer, or with greater functional disabilities. Other depressive diagnoses (dysphoria, adjustment disorders) have been found in 18–26% of hospital patients (Koenig & Blazer, 1992).

Depression is also quite common among medical outpatient samples. Between 12 and 20% of older patients seen in primary care meet diagnostic criteria for a depressive disorder, and perhaps another 10% have clinically significant depressive symptoms (Lyness, King, Cox, Yoediono, & Caine, 1999; Robison et al., 2003). Rates are especially high among recent immigrants and people with more social stress (Robison et al., 2003). Katzelnick and his colleagues (2000) found that 32% of high users of outpatient medical services met diagnostic criteria for depression.

Nursing home patients are particularly at risk for depression. In perhaps the most thorough study of depression in this population, Parmalee, Katz, and Lawton (1992) reported that 16% of residents of long-term care facilities met criteria for MDD and another 16% had significant depressive symptoms. A 1-year follow-up on this sample indicated a 6% incidence of new cases of MDD and a 6% incidence of minor depression. About one-half of people with either MDD or depressive symptoms at baseline were still symptomatic a year later.

Unfortunately, depression in both patients who are medically ill and those who are in nursing homes is often underdiagnosed (e.g., Stek, Gussekloo, Beekman, van Tilburg, & Westendorp, 2004). Diagnosis is complicated by the fact that depression and medical illnesses can present with similar symptoms. Depressed people often have somatic complaints, such as poor sleep and appetite, fatigue, and muscle or skeletal pain. In a younger patient with few medical problems, it is often easy to establish that these complaints are part of the depressive disorder. The situation is frequently more ambiguous among older people, who may suffer from one or more chronic health problems that could be the source of the symptoms.

Further complicating the situation, some changes that occur normally with aging are similar to symptoms of depression. Complaints of decreased sleep and frequent awakenings are common in both old age and depression. In other words, sometimes depression contributes to and perhaps exacerbates these sleep problems, and sometimes these problems occur without accompanying depressive symptoms. Likewise, some older people have poor appetites because of age-related changes in taste and smell or of dental problems, sometimes because of depression, and sometimes because of the cumulative effects of all these problems. There is no easy formula for differentiating the effects of aging and chronic illness from depression in the elderly; rather, clinicians must always keep in mind the possibility of comorbidity. As in the example of Henry at the start of the chapter, new symptoms even in a patient with a chronic history of depression may be part of an undiagnosed or untreated medical problem.

Table 4.1 summarizes the common medical conditions associated with depression. Disorders with high rates of depressive symptoms include age-related vision loss (Horowitz, Reinhardt, & Kennedy, 2005), dementia (Logsdon & Teri, 1995; Reifler, Larson, & Hanley, 1982), PD (Cole et al., 1996; Nuti et al., 2004), and a variety of other neurological disorders (see Cummings & Mega, 2003, for a review). Cerebrovascular disease, particularly stroke and white-matter lesions, may play a particularly important role

**TABLE 4.1. Common Medical Problems
Associated with Depressive Symptoms**

- Alcohol and drug abuse
- Alzheimer's disease
- Cancer
- Cardiac illness
- Cerebrovascular disease
- Cerebral neoplasms
- Chronic pain
- Central nervous system infections (e.g., Lyme disease)
- Endocrine disorders (e.g., hypothyroidism)
- Inflammatory diseases (e.g., lupus)
- Multiple sclerosis
- Nutritional deficits (e.g., vitamin B_{12} deficiency)
- Parkinson's disease
- Stroke
- Vascular dementia
- Viral and bacterial infections
- Vision loss

Note. Data from Blazer (2002) and Cummings and Mega (2003).

in the onset of late-life depression (Alexopoulos, 1994; Alexopoulos, Young, & Shindledecker, 1992; Devanand et al., 2004; Leuchter, 1994; Lyness, 2002; Mast, Onefold, MacNeill, & Lightener, 2004; Tiemeier et al., 2004; Whyte, Mulsant, Vanderbilt, Dodge, & Ganguli, 2004).

Etiology of Depression in Later Life

Biological influences, early life experience, stressful events, loss of positive reinforcement, and cognitive style may all play a role in the etiology of depression. Before discussing specific theories, however, we want to mention two overriding issues: the importance of avoiding simple dualities and the heterogeneity of depression in older populations.

Theories of the cause of depression often stress a single risk factor—biological, psychological, or social. A more promising approach, however, is to look at the possibility of multiple risks for depression. Rather than constituting competing theories, biological, psychological, and social processes represent different dimensions that can each contribute to the etiology of depression, with complex concurrent and reciprocal relations among them. Biological correlates are usually accorded the primary role in the etiology of depression, yet research has not established clearly whether biological differences are the cause or outcome of behavioral or cognitive patterns found in people with depression. Furthermore, even if one domain has a primary role in etiology, successful treatment may occur in any domain. For example, treatments that emphasize learning new patterns of behavior may be effective because changes in overt behavior lead to modification of underlying biological processes. Even biological treatments are heterogeneous—that is, drugs acting on different neurotransmitters have similar outcomes in relieving depression symptoms. As Akiskal and McKinney (1973) proposed in their classic work, depression is most likely the common outcome of many different pathways, with biological, psychological, and social processes contributing in varying degrees.

The second overriding issue is that older people who are depressed are quite heterogeneous. The "depressed" elderly includes people who have been troubled by depression intermittently throughout their adult lives, as well as individuals for whom depression is a new experience in later life. The particular etiological risk factors may differ depending on age of first onset. As we discuss in later chapters, biomedical risks are more likely to be involved when depression occurs for the first time in late life. How risk varies across different groups in the population—women, minorities, people with low socioeconomic status—add to the complexity of understanding the origins of depression.

Twin and family studies have found genetic influences on MDD and bipolar disorders (e.g., Gatz, Pedersen, Plomin, Nesselroade, & McClearn,

1992; Jang, Livesley, Taylor, Stein, & Moon, 2004; Jansson et al., 2004). Genetics may play a more important role for people who first experience depression early in life (Alexopoulos, Young, Abrams, Meyers, & Shamoian, 1989; Devanand et al., 2004).

Discoveries of the role of neurotransmitters have greatly increased our understanding of depressive disorders. Several neurotransmitters have been implicated in depression—notably, serotonin and norepinephrine—but other neurochemicals such as dopamine, histamine, gamma-aminobutyric acid (GABA), glutamate, glycine, and acetylcholine may play a part (Shuchter, Downs, & Zisook, 1996). Antidepressant medications block the reuptake of serotonin and norepinephrine by brain neurons or, in the case of monoamine oxidase (MAO) inhibitors, block the chemical that deactivates norepinephrine uptake at nerve endings. The result is to increase the levels of these neuro-transmitters available for brain cells.

Significant age changes have been found in the neurotransmitter systems associated with depression (for reviews, see Bisette, 2004; Ferrier & McKeith, 1991; Morgan, 1992). Serotonin, norepinephrine, and dopamine all have been found to decrease with aging. It has been speculated that both the amounts of various neurotransmitters and the balance among them contribute to late-life depression (Cohen, 1992).

Medical illness can play a role in the etiology of depression in two different ways (Koenig & Blazer, 1992). First, depressive symptoms can be part of a psychological reaction to medical illness, disability, and/or discomfort (e.g., Lyness, King, Conwell, Cox, & Caine, 2000; Zeiss, Lewinsohn, Rohde, & Seeley, 1996). Second, a variety of illnesses and medications are associated with physiological changes that increase the susceptibility to depression. These two factors can, of course, interact. For example, depression is a common feature of PD. A patient with PD may be depressed because of disease-related changes in levels of dopamine *and* because of his or her growing disability and poor prognosis.

The higher rates of depressive symptoms among women than men may be due to an interaction between biomedical and social factors. In a study of unlike-sex twins between the ages of 70 and 80, Takkinen and her colleagues (2004) found that sisters had higher rates of current depressive symptoms and past depression diagnoses than their brothers, despite the similarities in early childhood environment. These differences could partly be accounted for by the fact that women had lower socioeconomic status as adults than their brothers and also had more current health limitations. Estrogen and other hormones may also have played a role in women's greater vulnerability.

Psychosocial theories address in varying degrees the role of stress, behavioral factors, and cognitive dimensions in the etiology of depression. Stressful life events have long been regarded as a precipitant for depressive episodes (e.g., Brown, Bifulco, & Harris, 1987; Paykel, 1974, 1982). Rates of depression increase in the 6 months following negative life events (Paykel, 1982). The number of stressful life events and daily hassles have been found to be related to depression in samples of older people (Lewinsohn, Rohde, Fischer, & Seeley, 1991).

The psychological, social, and biological implications of stress and loss may result in increased vulnerability to depression. The role of stressful events as a precipitant, however, is complex. On the one hand, most depressed people identify negative events as triggers for the current episode. At one time, it was thought that a more biological (endogenous) form of depression did not have environmental precipitants. But individuals with so-called endogenous depression were more severely depressed and were poor reporters of their past histories. More careful interviewing of these individuals has led to identification of triggering events in most cases (Goodwin & Bunney, 1973). On the other hand, most people who experience negative life events do not become clinically depressed. Specific losses, such as retirement, loss of friends, and, particularly, death of a spouse, can be very stressful but do not necessarily lead to depression. Stressful events, then, may create a vulnerability to depression, which unfolds depending on other factors, such as a biological predisposition, the meaning of the loss to the person, social support, and coping resources.

A behavioral model of depression has been elaborated in a classic series of studies by Lewinsohn and his associates (e.g., Lewinsohn, 1975; Lewinsohn, Biglan, & Zeiss, 1976; Lewinsohn & MacPhillamy, 1974; Lewinsohn et al., 1991; Teri & Lewinsohn, 1982). These studies found that depressed people engage in fewer behaviors and receive lower levels of positive reinforcement than people who are not depressed. Several factors contribute to a decrease in positive reinforcement, including losses of significant people in one's life, erosion of positive exchanges with other people, or lack of skills to elicit positive responses from other people (Lewinsohn et al., 1976). Decreases in positive reinforcement then set off a vicious cycle: The person decreases the output of behavior, which further reduces the amount of reinforcement, which lowers mood, behavior output, and so forth. From this perspective, people who experience common losses in later life, such as becoming widowed or disabled, are at risk for depression because of decreased opportunities for obtaining positive reinforcement.

To examine the relation of depression and behavior, Lewinsohn and his colleagues developed the Pleasant Events Schedule, an instrument that assesses the extent to which people engage in behaviors that are reinforcing or enjoyable to them (Lewinsohn & MacPhillamy, 1974). As might be expected, people with depression—both younger and older—engage in fewer pleasant activities and find fewer activities potentially enjoyable. A version of the Pleasant Events Schedule has been developed specifically for use in assessment and treatment of older people (Teri & Lewinsohn, 1982).

Beck and his colleagues (Beck, 1976; Beck, Rush, Shaw, & Emery, 1979) have articulated a compelling model of the role of cognition in depression. As with Lewinsohn's behavioral approach, the cognitive model begins with observation—in this case, of what depressed people think. Depression is associated with specific patterns of thinking, in which people hold exaggerated, negative views of themselves, other people, and the future. As a result of negative appraisals of themselves and their experiences, people feel depressed. They may not, however, be aware of these negative beliefs. In fact, these cognitions are termed "automatic thoughts" because they constitute rapid and habitual ways of evaluating information.

A key feature of this model is that these negative beliefs are distortions produced by faulty logical patterns that emphasize the negative features or implications of any event or experience. These logical errors cause events to be interpreted consistent with a core set of beliefs about the self as worthless, unlovable, incompetent, and so on. The therapist's role is to help patients identify and question their automatic thoughts and develop alternative ways of looking at themselves and the world that are both realistic and positive, leading to a decrease in depressive cognitions.

As with other theories of depression, the cognitive theory would predict increased rates of depression in later life. Old age is associated with a variety of negative stereotypes and expectations, as well as real losses. The extent to which people incorporate negative cultural views of aging into their self-images and to which losses activate negative belief systems may predict increased depression. One of the keys to using cognitive therapy effectively in treatment of older adults is learning to identify the distortions in a person's beliefs. Bad things may indeed have happened to the person, but his or her beliefs may still be exaggerated and contribute to feelings of depression. We return to this point when discussing treatment of depression (Chapter 9).

Theory and practice overlap considerably in these approaches to depression. Similar features can also be found in other models, such as the interpersonal psychotherapy of depression (IPT; Klerman, Weissman, Rounsaville, & Chevron, 1984) model and Seligman's (1975, 1991) theory of learned helplessness and depression. Although each gives somewhat different weight to stressful events, cognitions, behavior, and social relationships, each approach incorporates all these dimensions in its theory and approach to treatment. Lewinsohn's behavioral treatment, for example, addresses negative thought patterns and social behavior as important dimensions. Beck's cognitive therapy emphasizes behavioral tasks as a useful way to generate and challenge negative cognitions. IPT uses behavioral and cognitive strategies in building improved social behavior and social relationships. The commonality among all of these approaches is an emphasis on identifying a client's immediate and habitual patterns of response that are associated with depression and then implementing strategies in a direct manner to change these usual responses. The result is a highly effective set of treatments that have outcome rates similar to those of antidepressant medications with younger patients (Robinson, Berman, & Neimeyer, 1990) and that have all been found to be effective in controlled trials with older adults (Gallagher-Thompson & Thompson, 1996).

Is Depression Different in Later Life?

Finally, we want to address the question of whether depression is different in later life. To address this question, we need to consider both the age of the person and the history of his or her disorder. For many people, a depressive disorder in later life is part of a recurrent pattern that was established early in life. Prognosis and treatment are likely to be similar to those for younger people. Treatment, however, should be informed by an understanding of geriatric issues, including the possible role of illness in the etiology of depression, the increased sensitivity of older people to medications (see Chapter 9), and how psychosocial issues such as retirement and bereavement may contribute.

For some people, however, depressive disorders occur for the first time in later life. Several differences in presentation of symptoms have been noted when the onset occurs after age 60 (for reviews, see Caine et al., 1994; Koenig & Blazer, 1992). These differences include more frequent occurrence of psychotic or delusional symptoms (Meyers & Greenberg, 1986), more hypochondriacal symptoms (Brown, Sweeney, Loutsch, Kocsis, & Frances, 1984), and a greater likelihood of cognitive problems, particularly in executive functioning (Alexopoulos et al., 2000). These differences may in part be due to the role that vascular disease plays in many cases of late-onset depression. Vascular changes, such as white-matter abnormalities in the frontal region of the brain, may also be associated with a poorer treatment response (Alexopoulos, Kiosses, Choi, Murphy, & Lim, 2002). By contrast, older people with recurrent depression who had a first onset early in life respond as well to treatment as do younger people (Alexopoulos et al., 1996).

Cross-sectional comparisons have suggested differences in the types of depressive symptoms reported by young and old. Using a community sample of people ages 20 to 98, Gatz and Hurwicz (1990) looked at the relationship of age to four dimensions of depression: depressed mood, psychomotor retardation, lack of well-being, and interpersonal difficulties. These factors were derived from a commonly used screening instrument, the Center for Epidemiologic Studies Depression Scale (CES-D; Radloff, 1977). Younger people reported more depressive feelings, whereas older respondents reported lower rates of positive feelings. In a longitudinal study, Newmann, Engel, and Jensen (1991) found that older women reported fewer depressive symptoms over time but also showed a decrease in positive emotions. These findings raise the possibility that depression in later life might be marked more by an absence of positive affect than by overt depressive emotions.

In summary, although estimates of the prevalence of depression vary, the consensus is that depressive symptoms are a frequent problem in later life. Rates of depression are particularly high in certain populations, notably people with medical illnesses who live in nursing homes. Both age and age of onset may affect the pattern of symptoms and response to treatment. Depressive symptoms are best viewed as the outcome of multiple processes involving biology, behavior, and cognition. As we discuss in Chapter 9, interventions can be made at any of these levels and can result in considerable improvement for older depressed people.

BIPOLAR DISORDERS

Bipolar disorders should be considered as part of a differential diagnosis when an older person presents with depressive symptoms or with manic features. Onset of bipolar symptoms usually occurs around age 20 (Burke et al., 1990), with symptoms recurring as people grow older. Late-onset cases have been reported but appear to be infrequent. Bipolar disorders may be found in as many as 25% of older patients seen in outpatient mental health clinics (Koenig & Blazer, 2004). Rates among patients in nursing homes referred for mental health evaluations are also high.

Recognizing bipolar disorders may be more difficult in later life. Patients who are experiencing a manic episode often present with less euphoria and more dysphoric mood and cognitive symptoms than younger patients (Gildengers et al., 2004; Koenig & Blazer, 2004). Poor impulse control can indicate a manic episode in an older patient, even though other indicators are not present. Besides bipolar disorders, mania also can frequently be part of a delirium or can have other organic causes.

ANXIETY DISORDERS

Anxiety disorders comprise several different diagnoses, which are shown in Table 4.2. Rates of these disorders are as high as or higher than those of depression. The most comprehensive investigation of the prevalence of anxiety in later life remains the Epidemiologic Catchment Area (ECA) study (Regier et al., 1988). Anxiety disorders, including phobias, panic attacks, and obsessive–compulsive disorders, were found to have a 1-month prevalence of 7.3% among older people (Regier et al., 1988). An additional 2.2% of the sample met diagnostic criteria for generalized anxiety disorder (Blazer, George, & Hughes, 1991). As with depression, however, rates of anxiety are higher among younger than older people. Also similar to depression, anxiety disorders are almost twice as high among women as men at every age.

TABLE 4.2. DSM-IV Anxiety Disorders

- Panic disorder without agoraphobia
- Panic disorder with agoraphobia
- Agoraphobia without history of panic disorder
- Simple phobia
- Social phobia
- Obsessive–compulsive disorder
- Posttraumatic stress disorder
- Acute stress disorder
- Generalized anxiety disorder
- Anxiety disorder due to a medical condition
- Substance-induced anxiety disorder
- Anxiety disorder not otherwise specified

As with depression, the first onset of anxiety symptoms usually occurs in adolescence or young adulthood, and the subsequent course is recurrent (Blazer et al., 1991; Kessler, Walters, & Wittchen, 2004). Cases of late-life onset of anxiety symptoms, including phobias and generalized anxiety, have been reported (Lenze et al., 2005; Stanley & Beck, 2000) and may be more common than indicated in epidemiological studies. Older people may not receive a diagnosis because they underreport symptoms or express anxiety through somatic symptoms (Beck & Averill, 2004).

People who are anxious often display comorbidity with other mental health symptoms, particularly depression. Many types of illnesses and medications can cause anxiety symptoms, as shown in Table 4.3. As is the case with depression, medical diseases can lead to physiological changes that increase susceptibility to anxiety. In turn, the psychological threat posed by illness and hospitalization may increase anxiety and worry. Patients with brain disorders, including AD and PD, frequently have anxiety symptoms (Cohen, 1992). Anxiety is associated with hearing and vision loss. Anxiety may also present as part of a syndrome of somatic symptoms that have no apparent underlying medical cause (Gurian & Miner, 1991). An older person may complain of headaches, chest pains, fatigue, or gastrointestinal symptoms that are primarily psychological in origin. Many common substances, such as alcohol and caffeine, contribute to anxiety. The challenge facing clinicians is to identify whether anxiety symptoms are due primarily to medical or to psychological causes or to an interaction of both.

Given the frequent overlap of depressive and anxiety symptoms, the question has been raised as to whether they represent different problems or part of a similar spectrum of disorders. Wetherell, Gatz, and Pedersen (2001) present an interesting hypothesis: that anxiety represents a stable personality characteristic that increases the risk of depressive symptoms. Using data from a longitudinal study, they found that anxiety symptoms

TABLE 4.3. Medical Disorders and Medications Associated with Anxiety

Medical disorders	Substances
Cardiac	**Over-the-counter medications**
Angina	Caffeine
Cardiac arrhythmias	Stimulants
Congestive heart failure	
Hypertension	**Prescription medications**
Mitral valve prolapse	Anticholinergics
Myocardial infarction	Psychostimulants (e.g., methylphenidate, amphetamine)
Endocrine	Sedative–hypnotics (withdrawal)
Cushing's syndrome	Steroids
Hypoglycemia	Sympathomimetics
Hypo- or hyperparathyroidism	
Hypo- or hyperthyroidism	**Other Substances**
Menopause	Alcohol
Premenstrual syndrome	Cocaine
	Hallucinogens
Neurological	Narcotics
Cerebral arteriosclerosis	
Complex partial seizures	
Delirium	
Early dementia	
Huntington's disease	
Meniere's disease	
Migraine	
Multiple sclerosis	
Postconcussion syndrome	
Vestibular dysfunction	
Wilson's disease	
Neoplastic	
Carcinoid syndrome	
Cerebral neoplasm	
Pheocromocytoma	
Pulmonary	
Asthma	
Chronic obstructive pulmonary disease	
Hypoxic states	
Pulmonary embolism	
Other	
Porphyria	

Note. From Beyer (2004). Copyright 2004 by Oxford University Press. Adapted by permission.

can trigger depressive episodes but that depressive symptoms did not lead to anxiety.

Clinical observations also suggest that anxiety often is a stable characteristic in people's lives. Older people with anxiety disorders have perfected rituals and routines that keep their anxiety sufficiently in check so that they can function adequately in their daily lives. They see tension, worry, and other symptoms as normal reactions to a threatening world. Anxious people seek treatment only when a stressful life event or illness disrupts the defenses they use to contain their anxiety. Even then, anxiety may not be the main presenting problem; instead, they focus first on whatever problem has upset their balance. It is only as the clinician obtains a full picture of how this person has functioned in the past that a long history of anxiety symptoms emerges. Clients themselves often do not view these symptoms as a problem, because they have always functioned in the world in that way and do not imagine that there is an alternative.

There has long been speculation that fears about death and dying might trigger anxiety in older people. Fear of death, however, is not more common among the elderly than in other age groups and may actually lessen with advancing age (see Gurian & Miner, 1991, for a review). Older people are concerned about the circumstances of how they might die—for example, dying alone or being put through painful medical procedures—but not about dying itself. Studies of everyday worries have also suggested that older people are not more preoccupied with worries about their health or other life domains than are younger people (Neikrug, 2003). The highest rates of worrying were found among people ages 45–64.

At a biological level, anxiety symptoms are believed to have their origins in the classic fight-or-flight response. Epinephrine and norepinephrine are critical in anxiety reactions. Serotonin functioning has a complex relation to anxiety, sometimes leading to increased symptoms and sometimes to lowered symptoms. The changes in these neurotransmitters with aging probably do not place older people at increased risk of anxiety (Sunderland, Lawlor, Martinez, & Molchan, 1991).

Psychologically, anxiety symptoms have been linked to cognitive processes (see Beck & Averill, 2004, for a review). Aaron Beck and his colleagues (Beck, Emery, & Greenberg, 1985) propose that people prone to anxiety have cognitive schemas that selectively attend to and focus on perceived threat. As with the cognitive theory of depression, the amount of threat is exaggerated. Anxiety and worry have been linked with poor problem-solving ability, as well as the perception of having little control or efficacy in solving problems (Davey, 1994). It has also been proposed that anxiety and worry are ways of avoiding stronger negative emotions such as depression, though this avoidance carries a substantial psychological cost (Borkovec, Roemer, & Kinyon, 1995).

ADJUSTMENT DISORDERS AND GRIEF REACTIONS

Adjustment disorders, especially those characterized by a depressed, anxious, or mixed affective state, are one of the most frequent diagnoses for older clients seen in private practice and in other outpatient settings. People with adjustment disorders have fewer and less severe symptoms than those found in affective or anxiety disorders, and their symptoms occur in reaction to specific life events. Adjustment disorders can develop following major losses, such as chronic illness, retirement, or taking care of a severely disabled spouse. Grief from the death of a spouse or other relative often triggers similar feelings but is categorized separately in the DSM-IV (American Psychiatric Association, 1994).

Despite the prevalence of adjustment disorders in the elderly, little systematic investigation has been done. No epidemiological data exist on incidence and prevalence of adjustment disorders in later life. Rates of diagnosis of adjustment disorder, however, are high in specific settings—for example, in a consultation liaison service (Smith, Clarke, Handrinos & Dunsis, 1998)—and among medically ill populations (see Thompson, Kaye, Tang, & Gallagher-Thompson, 2004, for a review).

Retirement has historically been viewed as a cause of emotional distress in later life, but a more positive view of the transition to retirement has emerged in recent years. As an indication of this shift in perspective, an issue of the journal *Generations* that was devoted entirely to retirement contained virtually no mention of an increased risk of emotional or mental health problems (Ekerdt & Dennis, 2002). Several trends contribute to this new perspective. First, many older people are financially secure, with disposable income that they can use for engaging in enjoyable and meaningful activities in retirement. The picture is not completely positive, however, and certain groups are more likely to be represented among the financially vulnerable—single and widowed women, the oldest old, and people from ethnic and racial minorities (Stanford & Usita, 2002). A second trend that has changed the nature of retirement is that many people who prefer to work have opportunities to do so. With only a few exceptions (airline pilots, police officers, firefighters, and prison personnel), people in the United States do not have a mandatory age for retirement. Other countries have adopted flexible policies that allow partial retirement. Third, it may not be the event of retirement that leads to emotional difficulties but problems that retirees encounter over time in finding meaningful activities. Freedman (2002) suggests viewing retirees as social capital, people who can be involved in community and public service activities. In that way, they can find opportunities for meaningful engagement while providing valuable assistance in the community.

We have increasingly addressed social and psychological aspects of retirement planning with our clients. Two useful planning guides that we use with clients are *Too Young to Retire: 101 Ways to Start the Rest of Your Life* (Stone & Stone, 2004) and *Second Acts: Creating the Life You Really Want, Building the Career You Truly Desire* (Pollan & Levine, 2004). Both books can be incorporated into therapy or can serve as the basis for educational groups or classes on retirement planning. Referral to specialists who provide financial planning can be an important step (Dennis, 2002).

The experience of a loss of a loved one can occur at any time during the life course, but the likelihood increases in later life. A certain amount of grief and sadness after a death is expected and normal and usually resolves within 3–12 months, though spouses may always have some feelings of loss (Thompson et al., 2004). At least some widows and widowers experience long-term difficulties. In one of the few prospective studies conducted, Wilcox and colleagues (2003) found that women who were widowed suffered from more changes in social functioning and increased depressive symptoms over a 3-year period than women who had not become widowed. Aneshensel and colleagues (1995) found that caregivers of people with dementia usually showed a pattern of recovery following the death of the person they were caring for, but one-fourth of the sample still experienced significant mental health symptoms 4 years later. Widowers in particular are prone to increases in alcohol use and suicide risk.

The normal grieving process is identified with a V code in DSM-IV (American Psychiatric Association, 1994), which indicates that people may need treatment but are not suffering from a mental disorder. People whose symptoms become more pronounced and disabling may meet the criteria for specific diagnoses. Depressive and anxious symptoms are prevalent among widows and widowers in the first 2 years following the death of a spouse (Zisook, Shuchter, Sledge, Paulus, & Judd, 1994). Interventions are warranted when grief reactions are unusually pronounced or disabling in the period immediately following a loss or when symptoms of anxiety and depression persist or worsen rather than diminish over time. Treatment should be considered when a person has persistent difficulties adjusting to everyday life more than 3 months after a loss.

SUICIDE

Older adults commit suicide at a much higher rate than any other age group. The rate for suicide in the United States is about 10 cases per 100,000 in the population; for the elderly, the rate is 15 per 100,000 (U.S. Department of Health and Human Services, 2003). Though they make up only 13% of the population, older people account for 20% of all suicides (Conwell, 1994; McIntosh, Santos, Hubbard, & Overholser, 1994; Moscicki, 1995).

The increase in suicide rates in later life is due solely to the high rates found among older men (see Figure 4.1). Women commit suicide at a lower

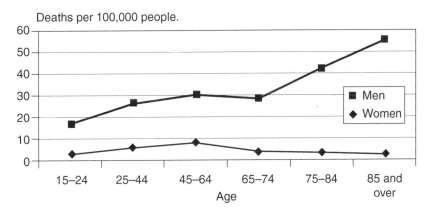

FIGURE 4.1. Death rates from suicide in the United States, 2001. Data from U.S. Department of Health and Human Services (2003).

rate than men at every age. The rate for women reaches a peak in the decade of the 50s and then declines slightly thereafter. Men, on the other hand, show a dramatic increase in suicides beginning in the late 50s, with the highest rate, 55.0 suicides per 100,000 people, found among men over age 85.

Suicide rates also vary by race and ethnicity. Rates of suicide increase with age for white, Hispanic, and Asian men in the United States. For African Americans and Native Americans, however, the peak for suicides occurs between ages 15 and 44, with a decline at later ages (U.S. Department of Health and Human Services, 2003). Similar effects of culture and ethnicity are found in other countries as well. In Great Britain, for example, older English-born white men have an increasing rate of suicide with aging, but male immigrants from the Indian subcontinent do not (Dennis & Lindesay, 1995).

Suicide attempts, compared with completed suicides, follow a different pattern. Young adults attempt the most suicides, and the rate of attempts declines with advancing age (Bille-Brahe, 1993). Women also make more attempts than men at every age, though the differences have narrowed both in young adulthood and again after age 65. These findings suggest that older men are more likely to make suicide attempts with more lethal means and greater intent to end their lives.

In contrast to rates, the methods of suicide do not vary much with age (McIntosh et al., 1994). The most common method is use of firearms, followed by hanging. Use of gas or poisons (including medication overdose) is the third most common method. Women are less likely to use firearms than men and more likely to use poisons, but firearm use by women is increasing.

A related problem is self-destructive behavior. Examples include inappropriate use of prescription medications or alcohol, delaying medical treatment for a life-threatening condition, or risk-taking behavior, such as driving recklessly. Little systematic information is available on this type of indirect suicide. Estimates suggest that self-destructive behaviors are more common at younger ages, although that finding might partly reflect the reluctance of physicians or medical examiners to subject the families of an older person to an extensive and potentially embarrassing inquiry about cause of death (McIntosh et al., 1994). The methods of self-destructive behavior the elderly use may also be more subtle than those chosen by younger people—for example, taking too much of a prescription medication or taking none at all.

The two foremost risk factors for suicide are physical illness and depression, typically in combination (Conwell, 1994; Heikkinen & Lönnqvist, 1995; McIntosh et al., 1994). Suicides often follow hospitalization for medical or psychiatric problems (Erlangsen, Mortensen, Vach, &; Jeune, 2005; Erlangsen, Vach, & Jeune, 2005). Among psychiatric disorders, depression plays an even greater role in suicides of older people than of younger (Conwell & Brent, 1995). The other psychiatric problem frequently associated with suicide in later life is personality disorder (Harwood, Hawton, Hope, & Jacoby, 2001). The somatic illnesses of people who commit suicide do not necessarily pose an imminent threat to life. More typically, they are diseases that involve pain or discomfort. They also tend to have a poor prognosis—that is, the condition will only get worse, not better.

AD is not related to higher risk of suicide. As a result of their cognitive deficits, people with dementing disorders are limited in their ability to formulate or follow through on a suicide plan (McIntosh et al., 1994). As would be done with any other client, however, someone with dementia should be assessed for suicide risk and appropriate precautions taken when suicidal ideation or behaviors are identified. A more likely concern with people with dementia is assisted suicide. Suicide pacts and double suicides by older couples get considerable media attention. The motivation usually involves preventing further suffering—for example, when the husband of a patient with AD kills his wife and then himself. When working with couples on issues of chronic illness or disability, clinicians should assess whether a suicide or homicide–suicide risk exists.

Marital status is also associated with suicide. Widows, widowers, and divorced men are more likely to commit suicide than married persons, especially if they have a weak social network (Conwell & Brent, 1995; McIntosh et al., 1994). The risk for men is greatest in the first year after their wives have died (Erlangsen, Jeune, Billie-Brahe, & Vaupel, 2004). Other factors associated with increased risk include alcoholism and recent losses. Retirement does not have a direct relation to suicide, but the long-term social, emotional, and economic consequences of retirement may contribute to some suicides. Finkel and Rosman (1995) suggest that knowing someone who committed suicide may be an important predisposing factor.

One of the most important factors in identifying risk is a history of prior suicide attempts. Older people are less likely to have made prior attempts or to have talked about committing suicide (Carney, Rich, Burke, & Fowler, 1994; Conwell, 1994). Many, however, have made visits to health professionals in the immediate past. In one large sample of older people who committed suicide, over one-half had seen a health professional in the preceding 30 days (Carney et al., 1994). Another study found that 40% of people who committed suicide had seen their primary care physicians in the preceding week (Conwell, Olsen, Caine, & Flannery, 1991). The medical visits may have triggered feelings of hopelessness over their medical conditions. Whether the health professionals involved might have been able to detect indirect evidence of suicide risk in the patient's behavior or demeanor or whether inquiry into the patient's mood might have identified the suicide risk cannot be determined. These findings, however, underscore the importance of monitoring older clients for suicidal thoughts, especially individuals in high-risk groups—men and people who are depressed or chronically ill.

We also want to note that some suicides occur in nursing homes and other institutional settings (McIntosh et al., 1994). It is usually difficult to gain access to the means to commit suicide in a nursing home, but some patients are able to develop and carry out a plan. As with other suicides, these residents tend to have better cognitive functioning and no dementia. A case in point is psychologist Bruno Bettelheim, who ended his life in a nursing home by taking an overdose of medications and tying a bag over his head (McIntosh et al., 1994). Anticipation of being placed in a nursing home or any other unwanted move can also increase risk of suicide.

One consequence of suicide may be feelings of embarrassment and shame among friends or relatives. Close relatives of older people who commit suicide may have greater difficulties in grieving and resolving their grief than they would if the person had died of natural causes. They also may receive less social support in the period following their relative's death than do mourners whose relatives died of natural causes (Farberow, Gallagher-Thompson, Gilewski, & Thompson, 1992).

CONCLUSIONS

Depression and anxiety represent the most common psychiatric disorders in later life. Despite their prevalence, these problems frequently are not recognized or treated. In many ways, depression and anxiety characterize the classic challenges of working with older people. There are high rates of comorbidity with other psychiatric problems and particularly with medical illnesses and medications. The life history of the person also matters. Many people experience recurrent depression and anxiety over the life course. Etiology and treatment could well vary depending on age of first onset. Adjustment disorders represent milder manifestations of anxiety and depressive symptoms that have occurred as a reaction to specific events. Emotional distress, particularly depression, increases the risk for suicide.

The challenges for clinical practice are to identify anxiety and depressive symptoms, to determine the extent to which comorbid conditions may be contributing to the symptoms, to assess for suicide risk, and to plan an effective treatment. Better identification and treatment of these problems can lead to improvements in the lives of many older people and their families.

CHAPTER 5

Other Common Mental Health Problems in Later Life

We conclude our review of disorders in later life by focusing on a heterogeneous group of problems that clinicians are likely to encounter in practice and that need to be considered as part of the process in differential diagnosis. These disorders include the Axis I diagnoses of schizophrenia and alcohol and substance abuse and the Axis II category, personality disorders.

The problems discussed in this chapter usually have their onset early in life, although late-onset forms have also been described. Disorders that occur for the first time in adolescence or young adulthood may become chronic or recurrent over the life course. Older people with chronic disorders may seek treatment to try to get relief from their ongoing problems or because of a recent worsening in symptoms. Often, psychotherapeutic interventions can help stabilize the situation. Progress in treatment, however, will be slow, and the gains may ultimately be limited, not because of the person's age but because of the intractability of the disorder. Sometimes, however, the person's chronic disorder is not the reason for seeking treatment. Instead, an individual may be looking for help for typical age-related problems such as failing health or memory. When assessing someone with a chronic mental disorder, it is especially important to get beyond the diagnostic label that the person carries and to identify problems or concerns that may be treatable.

SCHIZOPHRENIA

Schizophrenia is a heterogeneous category at any age and particularly in later life. The majority of older patients with schizophrenia experienced the first onset of the disorder in their teens or early 20s. Their symptoms are usually chronic and recurrent. In some cases, however, the first onset of symptoms occurs in middle or old age. Over the years, many researchers have debated whether these later-life forms of schizophrenia represent a variant of the disease that happens to occur later in life or a different disorder. The current consensus is that schizophrenia can be divided into three broad categories based on age of onset: (1) adolescence and young adulthood; (2) after age 40, called "late onset"; and (3) after age 60, called "very late onset" (Howard, Rabins, Seeman, Jeste, and the International Late-Onset Schizophrenia Group, 2000). As we shall see, symptoms and risk factors vary with age of onset. Age of onset also makes a difference for treatment, with patients with earlier onset likely to have more limited social and community support and a poorer occupational history.

The prevalence of all types of schizophrenia is low in later life. The Epidemiologic Catchment Area (ECA) studies found rates of 0.1% among people over age 65 compared with 0.8% for 18- to 24-year-olds and 1.1% for 25- to 44-year-olds (Regier et al., 1988). Studies in the United Kingdom have found a similar prevalence among people over age 65 (Copeland et al., 1998). About 80% of older people with schizophrenia experienced the first onset of symptoms early in life (see Jeste, Wetherell, & Dolder, 2004, for a review).

Several factors may account for the low prevalence of schizophrenia among people 65 and older. First, community surveys may underestimate prevalence. At least some people with chronic schizophrenia are likely to reside in institutional settings—particularly in nursing homes (e.g., Meeks et al., 1990). Gurland and Cross (1982), for example, estimated the prevalence of schizophrenia in nursing homes at 12%. Second, late-onset and particularly very-late-onset cases are more likely to involve paranoid symptoms and suspiciousness. These people are likely to refuse to be interviewed in a community survey. Third, as we discuss, at least some people experience a remission of symptoms with aging. Finally, life expectancy is somewhat lower for people with early-onset schizophrenia than for the general population (Jeste et al., 2004).

Early-Onset Schizophrenia

Despite progress in its treatment, schizophrenia remains a devastating and often intractable disorder. The person who grows old with schizophrenia often has had a lifelong accumulation of problems and disappointments, including inadequate interpersonal relationships and poor connections to the community. Work history often has been disrupted. Symptoms force many afflicted individuals to the social and economic margins of society.

The classic view of schizophrenia is that it involves an unremitting, deteriorating course. Current evidence suggests, however, that the majority of people with schizophrenia stabilize in their functioning and that at least some people experience partial or complete remission of symptoms over time

(Huber, 1997). There is little indication of the old pattern of "burnout," an emotional blunting that in part may have been due to the effects of poor care and chronic institutionalization. The book and film *A Beautiful Mind* (Nasar, 1998) provide a compelling portrait of the severe disruption caused by schizophrenia, as well as the possibility of remission.

The lifetime course of schizophrenia has been documented in several longitudinal studies. These studies differ on key methodological issues, such as how the diagnosis was confirmed and when and how follow-up information was obtained, but they provide a consistent picture of long-term outcomes. The results of these studies suggest that between one-fifth and one-half of people with a documented schizophrenic episode recover completely or have only minimal and occasional symptoms in later life. (e.g., Ciompi, 1987; Clausen, 1986; Harding, Brooks, Ashikaga, Strauss, & Breier, 1987; Huber, 1997; Strauss, 1987; Tsuang, 1986). Improvement may occur in one area of functioning, for example, work or social relationships, but not in other domains (Huber, 1997; Strauss, 1987). Most people experience at least some improvement as they age (Huber, 1997). Despite these positive trends, some individuals show little or no diminution of symptoms over time, and perhaps as many as 20% get worse (Jeste et al., 2004).

The results from a particularly well-conducted study in Lausanne, Switzerland, illustrate these outcomes (Ciompi, 1987). In this study, people who had been hospitalized for schizophrenia 30–40 years earlier were located and interviewed. Hospital records were evaluated to confirm that they would have met current diagnostic criteria for schizophrenia at the time of the original hospitalization. Age at follow-up ranged between 65 and 97 years. Among survivors, 20% had been free of symptoms for a period of at least 5 years, and another 43% were markedly improved compared with earlier functioning. The study also found that former patients had higher mortality than the normal population, raising the possibility that the survivors are a select group—that is, those with a more benign course might have been more likely to survive.

In a critique of schizophrenia outcome studies, Cohen (1990) has argued that some types of symptoms have been emphasized and others ignored. Grouping symptoms into three broad categories—psychopathological symptoms, organic factors, and social functioning—Cohen reviewed evidence of changes with aging for each domain. Psychopathology, including both positive symptoms (hallucinations, delusions) and negative symptoms (emotional blunting, avolition, inattention) diminishes with aging. In contrast, patients at every age had more indications of cognitive deficits and brain abnormalities such as ventricular enlargement than normal populations, though it is not clear whether these differences remain stable or increase with aging (Hijman, Hulshoff, Pol, Sitskoorn, & Kahn, 2003). Patterns of social functioning are more complex. People with schizophrenia generally have smaller social networks than other people, and their networks contain a higher proportion of kin than nonkin. These trends are accentuated in older patients, though that may reflect age-related factors rather than schizophrenia. On the other hand, improvement may occur with aging in some social domains, including quality of relationships and vocational activities.

Despite encouraging evidence about remission of symptoms, people with schizophrenia are more prone to certain adverse outcomes. They are disproportionately represented in the poorest levels of society, becoming homeless or living in single-room-occupancy hotels or nursing homes. They may also suffer from the neurological side effects of neuroleptic medications, especially tardive dyskinesia. At least one-quarter of patients may experience tardive dyskinesia, with the rate increasing with continued use of medication and possibly also with aging (see Jeste et al., 2004, for a review). Risk of suicide is also higher among patients with schizophrenia than among the general population, a trend that continues into old age (Barak, Knobler & Aizenberg, 2004).

Older people with schizophrenia may seek treatment for a variety of reasons. They may, of course, seek help for management of symptoms. In other instances, they may be concerned with age-related issues, such as the impact of an illness, and their schizophrenia may be only a background issue.

One of the most critical issues for many older people with schizophrenia is family support. Although some patients with schizophrenia have become relatively isolated and have lost contact with their families as they aged, others continue to receive routine help, as well as assistance in a crisis (Meeks et al., 1990). Parents and sometimes siblings may provide financial help and may be the main source of social contact. As parents age, however, their own ability to provide help may diminish. Clinical work with older adults with schizophrenia often begins with a focus on management of symptoms, but in some cases it turns quickly to how to cope with the diminishing resources of an aging parent to provide care. Some older parents are able to make plans for the care of their children when something happens to them, but others either are unable to plan or have unrealistic hopes that other relatives will take their place (Smith, 2004).

Late-Onset Schizophrenia

Late-onset schizophrenia refers to the development of a schizophrenia-like disorder between ages 40 and 60. Between 20 and 30% of cases of schizophrenia are believed to have their onset during this age period (Jeste et al., 2004). Compared with early-onset cases, a greater proportion of people with late-onset schizophrenia are women and have paranoid symptoms. Negative symptoms, such as emotional blunting, are less pronounced than in early-onset cases. Cognitive deficits are also less prominent than they are in early-onset cases, particularly in the areas of attention, abstract reasoning, and flexibility. Neuroimaging studies have identified possible risk factors for late-onset schizophrenia, including enlarged ventricles and increased prevalence of white-matter hyperintensities (Jeste et al., 2004). Besides gender, other risk factors include a family history of schizophrenia and of sensory deficits, particularly bilateral hearing loss. Differential diagnosis must rule out affective disorders and focal or degenerative brain pathology as the cause of symptoms (Howard et al., 2000).

The large sex difference in late-onset cases has led to speculation about the possible role of estrogen. Specifically, some researchers have hypothesized that estrogen may have a protective role for women who are at risk for schizophrenia and that lower levels at midlife might contribute to the emergence of symptoms (Jeste et al., 2004; Salokangas, Honkonen, & Saarinen, 2003). Clinical trials of estrogen replacement as an adjunct in treatment of late-onset schizophrenia have had mixed results (e.g., Huber, Borsutzky, Schneider, & Emrich, 2004; Louza et al., 2004).

As was the case with early-onset schizophrenia, the main implication for geriatric practice is that people with late-onset symptoms grow older, and they often have fewer social, emotional, and economic resources for coping with other age-related changes than an average older person does.

Very-Late-Onset Schizophrenia

Very-late-onset schizophrenia (onset after age 60) is similar to late onset in that patients are predominantly women and symptoms are more frequently paranoid (Jeste et al., 2004). Historically, various terms have been used to describe paranoid and other schizophrenic-like symptoms in later life, including "late-life paraphrenia" and "late-life paranoid disorder." Very-late-onset cases are both similar to and different from early- and late-onset cases (see Howard et al., 2000, for a review). Hallucinations and delusions are more florid with very late onset—that is, they tend to be vivid and dramatic. In a series of patients with very late onset, 69% had auditory hallucinations, 29% had visual hallucinations, and 26% had tactile hallucinations (some had more than one type of hallucination), and all showed evidence of delusions (Rabins, McHugh, Pauker, & Thomas, 1987). People with very-late-onset schizophrenia also show less evidence of thought disorder or flattening of affect.

Roth (1987) proposes that onset typically occurs in two stages. During the first stage, which may last for 6 to 18 months, a gradual increase in suspiciousness, irritability, and hostility occurs. During this period, people become more reclusive, develop ideas of reference about other people, and may begin making frequent complaints to the police or other authorities. The second stage involves the eruption of visual and auditory hallucinations. This second stage may be precipitated by stressful life events, but often the events are of a trivial nature. Patients, however, regard these events as highly significant, interpreting them within the framework of their delusions.

Compared with onset at earlier ages, people with very late onset are less likely to have a family history of schizophrenia (Jeste et al., 2004). Two predisposing characteristics have been identified in very-late-onset schizophrenia. First is a pattern of a lifelong history of marginal adjustment, particularly in the area of interpersonal relationships (Kay, Cooper, Garside, & Roth, 1976; Post, 1966, 1980; Rabins, 1992). These individuals may have been employed but did not marry or had brief, unsuccessful marriages. Symptoms are sometimes precipitated by an increase in social isolation, such as following retirement or the loss of a key family member or friend. This pattern occurs more frequently among women than men. In the second pattern, sensory loss plays a central role in the development of symptoms. People with hearing loss, particularly bilateral hearing loss that develops in midlife, are prone to development of paranoid disorders. Some association with vision loss has also been reported (Cooper & Porter, 1976). There are fewer predisposing personality and social factors in paranoid patients with sensory loss than in those without it (Cooper, Garside, & Kay, 1976).

The following example illustrates the first pattern of very-late-onset schizophrenia: marginal premorbid adjustment with increasing social isolation.

Very-Late-Onset Schizophrenia

Joan was a woman in her early 70s who sought help at an outpatient program serving the elderly because she believed that her landlord was using extrasensory perception (ESP) to stimulate her sexually. She provided a detailed life history. Joan was the unwanted only child of older parents. She described an upbringing devoid of attention. Her mother raised her with an odd set of beliefs, which combined psychoanalysis and astrology in an idiosyncratic way and emphasized that sex and elimination were disgusting processes. Joan still maintained these beliefs. She had married at age 40, shortly after her mother's death. Almost immediately after the marriage, she had a hysterectomy. She and her husband soon drifted apart, though she maintained occasional contact with him. During her adult years, Joan worked continuously as a salesperson in department stores. She had never had a psychiatric hospitalization, but she described one apparent psychotic episode 20 years earlier. This incident occurred in a dentist's office, and during it either she had felt sexual feelings toward the dentist or he had made sexual advances toward her. This story, however, was jumbled, and it was not possible to tell what had happened. It is possible that there had been other, similar episodes, but Joan did not volunteer information about them. Since she had retired a couple of years earlier, she had lost contact with the few friends she had had at work and lived a largely isolated life.

Joan's current symptoms had begun a few months earlier. She lived in a small apartment building built around a courtyard and could see her landlord's apartment from her window. Joan had been friendly with him, conversing with him when they met in the courtyard. One time she invited him to dinner, but he responded with a noncommittal answer. She concluded that he had signaled her that he was coming to dinner by moving the blinds in his window in a particular way. When he did not show up for dinner, Joan became very upset. She confronted him, but he treated her in a dismissive way. After that incident, she began experiencing sexual discomfort at night, which she believed was caused by ESP. Joan's symptoms included both revulsion at being violated and attraction toward her landlord.

This case is typical of many late-life paranoid disorders. Joan had functioned adequately during her adult life, particularly in her work role, with possibly only one previous psychotic episode. Symptoms developed following a period of increasing social isolation and after an incident in which she felt rejected and humiliated. Her symptoms were dramatic and florid. Despite these symptoms, she was continuing to function adequately and did not exhibit any other obvious problems. This case also illustrates the possible overlap between the late- and very-late-onset categories, as there had been at least one possible prior episode in midlife.

In cases involving sensory loss, symptoms often revolve around the disability. People with hearing loss may fill in what they think others are saying. They assume people are talking about them, saying negative things or making threats. In cases in which vision loss is involved, visual sensory input can be distorted, for example, seeing a threatening stranger in the mirror or believing someone is coming into the house and stealing things or rearranging the furniture.

Another pattern of symptoms involves paranoid or other delusional symptoms but no auditory or visual hallucinations. These cases do not meet diagnostic criteria for schizophrenia and instead are grouped together in the category of delusional disorder.

Issues in Differential Diagnosis of Schizophrenia in Later Life

When paranoid and other schizophrenia-like symptoms emerge in later life, differential diagnosis includes evaluating for a past history of schizophrenia, as well as ruling out conditions that can cause similar symptoms. Delirium, in particular, can be mistaken for schizophrenia because of the presence of hallucinations and delusions. According to Cummings and Mega (2003), many older (65+) patients with paranoid and other psychotic symptoms have a primary medical problem. Medications often trigger these symptoms. History and a careful medical examination can differentiate schizophrenia from delirium. Of course, it is important to keep in mind that a person with a history of schizophrenia early in life can also develop a delirium or dementia in old age.

Clinicians need to be alert to the emergence of new and potentially treatable medical, psychiatric, or social problems unrelated to the schizophrenia.

Paranoid symptoms can also be part of a variety of other syndromes, including depression, dementia, and obsessive–compulsive disorders. In contrast to schizophrenia, symptoms in dementia are often less elaborate or developed. People with dementia may fill in the gaps in their memories with paranoid thoughts—for example, patients who misplace a wallet or purse may complain that someone is stealing their money.

Finally, we want to note that we have encountered situations in which an initial complaint that sounded paranoid turned out to have a basis in fact: A son or daughter was, in fact, trying to get their mother's money. Some older clients can also present with loose and tangential thinking that suggests psychotic thought processes but that turn out to be part of an idiosyncratic conversational style (see Chapter 8).

PERSONALITY DISORDERS

Personality disorders are disturbing, disruptive, and difficult to treat. DSM-IV, in its definition of personality disorders, describes them as rigid and inflexible (American Psychiatric Association, 1994; Tyrer, 1995). People with personality disorders often have fragile and conflicted family relationships and may function poorly at work. Disorders are typically grouped into three clusters. Cluster A is characterized by odd and eccentric behaviors and includes schizoid, paranoid, and schizotypal diagnoses. Cluster B involves dramatic and impulsive behavior and includes histrionic, narcissistic, antisocial, and borderline diagnoses. Cluster C is marked by anxious and fearful behaviors and includes obsessive–compulsive, avoidant, and dependent diagnoses.

By definition, personality disorders have their onset in adolescence or early adulthood (American Psychiatric Association, 1994), so older clients with diagnoses of personality disorders typically have long histories of symptoms and problems. There are, however, two exceptions to this pattern. First, a personality disorder may be "uncovered" by a loss or other change in later life (Sadavoy & Fogel, 1992). As an example, a woman with a dependent personality functioned adequately during the adult years because of the efforts made by her husband, but after he died, she was unable to cope with even elementary tasks in everyday life. In these types of cases, a careful history will reveal features of personality disorder that were present throughout adulthood but that were contained by a supportive relationship or work. In the second exception, personality traits become exacerbated by other psychiatric problems such as depression or brain disorders. In these cases, the patient may meet most of the criteria for a personality disorder, but the symptoms are secondary to another problem.

Lifelong Personality Disorder with Some New Twists in Old Age

Brenda, age 70, was a divorced professor who had retired after her first stroke. She sought treatment from me because she had become anxious and fearful since her stroke, although she had regained most of her cognitive and physical functioning. Brenda lived alone in a large house and was afraid that she would have another stroke and no one would find her. She had hired a live-in helper, Donna, who essentially provided her with company. Brenda had become dependent on Donna, who would come whenever she called out, even in the middle of the night.

Brenda was the younger of two children, born in England. Her family lived a humble life, but her mother always encouraged her to pursue an education. Brenda had been a shy, backward child and did not have many friends growing up. Instead, she threw herself into school and sports, particularly tennis. She did so well in school that she won a scholarship to Oxford, where she studied hard and became a professor. Brenda married a fellow teacher, but that marriage ended after only a few years. She was never sure why, except that she felt somehow inadequate to hold his interest.

Brenda had a very successful career. She had depended on her work colleagues for company, so when she retired, she found herself quite alone. She acknowledged that dependency was a lifelong trait and that she liked to have other people take care of the details of her life, much as her secretary had done when she worked. Donna had stepped in and filled that void, but now the situation was not working well.

Brenda continued to worry about her health and saw her family practice doctor almost weekly. She had crises in which she would become overwhelmingly anxious, often about whether or not she would be able to fall asleep. On several occasions, Brenda ended up in the mental health unit of the community hospital because she had gone to the emergency room in such an anxious state that they felt that they had to admit her. She was put on an antidepressant, an atypical neuroleptic, and a minor tranquilizer. Brenda quickly became addicted to the minor tranquilizer and had a very hard time weaning off it. In the midst of this, she was behaving in a very dependent manner in therapy, asking for extra sessions and telephone calls and occasionally e-mailing questions to me. Brenda saw two different substitute therapists while I was on vacation and expressed dissatisfaction with each. The next time I went on vacation, more than a year later, Brenda cancelled all future appointments and refused to answer her telephone to discuss it. One month later, a release arrived asking for records to be sent to a new therapist.

Brenda had elements of both obsessive–compulsive and dependent personality disorders that were long-standing characteristics and that made her adjustment to her stroke more complicated. Despite her occupational accomplishments, she presented as somewhat immature and child-like. It was very important for Brenda to feel that she was the "teacher's pet," or favorite patient, and she could not tolerate having to share her therapist. These lifelong traits served her well in her work but not in personal relationships. These characteristics guarantee that Brenda will have to move from therapist to therapist, as each one inevitably disappoints her.

Personality disorders are difficult to diagnose reliably at any age. One source of unreliability is the fact that diagnosis depends, in part, on making inferences about the personality structure that underlies overt behavior (Sadavoy & Fogel, 1992). Another problem in developing reliable diagnostic criteria is that personality disorders overlap considerably; patients often show characteristics of two or more disorders (Tyrer, 1995; Widiger & Sanderson, 1995). As an alternative to traditional diagnosis, a dimensional model has been proposed that classifies people based on scores on standardized personality assessments (Widiger & Sanderson, 1995; Widiger & Simonsen, 2005). From a dimensional perspective, personality disorders represent a blending together of traits in unique patterns, which are captured only in part by current diagnostic categories. As yet, this type of dimensional approach has not been widely adopted.

There are also questions about whether the criteria for diagnosis, which have been established and validated on younger samples, are appropriate for people who are older (Agronin & Maletta, 2000; Clarkin, Spielman, & Klausner, 1999; Segal, Hersen, Van Hasselt, Silberman, & Roth, 1996). In particular, behaviors such as criminal activity and sexual promiscuity may decrease as part of a general trend with aging or due to more limited opportunities, but whether those changes represent improvement or a shift in problems to other domains has not been determined.

It is not surprising, then, given the difficulties in diagnosis, that estimates of the prevalence of personality disorder vary widely from study to study. Surveys of community populations have found prevalence to range from less than 1 to around 15% of the population (Girolamo & Reich, 1993; Grant et al., 2004). In a study conducted at the Baltimore ECA site, specific assessments were made using DSM-III (American Psychiatric Association, 1980) diagnostic criteria to identify personality disorders (Samuels, Nestadt, Romanoski, Folstein, & McHugh, 1994). Personality disorders occurred at a rate of 5.9% in that sample. Including people with provisional diagnoses of personality disorders increased the rate to 9.3%.

Despite the variability in estimates of prevalence, the consensus is that rates of personality disorders are lower in older than in younger individuals (Ames & Molinari, 1994; Cohen et al., 1994; Engels, Duijsens, Haringsma, & van Putten, 2003; Grant et al., 2004). Studies of patients with Axis I diagnoses show much higher rates of personality disorders at every age than are found in the general population (Abrams & Horowitz, 1999). In terms of specific diagnoses, older people are less likely than younger individuals to have Cluster B disorders involving antisocial and impulsive behavior (Cohen et al., 1994;

Engles et al., 2003). Cluster C disorders, however, become relatively more frequent in older people (Agbayewa, 1996).

There are several hypotheses about the overall decrease in prevalence of personality disorders with age. One possibility is selective mortality, that is, that people with these disorders tend to die at younger ages. Another theory is that the effects of aging may mitigate some symptoms, particularly antisocial and impulsive behavior and emotional outbursts (e.g., Agbayewa, 1996; Agronin & Maletta, 2000; Clarkin et al., 1999; Engels et al., 2003; Tyrer & Seivewright, 1988; Zweig & Hillman, 1999). Decline in these behaviors may account for the fact that fewer people meet the criteria for a Cluster B diagnosis. This decline is offset in part by an increase in schizoid and obsessive–compulsive symptoms (Engels et al., 2003). Clarkin and associates (1999) proposed a framework for examining age changes in personality disorders. They suggest that activity, emotionality, and cognition are all components of personality and that age-related changes in each of these domains account for developmental patterns in personality disorders. Specifically, activity and emotional expression are reduced, and mild cognitive changes associated with aging can lead to more errors in processing information and hence more unusual or distorted thoughts.

Another theory is that problems remain severe but that opportunities to engage in some behaviors decline (Agronin & Maletta, 2000). Our clinical observation of people with histories of histrionic or borderline disorders is consistent with that theory. These individuals continue to be troubled with the types of problems, particularly in work and relationships, that they had earlier in life, but the frequency of outbursts is somewhat reduced. That is mainly due to reduced opportunity. Their social networks have eroded due to the corrosive effect their behavior has on relationships.

There is also some evidence that personality disorders can worsen in later life, exacerbated by losses and other stressors. For example, a person concerned with issues of trust who experiences losses may brood excessively on them and become increasingly isolated, suspicious, and paranoid. Clinical observations suggest that features of a personality disorder can shift with age toward somatic and depressive preoccupations and conflict with children or other close relations (Sadavoy & Fogel, 1992).

Longitudinal data would be very useful in clarifying the questions about the long-term course of personality disorders. It could be that some people diagnosed with personality disorders early in life make substantial improvements. Identifying the treatments and other conditions that lead to meaningful long-term change would be very helpful. Some people may also make gradual improvements as they age—particularly, as noted, in cluster B symptoms—whereas others may be vulnerable to stressors associated with aging. The lack of clarity in conceptualization and diagnosis, combined with the lack of long-term studies, leaves considerable uncertainty about the course of personality disorders over the lifespan.

One factor that is clear, however, is that the individual with a personality disorder remains difficult to treat in late life. As at earlier ages, the persistent problems of clients with personality disorders absorb a disproportionate amount of a clinician's time and energy. The person's relationship with the therapist is likely to be stormy and challenging and not offset frequently enough by signs of improvement. Adding to the usual treatment difficulties, lifelong interpersonal tensions may have eroded family support and left the person without other close relationships. The therapist may be the one supportive person in the client's life. The emergence of health problems in later life poses another challenge. The same behaviors that alienate family and friends may interfere with communication with physicians. As a result, people with personality disorders may find it particularly difficult to get adequate treatment for medical problems. Therapists often find themselves having to repair disrupted relationships between the patient with a personality disorder and other professionals. It is therefore important to instruct clients on how to present themselves to health professionals so that they will receive the care they need, rather than having it withdrawn in an angry reaction to their typical interpersonal style.

Personality disorders can be especially disruptive in institutional settings such as hospitals and nursing homes, taking up disproportionate staff time and evoking angry, punitive responses. The clinician's role in those circumstances is varied, sometimes providing treatment and frequently intervening with staff to prevent things from getting worse.

ALCOHOL AND SUBSTANCE ABUSE

Alcohol and substance abuse is another of the hidden problems of old age, frequently overlooked despite severe health and social consequences. These disorders are generally viewed as problems of the young, and although rates of alcohol and drug abuse are in fact much higher earlier in life, there is a significant and possibly growing prevalence in old age. Many people, however, cannot conceive that the elderly would abuse drugs or alcohol and so ignore the signs and symptoms of a problem. Even professionals in the substance abuse field sometimes mistakenly believe that these problems burn out or that abusers die before reaching old age.

One barrier to recognition is that older people with drinking problems often do not fit the stereotype of the down-and-out alcoholic. Instead, they may come from middle-class homes and communities and have a history of stable functioning. As a result, physicians and other health professionals are reluctant to look for alcohol or drug problems (Atkinson, 1990).

Another barrier to recognition is that symptoms can be wrongly ascribed to aging or senility. Problems associated with alcohol and drug abuse include falls, anxiety, depression, insomnia and fatigue, slurred speech, poor memory, diarrhea, urinary incontinence, weight loss or malnutrition, and a decline in personal hygiene and self-care (Egbert, 1993; O'Connell, Chin, Cunningham, & Lawlor, 2003). These symptoms can occur in dementia and many other age-related problems, so the role of drugs or alcohol can be easily overlooked.

Most of the available information focuses on alcohol abuse, but other types of substance abuse also need to be considered. With the aging of the baby-boomer generation, growing numbers of older people will have had experience with illegal drugs in their youth. It is not known how many of these individuals have continued at least occasional use or may increase use in retirement. A more obvious problem is abuse of prescription medications, though precise data are difficult to obtain.

Alcohol use is common and socially accepted, and so rates of abuse are considerable, even in later life. Prevalence depends on the criteria used for investigating the problem. Rates of heavy drinking (four or more drinks a day) range between 6 and 24% for community-dwelling older men and between 1 and 7% of older women (Atkinson, Ganzini, & Bernstein, 1992; O'Connell et al., 2003; Thomas & Rockwood, 2001). When considering only severe problems, such as alcohol dependence, rates range between 1 and 12% for older men and between 0.01 and 1% for women. The proportion of alcohol problems is higher in certain populations, including hospitalized and psychiatric patients (Curtis, Geller, Stokes, Levine, & Moore, 1989; Mangion, Platt, & Syam, 1992). In outpatient mental health programs, 10% of older clients have been found to have alcohol problems (Jinks & Raschko, 1990; Reifler et al., 1982), whereas rates in inpatient programs have ranged between 23 and 44% (O'Connell et al., 2003). A study of consecutive admissions of older people to a hospital emergency room identified 14% who were currently alcohol abusers (Adams, Magruder-Habib, Trued, & Broome, 1992). Their most common medical complaints are gastrointestinal problems. Physicians detected only about one-fifth of people with alcohol problems. High rates of alcohol use have sometimes been reported in retirement communities. A careful analysis of these findings suggests that many residents drink moderately (1 or 2 drinks a day) but that heavy drinking is rare (Adams, 1995). Finally, the possibility of alcoholism among residents of nursing homes and other congregate living situations should not be overlooked. Although they may have limited access to alcohol, nursing home patients may be able to obtain sufficient amounts from family or friends—or even staff—for it to be a problem.

Two distinct patterns have been identified among older alcoholics (Atkinson, Tolson, & Turner, 1990; Atkinson, Turner, Kofoed, & Tolson, 1985; Mishara & Kastenbaum, 1980). First are the lifelong drinkers, people who have been either regular or intermittent abusers of alcohol all their adult lives. This group constitutes about two-thirds of older alcohol abusers. The other third of older problem drinkers are people who increased their consumption of alcohol in later life, usually following a stress or loss. A common pattern is for an older man who becomes widowed to drink more heavily as a way of dealing with loneliness and social isolation.

Health problems may have a complex relation to alcohol problems. Drawing on findings from a 10-year longitudinal study, Moos and his colleagues (Moos, Brennan, Schutte, & Moos, 2005) reported that health problems increased the likelihood of abstinence but also increased the rate of drinking problems. In other words, some people respond to major health problems by stopping the use of alcohol altogether, but others increase their consumption to harmful levels.

Alcohol may become a problem in later life in part because older people are more sensitive to its effects (Blazer, 2004; DeHart & Hoffmann, 1997). Older people tend to have less body water, and so a similar amount of alcohol raises their blood levels more than in a younger person. As a result, older people can experience adverse consequences when consuming lower amounts of alcohol than younger problem drinkers do. Even moderate amounts of alcohol can lead to mild cognitive impairment among older people (Atkinson & Kofoed, 1982). A person who always had one or two drinks a day with little or no adverse consequences may begin having problems in functioning in later life without any increase in alcohol consumption.

One of the risks of alcohol in old age is the potential for interactions with prescription medications (Adams, 1997). Even people who drink moderately may develop problems due to the interaction of alcohol with prescription medications they are taking. Many medications can increase the impact of even small amounts of alcohol. In turn, alcohol may block the effects of certain medications, or the combination may produce significant adverse effects. (Common drug–alcohol interactions are described on the Internet at http:// pubs.niaaa.nih.gov.publications/Medicine/medicine.htm.)

Cognitive impairment is a major consequence of alcohol abuse. Although the role of alcohol in the development of dementia is controversial, at least some researchers believe that alcohol contributes to the onset in approximately 20% of cases (Carlen et al., 1994; Smith & Atkinson, 1995; Thomas & Rockwood, 2001). Certainly, alcohol use and drug–alcohol interactions are a major source of potentially reversible cognitive impairments.

Counterbalancing the risks of alcohol are claims that consumption of one to two glasses of wine a day may have health benefits, such as decreases in cardiovascular disease and stroke. These findings are drawn from large population surveys, and it remains to be determined whether the benefits are due to alcohol use or to other unmeasured differences between people who drink moderately and those who do not drink at all. The potential benefits also have to be weighed against the increased impact of alcohol with aging, as well as the risk of interactions with prescription drugs.

Drug abuse is much less of a problem for older people than is alcohol abuse, and it usually involves misuse of legal rather than illegal drugs. Prevalence is difficult to determine, but one study of psychiatric outpatients found that 5% of their sample were abusing prescription medications (Jinks & Raschko, 1990). The main type of drug abuse involves minor tranquilizers, such as lorazepam (Ativan) and diazepam (Valium; Finlayson & Davis, 1994; Task Force on Benzodiazepine Dependency, 1990). Dependency on tranquilizers can develop among elderly people even at low dosages due to decreased rates of metabolism and excretion of medications. The major consequences of dependency include falls and fractures, depression, and memory impairment (Ancill, Embury, MacEwan, & Kennedy, 1987). Some depressed older people also develop dependencies. In these cases it appears that physicians prescribed tranquilizers for complaints of anxiety and insomnia but failed to detect underlying feelings of depression (Finlayson, 1997).

Finally, we want to note that a variety of over-the-counter medications and commonly consumed substances, such as nicotine, caffeine, herbs, vitamins, and other nutritional supplements, can result in problems for older people. In sufficient quantities, these substances can lead to health symptoms or may interfere with therapeutic regimens of prescription drugs.

CONCLUSIONS

Because many chronic problems are unabated as people with mental disorders grow older, it is possible to encounter virtually any type of pathology in an older population. We have not provided an exhaustive review of all possible disorders an older person might have but have concentrated instead on those disorders that are likely to be encountered in typical treatment settings or that need to be considered when making a differential diagnosis.

Several conclusions can be drawn from this survey. First and foremost, we have only begun to form a true developmental perspective on mental disorders, one that examines age of onset, the course of symptoms over time, and how one's personal life history contributes to risk and recovery. In later life, we encounter clients with varying developmental histories and patterns. Some have had problems since early life, some have late-onset disorders, and some have had fluctuating or changing patterns of symptoms over the years. The practical significance of these differences in history is not fully understood at this time.

Another important issue is the critical role of comorbidity. Comorbidity should be taken into account when planning treatment. Treatment of psychiatric symptoms associated with medical illness can lead to improvement in both physical and mental health.

The overlap among syndromes calls attention to the limitations of current classification systems for mental disorders. These systems have been developed as a tool for generating reliable diagnoses for research purposes. It would be premature to assume that these categories are actually homogeneous and that all people with the same disorders have a similar etiology or will respond to the same treatment. As we learn more about the variability of genetic, physiological, and psychosocial contributions to mental disorders, it is likely that more precise and differentiated categories will emerge. The diagnostic system for older people is problematic for another reason—categories and criteria in the DSM-IV and ICD-10 have been established largely on the basis of patterns of symptoms found among younger people. As we have stressed, there are places in the current classification system that do not fit well with disorders of late life. It may also be that the idea of illness categories is not the best approach to psychiatric disorders. A better approach might be to describe dimensions of functioning that fall along a continuum (e.g., Widiger, 2005). At least some part of the spectrum of what we call anxiety and depressive disorders is probably better described that way, as are the personality disorders. In sum, current classification schemes provide a framework that, as experienced clinicians know, is useful but could be improved.

Finally, we want to reiterate that mental disorders can be encountered in any of the settings in which older people live. We have cited epidemiological studies that emphasize prevalence in community populations of older people. Nursing homes, however, have replaced mental hospitals as sites for care of older people with chronic mental health problems. It is not unusual for more than one-half of residents of nursing homes to have mental health problems, although often these symptoms are unrecognized and untreated. These problems include not only dementia and its consequences but also schizophrenia and personality disorders. Other settings, such as retirement communities, assisted living, and board-and-care homes, also have significant numbers of residents with mental health problems.

The disorders of aging, then, represent a complex array of problems that are found in many different settings. Chapters 3, 4, and 5 have described the characteristics of the most frequent disorders. Building on these descriptions, we now turn to the process of assessment and how late-life disorders can be accurately diagnosed.

CHAPTER 6

The Clinical Interview

Assessment is the most important clinical skill in working with older people. The starting point in many cases is a question about diagnosis. Clinicians need to sort out evidence to differentiate among dementia, delirium, depression, and other common disorders of later life. Clients are often referred because a diagnosis needs to be established or because the presenting diagnosis may need to be revised—for example, if a patient previously diagnosed with dementia has had a recent delirium episode. In addition to questions of diagnosis, assessment can identify strengths and limitations that are useful in planning treatment.

In this chapter, we begin our discussion of assessment with a review of the principles that guide us when conducting an assessment. We then focus on the first step in assessment: a clinical interview. The clinical interview is conducted with the dual goals of clarifying diagnosis and obtaining information useful for planning treatment. Components of the clinical interview include identifying presenting symptoms and problems, obtaining a history of current symptoms and problems, and mental status testing. The chapter ends with a discussion of how to utilize the findings from the patient's medical examination. In Chapter 7, we continue the discussion by describing the uses of psychological testing in differential diagnosis and in determination of capacity.

In conducting an assessment, clinicians draw on their knowledge of the normal aging process and of characteristics of the disorders of aging. Evidence is gathered in a systematic way from several sources, including a clinical interview with the client and his or her family, psychological testing, and a review of medical information. In evaluating this information, the clinician needs to navigate between the excessively negative expectations about aging that are sometimes held by physicians, families, and older people themselves and the real, catastrophic problems that can occur.

Clinicians trained in assessment can play a valuable role in determining the correct diagnosis. Diagnosis of the major psychiatric disorders of late life is based to a considerable extent on evaluation of behavior and cognition. These domains cannot be assessed accurately in a brief interview in a physician's office but require observation, testing, and discussion with clients and their families. In contrast to a busy physician whose day is structured into brief appointment slots, mental health professionals can and should take the time needed to conduct the kind of in-depth clinical interview and other clinical observations, such as a home visits, that can provide a full picture of current symptoms, their history, and opportunities for intervention. Psychological testing provides a systematic sample of behavior and cognition that can clarify current symptoms and problems. The use of normed and standardized tests makes it possible to evaluate older clients' symptoms in light of objective indicators of their overall functioning. By combining the results of psychological testing with information from systematic clinical interviews, it is possible to determine whether behaviors and cognitions meet criteria for a particular diagnosis or whether they fall within the boundaries of normal aging.

The emphasis in both this chapter and the next is on differential diagnosis. We focus on the central question in a geriatric practice: Is this person suffering from dementia? At each step of the process—gathering information about symptoms, history, and mental status and psychological testing—we show how dementia differs from delirium, depression, and normal aging. We also discuss how the pattern with focal brain damage, such as from a head injury, differs from dementia. Head injury is fairly infrequent and often overlooked in older people. In almost all cases of older people with head injuries whom we have evaluated, a health professional who has seen them has assumed that their cognitive problems are due to dementia. Of course, differential diagnosis requires consideration of the full range of conditions that might contribute to current symptoms. It would be exhaustive to discuss all the possibilities, and so we have concentrated on the most likely distinctions that clinicians will need to make and the principles that guide the decision-making process.

Another consideration is the possibility of comorbidity. In other words, in some instances the outcome of an assessment process is identification of two or more problems. A person with dementia may have depressive and/or anxiety symptoms, which complicate care but can also respond to treatment. Depressive and anxiety symptoms often occur together. People with chronic problems, such as schizophrenia or a personality disorder, can become cognitively impaired or have symptoms of anxiety and depression, and anyone might develop a delirium. These comorbidities are important to recognize because of their implications for treatment.

Many textbooks address assessment either by discussing diagnostic features disorder by disorder or by including a chapter that presents information on tests and other assessment tools in a general way without focusing on how to make clinical decisions. We believe that that approach does not demonstrate the decision-making process that is central to differential diagnosis. Our approach is to go through the steps of an assessment and discuss how the information that is obtained can be used in thinking about diagnosis and treatment planning. In doing so, we draw on the descriptions of clinical characteristics of disorders in previous chapters. In the end, it is how information is evaluated, rather than the use of any particular test or procedure, that leads to sound clinical decisions.

PRINCIPLES OF ASSESSMENT

We begin with a discussion of the goals and principles that underlie the assessment process. Clinicians will be asked to address a clinical question; for example, is this client suffering from dementia? The goal is to provide an answer to that question, but how clinicians carry out the assessment will make a difference for the outcome. We start without prejudging the outcome. An older person who is referred for an evaluation could be experiencing any of a wide range of disorders. Symptoms may result from a recurrence of a disorder first experienced earlier in life with an overlay of age-related issues or from a new disorder. Given the many different disorders that can occur in later life, an assessment must start with a broad focus and then narrow down the choices as information is gathered. Even after years in this field, we can still be surprised by the outcomes of assessments. We have evaluated many cases in which the initial reason for referral was dementia but the problem turned out to be psychological and vice versa. In other words, it is important not to reach a conclusion prematurely nor to be persuaded by the opinion of the patient's doctor or family, because that could lead to overlooking some important evidence that suggests a different outcome.

The most common reason that an older patient is referred for an assessment is the possibility of dementia. In those cases, the initial focus of the assessment should be to gather evidence that makes it possible to differentiate dementia from other disorders and from normal aging. The first step is to determine whether the evidence points conclusively to dementia. A diagnosis of dementia is really about the prognosis—that this person is expected to continue declining—rather than about cognitive impairment. Cognitive impairment can be caused by many other factors, some of which are reversible and some of which are troublesome but stable. Dementia, however, worsens over time. Once dementia has been identified, then it is possible to determine its type, based on symptoms, history, and medical and neuropsychological findings. This type of assessment is, in many ways, the hallmark of practice with older people. When a possibility of a cognitive disorder exists, it is critical to clarify that diagnostic question first before doing anything else.

Clients can be referred for many other reasons, or they may seek treatment themselves. Some clinicians would argue that a thorough assessment of cognition should be undertaken at the outset with any older client. This approach is warranted in certain settings, such as a teaching clinic or hospital. It can be very helpful as part of a student's training to use at least some cognitive tests with every client in order to learn to differentiate normal and impaired patterns of performance. Likewise, for inexperienced clinicians, screening every referral in a setting such as a nursing home is also helpful, because the rates of dementia can be quite high and questions about cognitive functioning are usually part of the reason for conducting an evaluation. But the issue is less clear-cut in other settings. We receive many referrals for psychotherapy. In these cases, concerns about memory loss may not be an issue, so it is sufficient to conduct a briefer assessment. In that situation, the risk of not conducting a thorough assessment has to be weighed against the expense of doing so, the commitment of the client's time and energy, and the ageist implications of presuming that the person might have a cognitive deficit. If evidence subsequently emerges that indicates the possibility of a cognitive problem, a more thorough assessment can be performed.

The decision-making process in differential diagnosis involves hypothesis testing. Because there are as yet no definitive markers of dementia, delirium, depression, or other disorders in later life, the clinician must go through a process of evaluating the evidence to determine the most likely explanation for current symptoms. This task entails gathering information from several sources—interview, reports from informants, observations, and psychological testing—and then deciding among competing possibilities. We continually ask ourselves whether the pattern of symptoms, test results, and other observations is more like one disorder than another. The results of this process are then examined in light of medical findings.

When there is a question of possible dementia and the assessment does not yield conclusive evidence one way or the other, we have two options. The first is to consider whether other tests or assessments might clarify the situation. The second is for the clinician to conduct another evaluation at a later date (see Chapter 7). The clearest evidence that mild cognitive symptoms are evidence of dementia is the worsening of those symptoms over time.

On occasion, a client may have been evaluated previously, and the information from that session can serve as a baseline to compare with a new assessment.

HOW REPEATED EVALUATIONS CAN CLARIFY DIAGNOSIS

I once supervised the assessment of a 50-year-old man who had been diagnosed with AD a year earlier following an episode in which he had gotten lost while driving and had no recollection of how he got to the place where he ended up. In the interview, I asked him to describe any memory problems he was having. He reported some episodes of forgetting, but the problems seemed mild and transitory, such as misplacing and then finding something at home, and not the sort I would expect with AD. Rather, the history and current symptoms were more consistent with possible depression. He mentioned that psychological testing had been performed a year earlier, at the time the diagnosis of AD had been made. I obtained the records and report from the previous testing and then administered the same tests. Performance had not changed during the year. Furthermore, performance at both times of testing was generally good. Putting the evidence together, this man's cognitive performance was in normal ranges at both times of testing and did not decline over the period of a year, suggesting that he did not have a degenerative disorder such as AD. In retrospect, the diagnosis seems to have been based on the occurrence of a single amnestic episode.

The availability of baseline testing in this case made it possible to rule out a degenerative process. Repeated testing can also reveal evidence for deterioration in cases in which the initial findings were inconclusive. In those instances, worsening performance over time provides strong evidence of dementia.

As there is no definitive sign or symptom for a diagnosis of AD or dementia, the potential for an incorrect diagnosis is always present. When the results of an assessment are not conclusive, it is better to err in the direction of a treatable disorder. If the findings show some evidence of depressive symptoms but the possibility of early dementia cannot be ruled out, it is better to treat the depression first and to see whether that resolves the cognitive problems. Opinion on this issue has changed in recent years with the development of medications specifically for AD and other dementias. Many physicians now want to start someone on a cholinesterase inhibitor as soon as possible in the disease process to obtain maximum benefit. Given the relatively limited benefits associated with the current generation of medications, we still believe that when sufficient evidence exists for a different explanation of current symptoms, other treatment approaches should be initiated first. The biggest error we have seen over the years is making a diagnosis of dementia without sufficient evidence. As in the preceding example, the diagnosis can be devastating and can lead to or worsen depression. Similarly, if there is any evidence of delirium or any other potential treatable cause of cognitive symptoms, those possibilities should be explored first before assuming that the case involves dementia.

REVERSIBLE COGNITIVE SYMPTOMS

Calvin, age 85, was referred by a geriatrician for a neuropsychological evaluation. The geriatrician who had been seeing Calvin for about a year and a half believed that he had mild memory impairment. He had had a cerebrovascular accident (stroke) 20 years earlier, with full recovery, and heart bypass surgery 4 years earlier. He was otherwise in excellent health, maintained a healthy weight, and walked 5 miles per day. Calvin's son initiated a visit to the geriatrician because he was concerned about his father's memory problems. In the physician's office, Calvin's complaints seemed vague and not out of line with the previously noted memory impairment. But the son's concern prompted the geriatrician to refer the patient for a more thorough evaluation.

The neuropsychological evaluation included interviews with Calvin and his son. Calvin had been retired from an accounting position for 20 years. Careful interviewing of his son revealed that Calvin, who had always managed his own investments and finances, had suddenly become unable to balance his checkbook. He asked his son for help, and the son was alarmed by the tangled mess in the checkbook. Calvin's handwriting had also become micrographic (very tiny). Because of the ominous suddenness of these changes, the evaluation was done immediately. The Wechsler Memory Scale—Revised (Wechsler, 1987) was given, as well as the Wechsler Adult Intelligence Scale—Revised (WAIS-R; Wechsler, 1981). Massive deficits were found on all tests, but particularly on calculations. The geriatrician was called, and a thorough medical examination was begun. Calvin's left carotid artery was found to be 99% occluded, and the right carotid was 75% occluded, placing him at high risk for another stroke. Magnetic resonance imaging (MRI) revealed several new areas of small infarcts, which were consistent with the specific deficits that were found. A carotid endardectomy was performed, and Calvin recovered fairly well. He did not, however, return to his prior level of functioning because of the infarctions. Still, if his memory problems had been ignored, he would have suffered either a massive cerebral vascular accident or such significant anoxia (lack of oxygen to the brain) that he would have been much more severely impaired. As it is, he was able to continue living independently with his wife in an apartment in a retirement community with minimal assistance.

As this case illustrates, every reasonable test and treatment should be tried before concluding that someone suffers from dementia. If the results of an assessment are ambiguous or conflicting, a conservative decision rule should be used to avoid overdiagnosis of dementia. When other causes of the symptoms can be ruled out, then it is appropriate to begin treatment for dementia.

Finally, we want to note that much of the research on assessment of older adults is based on samples of white Europeans or Americans of European descent. There has been an effort in recent years to include African Americans and other groups in research on a routine basis (e.g., Lucas et al., 2005b), but data remain limited. The lack of information on diverse populations means that the available norms and cutoff scores may not be accurate for them. Another caution is that the possibilities for misunderstandings are considerable when evaluating immigrants in their second language. These problems will be less when assessing native-born and middle-class members of a minority group, but even then subtle differences in culture and language may lead to a different presentation of symptoms for a particular disorder. Significant problems, such as moderate to severe dementia, will be obvious across various groups, but it is easy to make mistakes when problems are mild and subtle and the task is to differentiate behaviors from normal functioning. We have presented research findings and examples on diverse groups, where possible, but much work remains to be done to gain a better understanding of the variability in functioning due to ethnicity, nationality, social class, and other factors. With the growing diversity among the older population, clinicians have to be prepared to learn about their clients' cultures and beliefs to help in the assessment process, as well as for treatment.

CONDUCTING THE CLINICAL INTERVIEW

The clinical interview is used to develop rapport with an older client, to gather information about presenting problems and history, and to obtain a brief assessment of cognitive functioning. Topics covered include the client's reported complaints and symptoms, history of the onset and course of the problem, brief mental status testing, and, when appropriate, the perspective of a close relative or other informant. This information contributes to evaluating possible diagnosis and leads to development of a treatment plan. (For a thorough discussion of clinical interviews with older adults, see Scogin, 2000.)

Setting the Stage: Rapport, Confidentiality, and Other Issues

A clinical interview can be structured to put clients at ease and to obtain reliable and relatively complete information. As a preliminary step, it is essential to talk with clients about confidentiality and the conditions under which information can be released. This discussion is especially critical for clients living in institutional settings, who often have little privacy, a point we return to later (see Chapter 14).

The office setting should be a welcoming and comfortable place, not like a medical examining room. It should also convey professionalism—not messy or filled with distracting or inappropriate decorations. Choice of chairs for older clients is very important. Clinicians who work with older people should have at least one firm chair with arms that is easy to get in and out of. The clinician can guide a new client to that chair when it seems appropriate. The setting should also be able to accommodate someone in a wheelchair.

In conducting the initial interview, it is best to sit directly opposite and close enough to the older person to hear and be heard. Early on during the interview, I inquire about how well the person can see and hear and then make adaptations when necessary—for example, turning off the air conditioning when someone is having problems hearing. The office in which the assessment is conducted should be well lighted, without excessive glare. Older clients should not be positioned so that they are looking directly toward a window or a bright light.

Although I increasingly see older clients who have been in therapy in the past, many people who are referred have had little or no prior contact with mental health professionals. Often, these individuals are referred by their physicians. They are comfortable viewing me as an extension of their medical treatment. They prefer referring to me as "doctor." In turn, I establish my credibility by asking about current medications and obtaining a release for medical records or to talk with the referring physician. I also avoid using psychological jargon with them.

The pacing of the interview needs to be carefully balanced between giving clients sufficient opportunity to talk about their concerns and completing the assessment in a timely way. Rushing through an assessment undermines rapport. Clients need the time to tell their stories. Older clients, in particular, may take more time to get to the point, and they also have longer histories to relate than younger clients. Taking the time with older clients may be especially important because they may have no one who listens. Having grown up in an era in which a family doctor would take the time to discuss personal issues, they are often frustrated at how brief and rushed medical appointments have become. Of course, therapists need to hear only the more pertinent parts of the history, not every detail. Some clients are not good at selecting the relevant portions of their stories, or they believe that they have to relate everything to the therapist for the therapist to understand them. In these cases, the therapist needs to create a balance, listening to enough of the history so as to convey understanding and obtain sufficient clinical information to proceed with treatment but also moving clients along in a gentle way. Therapists can keep the pace moving by saying that they will come back to an issue later if there is time but that they need to get through some other things in order to be able to help the client.

It is important to gather a lot of information and to listen carefully to clients to sort out and make sense of the information. More than with younger clients, we have found that some older people initially present themselves and their experiences in a disorganized way. Their thinking may initially seem loose and tangential, suggesting a psychotic process or personality disorder. The problem, however, can turn out to be the way clients are describing their experiences rather than their underlying thought processes. By taking the time to get a full picture and not drawing conclusions about diagnosis too quickly, therapists can differentiate the idiosyncratic ways clients have of expressing themselves from a psychiatric disorder.

LEARNING TO RECOGNIZE THE COHERENCE IN A CLIENT'S STORY

Milly, age 70, told a story of a life event in her first session that sounded bizarre and possibly psychotic but that turned out to be more understandable once she provided more details. The incident had occurred when she was a teenager. Milly recounted that her high school principal had told her that her father had been convicted of a crime and that she had then bled all over the principal's office. Her unconnected way of telling the story suggested loose or even psychotic thought processes. Throughout the first session, Milly described other events in similarly unconnected ways. During the second session, she was more relaxed and less pressured in her speech. Milly talked about how she had had recurrent nosebleeds when she was a teenager and that her nose would bleed copiously when she was under stress. This information filled gaps in the story she told previously, when she had not mentioned nosebleeds. Milly also commented on the fact that she had felt nervous in the previous session. Although some of her stories remained tangential, it was clear once I got to know her better that she did not have a thought disorder.

This case illustrates how important it is not to reach a judgment about diagnosis based on one example. Some older people communicate in ways that can contribute to incorrect initial impressions. If they spend a lot of time alone, as Milly did, their initial recounting of stories may reflect thought processes that have become somewhat idiosyncratic. Accustomed to examining experiences only for themselves, they recount events without providing the context or connections for anyone else to make sense out of them. This manner of communicating creates the impression of loose and tangential thinking. The therapist must patiently sort through the information provided in order to determine whether it does, in fact, make sense. This is done by asking questions and also by learning to grasp a client's perspective and meaning. After a few sessions, it often emerges that the person's experiences and thought processes are quite normal but that he or she relates experiences in an unusual way.

Another source of misunderstandings is the fact that older people have different patterns of speech and vocabulary than younger people. They may use expressions that were contemporary many years ago but that a young therapist may not recognize.

There are times when it is appropriate to conduct the initial interview outside the office, for example, at a hospital, retirement or nursing home, or in the client's own home. In institutional settings, it is absolutely essential to find a private place where you will not be interrupted and where the client can feel comfortable talking about personal and confidential matters. An initial home visit can be very useful when a client is unable or unwilling to come to the office. Even when clients can come to the office, there will be times when a home visit is warranted as part of the assessment. A home visit can be very informative when there is a question about the competency of a person to remain at home. A patient with dementia, for example, may have a great deal of difficulty functioning in an unfamiliar setting but may still be able to perform everyday activities in a familiar setting. A good informant may obviate the need for a home visit, but in some cases, the opportunity to observe how a client actually performs activities and interacts with other people at home may make a home visit worth the effort.

The following example illustrates the value of a home visit. An older man had suffered a mild stroke while in the hospital, which left him incontinent and with limited speech. Staff members at the hospital were very concerned that he would not be able to manage at home but were willing to let him try. A nurse who accompanied him home to observe him described his adjustment this way: "He walked in, looked at the open fire, and said, 'Oh, isn't that nice?' He saw the cat and said, 'Oh, there is Whiskey,' and took the cat on his lap. He sought out the toilet when he needed it. He was a completely different man in the afternoon from what he had been in the morning" (Glasscote, Gudeman, & Miles, 1977, p. 140). Of course, not everyone responds so positively to being at home, but when there is a question about a client's ability to function at home, the best assessment is one that includes a home visit.

The Role of Informants

Sometimes an older person will be accompanied to the appointment by a family member who made the appointment and provided initial information about the client's problem. It is always helpful to get information from family members, when clients give permission to do so. This frequent use of an informant is one of the ways that assessment of older people differs from that of other adults.

In cases of dementia, it is almost always necessary to involve an informant. The client may be able to provide little or no information or may deny that there is a problem. In that situation, an informant can provide a picture of symptoms and history. Reports by family informants are usually reliable (e.g., Teri & Truax, 1994). But it is always necessary to weigh the possibility that an informant might be presenting a biased or even factually inaccurate version of events.

When dementia is not involved, the input from a family member is useful in other ways. We always find that we get a different story when talking with a family member. Clients edit what they tell clinicians. They present their stories in ways that are designed to persuade the clinician to see things the way they see them. But that way of looking at things may be causing their problems. They do not have the ability to step back to gain perspective on their problems or see their role in them. When a key family member has not been involved at the start of treatment, it is possible, with the client's permission, to invite that person to come in or to talk with the person on the phone. Sometimes a single session in which client and family member interact with each other tells us more about our client than several individual sessions (see Chapter 8).

Because families frequently initiate treatment for their older relatives and to some extent define the presenting problem, clinicians must consider the question "Whose problem is it?" In cases of dementia, for example, the patient may have little or no awareness of difficulties. Instead, the caregiver who is overwhelmed by the changes caused by the disease needs and can benefit from treatment. There can be situations not involving dementia, as well, in which a person's relationship with an older relative is causing distress but the relative refuses treatment. Again, treatment can be offered to the family member who initiated the contact and who is troubled by the older person's actions. The goal for treatment will be to identify what the person can do to make the situation better for him- or herself and for the older person.

Identifying Presenting Symptoms and Problems

After making the client comfortable, the clinician can begin the inquiry by asking the client to describe his or her current problems or symptoms. Some clients will talk freely, others need to be kept focused, and still others need to be prompted and encouraged to talk. The goal at this point is to get a clear description of presenting symptoms and problems, including specific examples of what happens when the problems occur, how often they occur, in what situations they occur, and possible triggering (antecedent) or reinforcing (consequent) events. These questions form the foundation of an assessment. When clients use such broad terms as "forgetting" or "depression," ask for examples. Likewise, if a client uses psychological jargon, such as "disorientation," probe for what he or she means rather than assuming that he or she is using the term in the same way you might. Part of the assessment is to observe clients describing their problems—whether they are direct, evasive, or vague or deny having any problems altogether.

An important part of the clinical interview is obtaining a medical history and information about current medications. It is often important to determine exactly which medications a client might be taking, and so we use the "brown bag" approach; that is, we ask clients to bring all their medications to the appointment in a bag. After noting what medications have been prescribed, it is important to determine which of the medications they are actually taking and in what dosage.

When there is a question of possible dementia, three types of symptoms are explored in detail: perceptions of memory and other intellectual deficits, delusions and hallucinations, and affect. The information obtained is critical for differentiating dementia from delirium, from other psychiatric disorders, and from normal aging.

Memory Complaints and Performance

Most older clients are concerned about their memories at least to some degree. If memory is part of the presenting complaint, the assessment should begin there. When memory is not mentioned in the referral or by the client, the clinician should still inquire about it during the course of the interview.

The first step is asking about the client's perception of memory functioning. Questions such as "Are you having any problems with your memory?" and "Have you noticed any changes in your memory in the past year or two?" are generally nonthreatening and provide valuable information about how clients (and informants) view the situation. Follow-up questions should determine what kinds of things the person forgets, how often this happens, and whether forgetting is more likely in certain situations or settings.

Ways in which people with various problems characterize their memory functioning are summarized in Table 6.1. Information about perceived memory problems is useful in the diagnostic process, but in a paradoxical way—people with good memories often report problems, whereas someone whose memory is poor may say he or she has little or no difficulty in remembering (Flicker, Ferris, & Reisberg, 1993; Kahn, Zarit, Hilbert, & Niederehe, 1975; Kaszniak, 1987). Patients with dementia are sometimes aware of their memory problems in the early stages of their illness, and complaints about poor memory are sometimes the first problem noticed by other people. As the disease progresses, however, people lose that awareness. They can provide little specific information about memory or any other area of functioning. Their answers to questions about their memories will be vague or even evasive. There may be an inherent adaptive tendency to deny problems in the face of massive brain dysfunction, or they may simply forget episodes of forgetting. Denial in the face of obvious problems suggests a significant cognitive problem.

There are exceptions. Some people have an awareness of their difficulties, even when suffering from fairly substantial amounts of cognitive impairment. Even though patients may verbally deny problems, they may still on occasions recognize their problems and communicate distress, either verbally or nonverbally. Awareness can be found in any type of dementia, but it is more common with vascular dementias, in which damage may be localized in specific regions in the brain, thereby sometimes sparing abilities lost in other dementias.

AWARENESS OF DEFICITS

George, who was in his early 70s and had a probable vascular dementia (VaD), showed recognition of his deficits throughout a testing session. In the past, he had been able to use mnemonic devices to assist him in learning people's names, but he was now unable to do memory tasks that had previously been quite easy for him,

TABLE 6.1. The Significance of Reports of Memory Problems

Dementia	Delirium	Depression	Nonprogressive brain injury	Normal aging
		Reported by patient		
May report problems, especially in early and mild cases. Some patients recognize that memory is poor but can provide no specific details. Awareness of problems may be greater in vascular dementia.	Usually denies problems or may confabulate	Usually complains of memory problems; may fear becoming senile	Depends on the location of the injury; if the damage is not too severe, the patient is usually aware of deficits.	May complain that memory is not as good as it used to be; forgets common things (e.g., forgetting to buy an item at the store), but problems do not interfere with everyday activities
		Reported by family		
Pronounced problems that interfere with carrying out everyday activities	Profound disruption of usual activities	Some absentminded-ness and preoccupation	Depends on location of injury	May report occasional forgetting that does not interfere with everyday activities
		Test results		
Evidence of significant memory loss	Memory may or may not be impaired	Little or no memory deficits except in severe depression	Depends on location and extent of damage	Little or no evidence of memory problems

such as learning novel word pairs. At one point in the session, George said to me, "Has anyone said they wanted to punch you?" He said this in a friendly way and with a smile, but it indicated his frustration. Later on he said, "You know who I really feel sorry for? I feel sorry for you having to do this [the testing] to people." In these comments, George was expressing awareness of his deficits, as well as embarrassment over having them brought out in testing.

In contrast to these patterns with dementia, many older people complain about failing memory, even though they do not have significant memory loss and do not go on to develop it in the next few years. Older depressed people often create a convincing picture of failing memory, even when no objective evidence of problems can be found (Kahn et al., 1975; Kaszniak, 1987; Niederehe & Yoder, 1989). When asked, they often say their memories are terrible, and they may even worry that they are becoming senile. These complaints are part of the exaggerated negative evaluations typical of depression.

Depressed older people usually have little or no objective cognitive loss. In instances of comorbidity of depression and dementia, the person often will complain of failing memory (e.g., Johansson et al., 1997; Kahn et al., 1975).

MEMORY COMPLAINTS AND DEPRESSION

Lloyd, who was in his early 60s, sought help because he thought his memory was failing. He said he could not remember anything anymore and believed he was becoming senile. He had recently been forced to retire because of health problems that interfered with his job, and he reported having no other interests besides his work. Lloyd's wife still worked, and he spent his days at home alone. When asked what he forgot, Lloyd said he watched daytime television and could not remember what he had just been watching. When asked whether he was paying attention, he said no. Besides his concern with memory, he reported feeling very depressed. Lloyd's cognitive test scores were in normal ranges and did not suggest dementia.

This case demonstrates the association of depression and memory complaints. Depressed patients are preoccupied with their own thoughts and do not attend to the events around them. When forced to do so, as in a structured testing situation, they can process information adequately, except in cases of severe depression. In this case, treatment for depression was initiated. As the client improved, his complaints of failing memory decreased. Studies of treatment of depression have found a similar decrease in memory complaints with improvement in mood (Popkin, Gallagher, Thompson, & Moore, 1982).

Concern about failing memory is very common among healthy older people who show no evidence of dementia. Normal older people often report memory problems, though complaints are less frequent and less severe than those found in depression.

Memory complaints may be present or absent in delirium, though patients with delirium tend to deny problems. Patients with nonprogressive brain trauma may or may not complain about failing memory, depending on the site and severity of their injuries.

Although complaints of failing memory do not by themselves indicate dementia or depression, clinicians can clarify the situation somewhat by asking for specific examples. If clients mention difficulties, we ask them to describe a specific episode when they forgot something. When they deny having problems, we will probe by asking whether their memories are as good as they used to be or whether there are any things at all that they have trouble remembering. It is possible to ask whether they can remember specific things, such as names of grandchildren, or whether they ever have trouble finding something around the house.

This type of questioning brings out qualitative differences between normal age-related forgetfulness and the memory problems associated with organic pathology. The more details a client provides about incidents, the better his or her memory. Healthy older adults will frequently say they are having memory problems and give many different specific examples of everyday lapses of memory, such as forgetting a name or forgetting to pick up an item at the store. These commonplace incidents of forgetting can occur at any age and do not by themselves indicate anything pathological. These incidents also do not interfere in any significant way with normal functioning. By contrast, dementia results in problems that typically go beyond everyday forgetting and interfere with functioning. As an example of this type of forgetting, a stockbroker who had always woken up and gone to work early to be in time for the opening of the markets was now going to work at 6:00 in the evening rather than 6:00 in the morning. This is clearly forgetting of a different magnitude than forgetting a name or losing one's glasses. These more severe types of problems are usually reported by informants.

Another useful question to ask is how often a problem has occurred. An incident, such as forgetting where you parked a car, that happens once or at infrequent intervals is not usually a sign that something is wrong. Anyone can do that. But forgetting repeatedly suggests that there may be a problem. A high frequency of misplacing objects in a short time frame, being unable to find those objects, and putting them in unusual places all point toward a more significant memory deficit.

Not all forgetting, however, is symptomatic. It is necessary to take into account whether this problem represents a change in functioning. Some people have always been absent-minded, misplacing objects, forgetting appointments, and otherwise paying little attention to everyday activities. These people already have a high baseline of everyday forgetting. A careful evaluation can usually determine whether the frequency and type of these absent-minded errors has changed. For example, a scientist in his late 70s sought help because of concerns about failing memory. He reported that his biggest problem was that he could not find what he was looking for in his office. This complaint, however, was not new or age related. Through his whole career, he had been the prototypical absent-minded professor, who always had difficulty finding things in his cluttered and disorganized office. In every other way, his functioning appeared normal. That is not to say that absent-minded people will never get dementia. Rather, the therapist needs to consider whether current functioning differs from how that person has typically functioned in the past.

In addition to memory problems, the client and any informant who is interviewed can be asked about other kinds of cognitive problems, such as word-finding difficulties, problems finding one's way around, not remembering how to do familiar tasks or to carry out a sequence of tasks, and failing to recognize familiar objects. These problems are more specific to dementia and other brain disorders and less likely to occur with any frequency in depression or normal aging.

When a person has significant memory problems, much of the detail about the kinds and severity of problems comes from family members or other informants. The clinician should ask informants a series of questions, beginning with a general question about the client's memory and then moving to specific inquiries about the types of things the person forgets, how often it happens, and whether the person remembers better at some times than others. It is important to go beyond any general terms the informant might use to describe the client, such as "senile," and ask for specific examples.

Although informants are usually reliable, some will be poor observers or will not have had sufficient contact with the client to provide adequate information. We sometimes encounter what we like to call the "out-of-town sibling" syndrome. In this situation, one child has assumed the bulk of care for an aging parent and sees the parent frequently. This child usually can give a reliable history, perhaps of gradual, steady decline. Then an out-of-town brother or sister swoops in for a visit and is horrified at the "sudden" changes in the parent and may even blame the local sibling for this condition. Old sibling rivalries, guilt over being so far away, and other family dynamics must be considered in evaluating the reliability of an informant.

On occasion, the discrepancy between subjective and objective memory functioning can be enormous. Knight (1992) reports a case in which a husband was concerned about what he believed was his own failing memory and the onset of dementia. He described his wife as physically frail but mentally alert. Tests did not reveal any evidence of dementia in the man. He was primarily depressed over a move to a new community and a loss of previous social supports. When his wife was subsequently brought into treatment, however, it was found that she had a moderately severe dementia.

When dementia is suspected, we also find it useful to have the family members complete the Memory and Behavior Problems Checklist (Zarit, Orr, & Zarit, 1985), which can be found at the end of this chapter in Appendix 6.1. This instrument identifies common problems associated with dementia, as well as behaviors that the family finds particularly troublesome or stressful. Families can complete this instrument in the waiting room while the patient is being interviewed. This instrument allows family members to identify and quantify specific memory and behavior problems, and most will take the opportunity to write down concerns that they do not want to bring up in front of the patient.

Hallucinations and Delusions

Whereas memory complaints are fairly common and generally nonspecific, hallucinations and delusions occur with a low frequency among older people but indicate a significant disturbance. Informants will often be the source of information about these problems. Clients may also report hallucinations and delusions when asked about the things that are bothering them. When an informant has mentioned these problems, or when there is some other reason to suspect that the person might be having hallucinations or delusions, it is possible to ask whether they sometimes see or hear things that turn out not to be there or whether they are having thoughts that trouble or worry them. As with memory complaints, when a hallucination or delusion is reported, it is important to ask for a specific description, the circumstances in which it occurs, and how often.

The diagnostic implications of hallucinations and delusions are shown in Table 6.2. The first consideration is the possibility of a delirium. Delirium typically involves a global distortion in perceptions, in which people cannot grasp or understand what they see (Lipowski, 1990). Patients may experience illusions, that is, mistaking one object for another. The changing light and shadows from a television screen might be perceived as a small animal running across the room. Hallucinations, or actual false perceptions, are quite common in delirium and are usually visual or visual and auditory. Full-blown delusional systems, in which clients believe there are plots and conspiracies against them, can also occur.

DISTORTIONS IN DELIRIUM

I was asked to evaluate Merle, a 103-year-old woman who had been moved to an assisted-living community 6 days earlier. Merle had lived independently until she was in her mid-90s and then lived with her one surviving daughter until she

TABLE 6.2. Implications of Hallucinations and Delusions for Diagnosis

Dementia	Delirium	Depression	Schizophrenia (early, late, and very late onset)	Personality disorders
		Hallucinations		
Low rates, except in Lewy body dementia and with a comorbid delirium and/or medication reaction. Late in the dementia, a person may experience illusions (e.g., an intruder or a small animal or child running across a poorly lit room).	Frequent	Very rare. Found only in very severe depression or with a comorbid diagnosis.	Frequent	Occasionally reported, especially during a crisis.
		Delusions		
Complains that someone is stealing money or valuables. Usually found in the middle stages of the disease	Frequent	Can occur, but fairly rare	Frequent	Common in some types of personality disorders

required more care and attention than her daughter could provide. After moving into the facility, Merle began telling her daughter that doctors and nurses were coming into her room in the middle of the night to give her rough gynecological examinations. Staff members confirmed going into her room to change a wet adult diaper. In her disorientation, however, Merle confabulated a more distressing but familiar explanation. On another occasion, she identified the assisted-living facility as a resort that she and her husband used to vacation at, and she said she had been to visit the gardens the previous spring. Merle had not, however, been to the facility prior to moving there.

These are classic responses that are typical of a delirium. In Merle's case, the delirium was probably due to her recent relocation, the presence of a hearing impairment, and perhaps mild cognitive impairment. As she settled into the routines at the facility, these experiences diminished.

Hallucinations and delusions can also occur in dementia, particularly dementia with Lewy bodies (see Chapter 3), but are less common than with delirium. A common pattern in dementia is paranoid delusions—for example, patients complaining that someone is stealing money or valuables from them. These types of delusions appear to be reactions to memory loss. Patients cannot remember where they placed valuables and assume someone must have stolen them. These delusions are often intermittent, but some people can become quite preoccupied with suspicions and accusations. When paranoid delusions become a prominent feature of dementia, it can be very disturbing to family and other involved persons. As dementia progresses to its later stages, these types of delusions gradually lessen. By contrast, illusory experiences, such as seeing imagined intruders, become more common, perhaps because of the patient's increasing difficulties perceiving and recognizing objects.

Other disorders should be considered when hallucinations or delusions are identified. The client might be suffering from schizophrenia or a paranoid personality disorder. Again, it is important to keep in mind the possibility of comorbidities; for example, someone with a lifelong disorder might develop dementia, delirium, or depression in later life.

Mood Disturbances

As shown in Table 6.3, anxiety and depressive symptoms can be part of many different disorders, including dementia and delirium. Mood can be assessed by asking people how they are feeling and by observing facial expression, voice, appearance, and other nonverbal indicators. Questions can also probe for somatic symptoms typical of depression and anxiety, such as sleep problems and poor appetite.

TABLE 6.3. Implications of Depressive and Anxiety Symptoms for Diagnosis

Dementia	Delirium	Depression	Anxiety	Normal aging
		Depression		
Common in early- to moderate-stage dementia	Depressive symptoms can precede the onset or be present in quieter phases	Depressed mood is the defining characteristic	Frequent	Some depressive symptoms are common
		Anxiety		
Can increase in some patients as dementia worsens	Frequent	Frequent	Anxiety is the defining characteristic	Anxiety and worries are common in some people

Depressed mood, of course, is the defining characteristic of depressive syndromes and may be accompanied by considerable anxiety. On rare occasions, depressed mood may be muted or absent, but the person will have pronounced depressive thoughts—hopelessness, helplessness, worthlessness. This type of pattern is sometimes referred to as a "masked depression."

Depression and anxiety can also be prominent features in dementia. Symptoms of depression in patients with AD can be sufficiently pronounced to warrant a diagnosis of major depression (Reifler, Larson, Teri, & Poulsen, 1986; Teri & Wagner, 1992). The depression of the patient with dementia often has a realistic component, awareness of one's own decline and disability. As the dementia worsens, depressive symptoms may lessen. In later stages of dementia, depressive symptoms may still occur, though now indicated by a sad appearance or crying. In contrast to depressive symptoms, anxiety can sometimes increase as the dementia progresses.

Anxiety is a common component in delirium, although depressed mood can be a prodromal symptom or can occur in quieter phases.

Assessing the History of a Disorder

An accurate and thorough history can probably contribute more than any other factor to correct assessment and diagnosis of an older person. Clinicians should gather information on the onset, course, and duration of symptoms, as well as whether there are fluctuations or situations in which symptoms are more pronounced or reduced. Another important piece of information is whether there have been similar episodes in the past. Clients, family informants, and medical records are all important sources of information about history.

As shown in Table 6.4, the histories of dementia, delirium, and depression usually are distinct from one another and differ from the course of normal aging. The main types of dementia also tend to differ from one another in onset and course.

AD has an insidious onset, a term that captures the terrible nature of this disease. By insidious, it is meant that the patient experiences ordinary sorts of forgetting, which gradually increase in frequency. Over time these incidents are noticed by other people and begin interfering with everyday activities. Progression is typically gradual. Families may not realize that something serious is going on until a major problem occurs, such as the patient getting lost while driving or walking or forgetting how to do a familiar activity. When the family is interviewed carefully, however, they can often identify other incidents that show a pattern of gradual onset and worsening.

By the time someone is referred for an evaluation, problems may have been going on for anywhere from a few months to several years. This difference in when families seek an evaluation partly depends on the point at which they recognize that the person's forgetting has become a problem or when forgetting begins to interfere with performance of everyday activities.

The rate of progression can also vary. Some people decline relatively rapidly, and others gradually, which is the more typical course. Symptoms can also fluctuate from day to day and even from one part of the day to another. Early in the disease families sometimes interpret these "good days" as a sign

TABLE 6.4. The Significance of History for Diagnosis

Dementia	Delirium	Depression	Nonprogressive brain injury	Normal aging
Alzheimer's disease and frontotemporal dementia	Sudden and recent onset. Dramatic daily fluctuations are possible. Symptoms may be more pronounced in the evening.	Symptoms develop over a few weeks' period, often in response to stressful life events. In contrast to dementia, functioning is stable, not deteriorating.	Deficits date to the time of the injury. Deficits are usually related to the site of the injury and do not progress.	Changes are apparent only over long periods of time (several years). Changes do not interfere with everyday functioning.
Insidious onset and gradual progression				
Vascular				
Onset can be abrupt, with stepwise progression and daily fluctuations				
Dementia with Lewy bodies				
Cognitive and motor symptoms appear at the same time or in close temporal proximity				

that nothing is really wrong with their relative, but then they are surprised or disappointed when the patient relapses the following day. Despite these fluctuations, there is a clear downward course, and good days become fewer and fewer.

ONSET AND PROGRESSION OF DEMENTIA SYMPTOMS

Sally, 71, was referred by a neurologist for evaluation of her memory problems. She was accompanied to the assessment by her husband, Morris. When asked whether she had memory problems, Sally said yes, but deferred to Morris to provide specific information. When asked how long the problem had been going on, he first said a few months. As we talked, Morris realized that he had first noticed her having problems 5 years earlier. At that time, Sally was performing in a play in a community theater and uncharacteristically forgot her lines. Everyone regarded the incident as stage fright, but in retrospect, it was the first notable change in her behavior. The changes had been occurring so gradually over the 5-year period, however, that Morris could not pinpoint the onset readily. With some gentle prompting, he was able to give a more complete picture of gradual onset and progression. During this period Morris had steadily been assuming responsibility for more and more household tasks. Sally no longer could cook, do the laundry, or clean the house. As in many AD cases, then, onset was insidious, progression was gradual, and the duration of symptoms spanned several years.

Frontotemporal dementia (FTD) also has an insidious onset and gradual progression, and it is differentiated from AD based on symptoms rather than history (see Chapter 3).

The onset and progression of VaD can vary somewhat, depending on the type of vascular changes that are present. Multi-infarct dementia has the most distinctive pattern. Onset can be relatively abrupt, with symptoms emerging in conjunction with a new infarction. Stroke-like symptoms, such as mild paralysis, may be observable for short periods of time, although more often there are no observable symptoms. The course is marked by a pattern of stepwise deterioration, that is, plateaus of stability followed by a sudden drop, which probably corresponds to a new stroke. As with AD, the rate of decline can vary. Daily fluctuations can be a little more pronounced in VaD than in AD.

Finally, the three parkinsonian syndromes—dementia with Lewy bodies (DLB), Parkinson's disease with dementia (PDD), and AD with parkinsonian symptoms—can be differentiated from one another and from other dementias based on onset. In DLB, cognitive and motor symptoms appear at the same time, or in close temporal proximity to one another. In PDD, dementia symptoms emerge several years after the onset of motor symptoms. The reverse occurs in AD with parkinsonian symptoms—that is, motor symptoms emerge several years after the first onset of cognitive problems.

There are exceptions to these patterns. Sometimes families provide a history of abrupt onset of symptoms associated with a stressful life event in cases that otherwise appear to be AD. Triggering events include surgery with a general anesthesia, death of a spouse, and moving to a new location. In a typical scenario, the family reports that the patient functioned with no apparent difficulty prior to the surgery. Immediately following the surgery, a delirium occurred, with considerable cognitive impairment. The patient improved somewhat as the delirium cleared but never regained prior levels of functioning. Subsequently, a gradual decline occurred. Surgery can result in brain damage, such as when an anoxia or other problem occurs (e.g., Roach et al., 1996; see also the case example later in this chapter). There has been speculation that this type of damage can be a trigger for AD. An alternative explanation is that the stress of the surgery uncovered a degenerative process that the family had not noticed previously.

Families often report a sudden onset of dementia symptoms following the death of the patient's husband or wife. In these cases, a more careful history usually reveals that the spouse who died had been covering up for the patient's cognitive lapses. Their children had not been aware of these problems until they were confronted with their surviving parent's behavior.

In contrast to dementia, a delirium typically has a recent and sudden onset. It develops rapidly, over a period of a few hours or days, and results in a dramatic change in functioning. There can also be dramatic fluctuations of symptoms. Patients can be extremely agitated and restless one hour and nearly comatose the next.

It is common for a delirium to become more pronounced in the evening. The term "sundowner's syndrome" refers to a pattern of mild delirium that occurs only in the evening (Evans, 1987). This pattern is frequently encountered in hospitals and nursing homes. Someone suffering from dementia is especially prone to sundowner's syndrome, but older people with normal functioning can develop this late-afternoon delirium in response to the multiple stresses associated with hospitalization—the unfamiliar setting, disrupted sleep, discomfort, and the effects of medications, as well as anxiety. Exposure to sunlight during the daytime and increased activity has been found clinically to reduce sundowner's syndrome in institutional settings.

The duration of a delirium is usually relatively brief, although, as noted in Chapter 3, some chronic cases have been reported. Resolution usually occurs within a few days to a few weeks, ending either in death or in recovery once its cause has been treated. Failure to treat the cause of the delirium may also result in permanent brain damage, for example, when it is due to malnutrition.

Most episodes of depression develop over a period of a few weeks. They are typically associated with stressful life events. Duration of a depressive episode is usually several months, but it can also be chronic. We have worked with some older people who have had symptoms of a major depression for a few years or longer. These chronic depressions can be differentiated from dementia by the fact that cognitive problems and ability to perform everyday tasks do not get worse over time. Depressed patients can also fluctuate in performance, typically functioning worse in the mornings than later in the day.

ONSET OF DEPRESSION IN LATER LIFE

Martha was a 65-year-old woman who had no prior history of mental health problems. She had managed to raise 10 children successfully. When her last child had left the home 6 months earlier, Martha's mood had plummeted. She became severely depressed and suicidal. It emerged from the history that the symptoms she was experiencing coincided with her child's leaving home. As in this case, it is almost always possible with depression to date the onset of symptoms by specific events.

In gathering the history, clinicians should ask about any previous mental health problems and about prior treatment, including hospitalization. Many problems are recurrent, and so current symptoms may be part of a new episode of an old problem. If there is a history of past problems, the first step in assessment is to rule out a recurrence before making a new diagnosis. As noted, however, it is important to keep an open mind and to consider whether the symptoms suggest a new problem.

RECURRENT EPISODES OF PSYCHOTIC SYMPTOMS

A neuropsychological evaluation was requested for Peter, a 67-year-old man in the stabilization unit of a psychiatric hospital. The psychiatrist wondered whether Peter might have AD. In reviewing the medical record, I noticed immediately that he had been diagnosed with schizophrenia while in his 20s and had functioned on neuroleptics (major tranquilizers) for the past 40 years, while working as a manual laborer. About 5 years before he had retired on disability. Peter was tested and was found to be hypomanic and to have pressured and tangential speech. There were no memory impairments per se. However, with further questioning, it became apparent that Peter would run out of money at the end of each month, fail to take his medication, and become delusional. Although his family was accustomed to this pattern, his behavior had come to the attention of local authorities, which led to the hospitalization. The chronicity of his schizophrenia had made him a poor historian. Peter also had performed poorly on a standard mental status examination, primarily because he was so caught up in his own thoughts that he did not pay attention to current events or to the specifics of his surroundings. Thus the psychiatrist mistook his chronic lack of interest in the world around him for memory impairment. Once the diagnosis was clarified, treatment was coordinated with the local mental health clinic. They were very familiar with Peter and agreed to redouble their efforts to be sure he had consistent supplies of medication available to him.

In contrast to dementia, cognitive deficits due to a nonprogressive head injury date to the time of the injury. Although these types of injury are relatively rare in an older population, they should be ruled out when conducting a history.

When there has been a brain injury, an important distinction is whether or not symptoms worsen over time. In most cases, people who have suffered a serious head injury have deficits that are stable or that improve somewhat over time. As was noted in Chapter 3, however, head trauma may be a risk factor for AD. We have seen cases in which the first symptoms of dementia followed immediately or soon after a head injury. Whether the injury was, in fact, a trigger for dementia or whether the damage caused by the injury served to uncover a dementia that was already in its beginning stages cannot be determined.

Surgery can result also in nonprogressive brain damage, as illustrated in the next case.

COGNITIVE SYMPTOMS FOLLOWING SURGERY

Sam was an 82-year-old man whom I had followed in therapy for a few years and who had good cognitive functioning. He was having a heart problem, and his physicians determined that he was a good candidate for bypass surgery. During the surgery, Sam experienced anoxia when oxygen was briefly cut off to the brain. When Sam awoke after the surgery, he was not himself. The changes were initially believed to be a delirium related to the anesthesia, but they did not clear up. I subsequently tested Sam and found that he had deficits in memory and other cognitive functions that were not evident before the surgery. These deficits were stable over time. The differences from dementia included an onset of symptoms dating from the time of the injury and a lack of progression.

Alcohol use is another problem to consider in the history. As noted in Chapter 5, even moderate consumption of alcohol can result in dementia-like symptoms in an older person.

The history of these disorders can be contrasted to the changes found in normal aging. A typical history of a healthy older person is one of very gradual changes in memory and cognition that span a long period of time. People may describe themselves as not being able to remember as much as they previously did, but their point of comparison may be 30 or 40 years earlier. There can also be fluctuations in functioning with normal aging. People will report more cognitive problems and other difficulties during and after stressful events or in association with depressed mood.

Mental Status Testing

Mental status tests can be used as part of the clinical interview to obtain a quick impression of cognitive functioning. They are widely employed in medical settings and may be administered by physicians, nurses, psychologists, or other health professionals. Mental status tests were developed from questions typically asked in clinical examinations to assess altered states of consciousness that are found in delirium and acute psychotic disorders such as schizophrenia. These tests typically assess recall of basic information that people with normal brain functioning rarely forget. Orientation questions, such as where the person currently is, the address, and the date, are a core part of these tests. Personal information such as age and birth date is typically included. General informational questions, such as name of the current and past presidents, and simple cognitive tasks, such as recalling three words or serial subtraction, may also be assessed.

The first systematic compilation of mental status items into a test was the 10-item Mental Status Questionnaire (MSQ; Kahn, Goldfarb, Pollack, & Peck, 1960; Kahn, Pollack, & Goldfarb, 1961). Other tests include the Short Portable Mental Status Questionnaire (SPMSQ; Pfeiffer, 1975) and the Blessed Information–Concentration–Attention Test (Blessed, Tomlinson, & Roth, 1968), which was adapted for use in the United States by Fuld (1978). A recently developed test is the 7-Minute Screen (Solomon et al., 1998). This instrument contains brief tests of four neuropsychological functions: Enhanced Cued Recall, Temporal Orientation, Verbal Fluency, and Clock Drawing. The 7-Minute Screen has good psychometric properties, as well as demonstrating the ability to differentiate well between dementia and normal aging.

The most widely used test is the Mini-Mental State Exam (MMSE; Folstein, Folstein, & McHugh, 1975), which supplements questions on orientation with single items that assess other cognitive functions, including language, recall, writing, and spatial orientation. Scores of 23 or below (out of a possible 30 points) are considered to indicate significant cognitive impairment. The MMSE has the advantage of being the instrument most likely to be known and used by physicians. The MMSE has been used in many different studies, and so considerable normative data are available (e.g., Crum et al., 1993; Uhlmann & Larson, 1991).

Cut-off scores on the MMSE and other mental status tests are often used to indicate impairment, but there are problems with relying on this single score to diagnose dementia or its absence. For one thing, patients should always have a medical evaluation to rule out delirium and other reversible causes of cognitive impairment, if that has not been done already. Furthermore, any particular test result may not be accurate. The MMSE, for example, may be particularly prone to false positive findings (that is, identifying someone as cognitively impaired who is not) among more poorly educated people and minorities (Anthony, LeResche, Niaz, Von Korff, & Folstein, 1982; Folstein, Anthony, Parhad, Duffy, & Gruenberg, 1985; Murden, McRae, Kaner, & Bucknam, 1991; see Tombaugh & McIntyre, 1992, for a review). Severe depression can also lead to a false positive finding (Rabins, Merchant, & Nestadt, 1984). People in the early stages of dementia, particularly those with college educations, often show false negative findings on the MMSE. They score above the cutoff of 23, even though other testing reveals significant cognitive impairment. Tests that have a greater degree of difficulty are needed to reveal early and mild deficits in dementia, especially among well-educated people (see Chapter 7).

Another limitation in relying solely on a quantitative score from mental status tests is that errors differ in their significance. People with good cognitive functioning are likely to miss certain items, for example, the serial subtractions of 7's task on the MMSE. Another common error is to miss the current date by a couple of days. That type of error is not as significant clinically as when someone cannot name the correct month or year. Similarly, we do not score the response to month incorrect on the first date of a new month, for example, if a client responds "July 31" on "August 1." On the other hand, a response of "March" in August or reporting the incorrect year (except soon after the first of the year) is more telling of a serious problem.

As a result of these limitations, the findings from mental status tests should *always* be viewed as an impression that should be followed up by additional neuropsychological tests, as discussed in Chapter 7. The results of mental status testing will suggest how much additional testing will be possible. When a client struggles on a mental status test, it may be possible only to follow up with a brief battery that can confirm the initial impression of impairment. When someone has performed on the mental status test without much difficulty, a full neuropsychological assessment can be administered. Rather than relying on a specific mental status score to make the decision about which tests to use next, it is better to make a clinical judgment based on how much difficulty the person had with mental status items.

As an alternative to the traditional mental status tests, we now usually rely on the orientation and information items that are included as part of more comprehensive batteries (see Chapter 7), which have better psychometric properties. Mental status tests may be used for three main purposes: as a requirement in a particular setting, as a screening that precedes more thorough evaluation, or as a repeat of a previously performed test in order to assess change.

A mental status score may not be useful for identifying delirium or differentiating delirium from dementia. Patients with a delirium may score above the cutoffs on mental status tests (Tune & Folstein, 1986). The presence of noncognitive symptoms (e.g., inattention, fluctuations, altered level of con-sciousness) is a better indication of the presence of a delirium than the total score.

Several mental status items, however, can elicit a type of response typical of delirium (Table 6.5). Errors in responding to these questions can be classified as denotative or connotative (Kahn & Miller, 1978). Denotative responses keep the same frame of reference as the question. Asked "Where are you?" a patient will reply "in the hospital" but will not know the name. This type of response is factually incorrect but represents an effort to respond to the explicit content of the question. A typical pattern with dementia is to not know or be unable to recall this information. Depressed patients can also make denotative errors on these items. Responses by severely depressed persons will typically be characterized by a lack of effort. These patients will appear too preoccupied with their own thoughts to respond. Incorrect answers made by a person who has pronounced depressed mood and appears distracted or preoccupied during the testing suggests potentially reversible cognitive impairment due to depression.

In contrast, when a patient is giving a connotative answer it is "as though he were responding in a different symbolic system, or that he is answering a different question than the one asked. Thus, if a person is asked where he is his response may actually answer the question of where he would like to be" (Kahn & Miller, 1978, p. 55). These kinds of errors are more likely to indicate a delirium or other acute, rapidly developing conditions. People who recently suffered a stroke or a severe blow to the head also frequently give these responses.

Some typical connotative responses involve misnaming or displacement. A hospital will be identified with a more benign term, such as "country club" or "hotel." It may be displaced spatially by being located near the person's home. The location may also be displaced temporally, for example, if the per-

---

TABLE 6.5. Mental Status Items Useful in the Assessment of Delirium

1. Where are you? (Use these probes if necessary: What place is this? What do you call this place? What kind of place is this? If the place is an institution the correct answer must include both the name and *kind* of place, e.g., hospital, nursing home.).

   Note: This item can substitute for the first item in the MMSE.

2. What is the address of this place? (or, What street is this place located on? Generally, the name of any street bordering the block in which the interview takes place is satisfactory.)

3. Have you ever been in another (name of institution, e.g., St. Vincent's Hospital) with the same name? (If yes, Where was that?)

4. Have you ever seen me before? (If yes, Where was that?)

5. What's my job called?

6. Where were you last night?

son identifies a hospital where he or she was treated successfully in the past. This type of response differs from a memory problem. The person may be able to give the address of this other hospital or location. When shown bedsheets or other items that show the current hospital's name, he or she will be able to read the name correctly but may insist the item is there by mistake. Patients may also claim that they are in a different institution from the one that they are in but that has the same name. They may ascribe a benign quality to this other institution, such as being the place where people recover or go for minor problems. Other connotative responses may include identifying the interviewer or his or her job as unconnected with the hospital or medical care (e.g., calling the clinician "an insurance salesman") and reporting an imagined journey the night before. These kinds of responses are usually accompanied by denial that anything is wrong (Kahn & Miller, 1978; Weinstein & Kahn, 1955).

The following example illustrates these kinds of connotative responses in patients with delirium.

LANGUAGE CHANGES IN DELIRIUM

Clancy, a 55-year-old man who had suffered a sudden heart attack a couple of days earlier was transferred from a medical floor to the psychiatric unit of a hospital because he could not be managed in the medical unit. He would alternatively try to escape or climb into bed with a woman patient. When first examined in the psychiatric ward, Clancy responded to the question "Where are you?" by saying he was in the county jail and then gave the correct address for the jail. Subsequently, he identified himself as being at work and gave his work address. Clancy denied having any problems and tried repeatedly to leave the unit, insisting he had to go to work. After a few days, during which the delirium resolved, he was able to correctly identify the hospital and its address.

This case illustrates the difference between recall of factual information and connotative responses in a delirium. The patient could provide factual information about the addresses of his workplace and the county jail. The issue was not memory per se but the metaphorical way in which reality can be transformed during a delirium. Inappropriate sexual behavior is also sometimes observed in a delirium.

New screening instruments have been developed that are specifically designed for the detection of a delirium (e.g., Inouye et al., 1990; Rockwood, Goodman, Flynn, & Stolee, 1996; Trzepacz & Dew, 1995). Robertsson (2002) and Laurila, Pitkala, Strandberg, and Tilvis (2002) present comprehensive reviews of various approaches. One of the most promising approaches, the Delirium Symptom Interview (Levkoff, Liptzin, Cleary, Reilly, & Evans, 1991), combines typical mental status items with questions and observations designed to match DSM-IV (American Psychiatric Association, 1994) criteria for delirium. Items for this questionnaire are shown in Appendix 6.2. The scale can detect the presence of delirium symptoms with about 90% accuracy without leading to high rates of false positive identifications. Interrater reliabilities are also very good.

In conclusion, mental status tests are widely used tools that can identify obvious cognitive impairment, but they should never be the only source of information on which a decision about diagnosis is made. When used in conjunction with other information about the individual, including education and performance on other psychological tests, they can provide valuable information about the likely presence of marked cognitive impairments.

What to Look for in the Medical Examination

The medical examination is, of course, a central part of the diagnostic process. We look for two types of results from medical assessments. First, have treatable illnesses and problems been ruled out as a cause of the patient's symptoms? This is particularly important with dementia, in which a myriad of illnesses and medications can cause cognitive symptoms, but it also applies to depression, anxiety, and other psychiatric symptoms. Second, when dementia is diagnosed, what type of dementia is it?

An evaluation should include assessment of all main systems and current medications. A recommended evaluation is shown in Table 6.6. Laboratory tests can uncover infections and endocrine, metabolic, and electrolyte disturbances. Nutritional deficits also need to be considered, as they can contribute to cognitive problems and delirium. Older people living alone are likely not to eat properly. Another consideration is pain. Patients sometimes do not report pain, so the possibility of an undetected fracture, fecal impaction, or similar disorder should be explored.

TABLE 6.6. Recommended Medical Tests in the Assessment of Possible Dementia

1. Complete blood count
2. Chem 21 panel, including electrolytes, kidney function, calcium, albumin, liver function, and glucose
3. Thyroid function tests
4. Vitamin B_{12} and folate levels
5. Tests for syphilis and, depending on history, human immunodeficiency antibodies
6. Urinalysis
7. Electrocardiogram
8. Chest X-ray

Note. Data from National Institutes of Health (1987), and Rabins, Lyketsos, and Steele (1999).

It is especially important to review medications for possible adverse effects. Medications are a common cause of reversible cognitive impairment and delirium (Chapter 3). They can also lead to symptoms of depression and anxiety and other mood changes. Both prescription and over-the-counter medications should be considered. Alcohol use, which can potentiate the effects of many medications, should also be evaluated. Caffeine can play a role in anxiety and sleep problems.

The assessment should also identify any natural remedies a person may be using. People are increasingly turning to natural substances such as vitamins, nutritional supplements, and homeopathic remedies for treatment of their health problems or for preventive purposes. Often they believe that these substances are not harmful because they are "natural," but that is not necessarily the case. Just like other medications, natural substances, including vitamins, can become toxic in high dosages or can produce adverse side effects by themselves or in combination with each other or with prescription medications.

Whenever a medication changes, whether a new drug is introduced or another is discontinued, the potential for an adverse reaction exists. Identifying the sequence of changes in medications and onset of psychological symptoms is very important, as shown in the following example.

HOW AN OVERLOOKED CHANGE IN MEDICATION
PRODUCED CATASTROPHIC RESULTS

Karen, age 58, had been in an automobile accident that necessitated many surgeries. She had sustained a mild traumatic brain injury as well but was recovering and continued to work. Another problem that stemmed from the accident emerged that required major surgery. She had taken a diuretic for many years for hypertension, along with potassium. While Karen was in the hospital for surgery, the potassium was discontinued and never restarted. She was not 100% cognitively alert while she recuperated, and gradually she became more disoriented. She then suffered a seizure-like fall and sustained a new head injury. Karen returned to the hospital, where it was discovered that she had dangerously low levels of potassium, which caused an electrolyte imbalance. Restarting potassium eliminated her cognitive problems.

A brain scan (CT or MRI) is recommended as part of an initial assessment when dementia is suspected. Scans generally can rule out other possible causes of symptoms, such as a brain tumor, stroke, or normal pressure hydrocephalus and point to the type of dementia. AD is marked by widespread atrophy. Specific findings on a scan that point to AD include enlargement of the sulci and ventricles and atrophy of the hippocampus. Widespread atrophy is also found in dementia with Lewy bodies (Mendez & Cummings, 2003). In frontotemporal dementia, atrophy is found mainly in frontal and temporal regions. Some healthy older people can display evidence of ventricle enlargement and mild atrophy. These findings alone, without other evidence of dementia, should not be used to make a diagnosis.

MRIs can identify multiple large-vessel strokes associated with multi-infarct dementia, as well as white-matter lesions (Román et al., 1993). Patients with vascular dementia will show less atrophy that those with AD (Mendez & Cummings, 2003). As discussed in Chapter 3, white-matter lesions alone are not sufficient to make a diagnosis in the absence of cognitive impairment or for a prediction that the person will become demented in the future.

The following case illustrates the importance of a careful medical examination in differentiating delirium from other conditions. It also demonstrates how a change in medications can have damaging effects.

"IF IT AIN'T BROKE, DON'T FIX IT"

Roberta was a 76-year-old woman who lived alone. She suffered from diabetes, high blood pressure, and emphysema but was otherwise in good health. Her physician had gone on vacation, and Roberta went to see one of the physician's partners for a minor complaint. Unrelated to her complaint, the partner decided to change Roberta's antihypertensive medication. Roberta had not been having any trouble with the antihypertensive she had been taking, but the physician thought the new drug would work better.

A few days later Roberta's niece visited and found that she was aphasic and had a right-sided weakness. Roberta was taken to the emergency room, where she was treated as if she had had a stroke. Findings from an MRI, however, indicated no evidence of a recent stroke. She was very difficult to manage in the emergency room and struggled with staff. Roberta was disoriented, delusional, and also incontinent. The neurologist who was called in on the case continued exploring other hypotheses besides a stroke. Blood work indicated severe sodium depletion (hyponatremia), which had apparently been caused by the new antihypertensive medication. Roberta had been monitoring salt in her diet very carefully, and the result of the new medication was to reduce salt levels too low. The emergency room treated her for the sodium depletion by giving her salt water and changing her medication. Within 2 days the delirium had cleared.

In this case, the onset and pattern of symptoms were consistent with a stroke. Changes in mental status and behavior suggested a delirium, but that could have been the aftermath of a stroke. When neuroradiological findings did not provide confirmation of a stroke, however, the neurologist looked for other causes and found the change in antihypertensive medication. As in many cases of delirium, the woman recovered fully.

OTHER ASSESSMENT ISSUES

We have focused on information that contributes to differential diagnosis. A full assessment should obtain a complete picture of all presenting symptoms and behavior, as well as other problems or strengths the client might have. Besides contributing to diagnosis, the assessment should provide information that will be useful in planning treatment. Some areas for assessment include:

1. *Activities of daily living.* We assess problems in everyday functioning, including performance of basic and instrumental activities of daily living (e.g., bathing, dressing, shopping, managing finances) and work and leisure pursuits. As emphasized, these activities are disrupted by dementia and delirium. People with severe depression may not perform usual activities, though from a lack of motivation rather than the inability to plan or carry out the activity.

2. *Resources.* What psychological or social resources or strengths does the patient have that can be brought to bear in treatment? A depressed client, for example, may have had good planning skills in his or her job. These skills could be used in developing and implementing a treatment plan.

3. *Deficits.* Besides the main presenting problem, what other deficits are present? A person who is impulsive and disorganized, for example, may have trouble with some features of highly structured therapy approaches.

4. *Social network.* Who are the people to whom the client can turn for support and help, and are there problematic relationships? The support provided by other people may play a critical role in the treatment plan. Conflict in personal relationships may also need to be addressed in treatment.

5. *Substance abuse.* Along with evaluation of prescription medications, it is important to find out whether an older client may be abusing alcohol or other medications (see Chapter 5).

6. *Suicidal and homicidal thoughts.* Clinicians need to determine whether an older client is thinking about suicide. In couples in which one person is disabled, the possibility of a double suicide or a homicide–suicide should also be evaluated.

7. *Sleep and appetite disturbance.* How well is the person eating or sleeping? Appetite and sleep problems are both indicators of the severity of psychiatric disorders and can contribute to making problems worse. We often find that part of the treatment involves restoring good sleep habits or addressing eating problems. In contrast to younger clients, overeating is a more frequent issue with older people than not eating enough. The effects of medications can be altered by when and what the person eats.

8. *Prior treatment history.* What prior treatment experience did the client have? Treatments that helped with similar problems in the past should be noted because they are likely to be effective again.

We expand on these issues and discuss treatment planning in detail in subsequent chapters.

CONCLUSIONS

In this chapter, we have looked at the principles underlying assessment of older people and the features of a clinical interview, including examination of presenting symptoms and problems, history, and mental status testing. This information contributes to differential diagnosis, as well as to treatment planning. We continue our discussion of assessment in the next chapter, focusing on psychological testing to complete the process of differential diagnosis and to determine capacity.

APPENDIX 6.1. The Memory and Behavior Problems Checklist

INSTRUCTIONS TO CAREGIVER

"I am going to read you a list of common problems that people with dementia can have. Tell me whether your relative has had any of these problems. If so, how often has the problem occurred during the past week?" Hand the person the card on which the frequency ratings are printed. Read through the choices for the first problem reported as having occurred. For each subsequent item, ask whether the problem has occurred and then how often.

REACTION RATINGS

For each problem that the caregiver reports as having occurred (codes 1 through 4), ask, "How much did this problem bother or upset you when it happened?"

Frequency ratings	Reaction ratings
0 = Never occurred	0 = Not at all
1 = Has occurred, but not in the past week	1 = A little
2 = 1 or 2 times in the past week	2 = Moderately
3 = 3 to 6 times in the past week	3 = Very much
4 = Daily or more often	4 = Extremely
9 = Don't know/not applicable	

Behaviors	Frequency	Reaction
1. Asks the same question over and over again	0 1 2 3 4 9	0 1 2 3 4
2. Mixes up past and present (e.g., thinking a deceased parent is alive)	0 1 2 3 4 9	0 1 2 3 4
3. Loses, misplaces, or hides things	0 1 2 3 4 9	0 1 2 3 4
4. Wanders or gets lost	0 1 2 3 4 9	0 1 2 3 4
5. Does not recognize familiar people	0 1 2 3 4 9	0 1 2 3 4
6. Forgets what day it is	0 1 2 3 4 9	0 1 2 3 4
7. Unable to keep occupied or busy by him- or herself	0 1 2 3 4 9	0 1 2 3 4

(continued)

Behaviors	Frequency	Reaction
8. Follows you around	0 1 2 3 4 9	0 1 2 3 4
9. Constantly restless or agitated	0 1 2 3 4 9	0 1 2 3 4
10. Interrupts you when you are busy	0 1 2 3 4 9	0 1 2 3 4
11. Spends long periods of time inactive	0 1 2 3 4 9	0 1 2 3 4
12. Talks constantly	0 1 2 3 4 9	0 1 2 3 4
13. Talks little or not at all	0 1 2 3 4 9	0 1 2 3 4
14. Is suspicious or makes accusations	0 1 2 3 4 9	0 1 2 3 4
15. Wakes you up at night	0 1 2 3 4 9	0 1 2 3 4
16. Appears sad or depressed	0 1 2 3 4 9	0 1 2 3 4
17. Becomes angry	0 1 2 3 4 9	0 1 2 3 4
18. Strikes out or tries to hit	0 1 2 3 4 9	0 1 2 3 4
19. Engages in behavior that is potentially dangerous to others or self	0 1 2 3 4 9	0 1 2 3 4
20. Sees or hears things that are not there (hallucinations or illusions)	0 1 2 3 4 9	0 1 2 3 4
21. Talks in an aggressive or threatening manner	0 1 2 3 4 9	0 1 2 3 4
22. Cries or becomes tearful	0 1 2 3 4 9	0 1 2 3 4
23. Problems eating: Eats excessively or not at all	0 1 2 3 4 9	0 1 2 3 4
24. Incontinent of bowel or bladder	0 1 2 3 4 9	0 1 2 3 4
25. Is uncooperative when you want him or her to do something	0 1 2 3 4 9	0 1 2 3 4
26. Any other problems (specify):	0 1 2 3 4 9	0 1 2 3 4

APPENDIX 6.2. Questions from the Delirium Symptom Interview According to Symptom Domain

DISORIENTATION

Have we ever met before today?
Can you tell me what time of day it is now?
Can you tell me where we are now?
Why are you in the hospital?
During the past day, did you think that you weren't really in the hospital?
Have you felt confused at any time during the past day?

DISTURBANCE OF SLEEP

Did you have trouble falling asleep last night?
After you fell asleep, did you wake up and have trouble falling back to sleep?
Did you wake up on your own too early this morning?
Were you sleepy during the day?
Did you have nightmares or vivid dreams that were intense or bothersome last night?

PERCEPTUAL DISTURBANCE

At any time during the past day have you experienced or imagined seeing, hearing, or feeling things that weren't really there?
(*Interviewer:* During the interview was there evidence of any of the preceding delusions; for example, did the patient think he or she was at home because things in the room looked like home?)
Now I want to ask you about objects that you have seen or sounds that you have heard that you may have misinterpreted; for example, sounds that you have heard that were not what they appeared to be.
Did you think that people were trying to harm you when they weren't?
(*Interviewer:* During the interview, was there evidence of any of the preceding misperceptions; for example, did the patient answer the intercom or think a spot on the wall was a surveillance camera?)

(continued)

Note. From Levkoff, Lipzin, Cleary, Reilly, and Evans (1991). Copyright 1991 by Springer Publishing Company, Inc. Reprinted by permission. This appendix does not include all questions from the Delirium Symptom Interview. For complete interview, write to Sue Levkoff, ScD, Harvard Geriatric Education Center, Division on Aging, Harvard Medical School, 643 Huntington Avenue, Boston, MA 02115.
*These are based on observations made of patients.

Now, I'd like to ask you whether things that you recognized correctly looked distorted or strange. For example, did:

things look bigger or smaller than they really were?
things move that were not really moving?
things seem as if they were moving in slow motion?
your body size, shape, or weight look different from what it is?
(*Interviewer:* During the interview, was there evidence of any of the preceding misperceptions; for example, did the patient think a light was swirling that wasn't?)

DISTURBANCE OF CONSCIOUSNESS*

Did the patient stare into space and appear unaware of his or her environment? Did the patient talk about something else; for example, did he or she change the subject suddenly (e.g., non sequitur) or tell a story unrelated to the interview?
Did the patient appear inappropriately distracted by environmental stimuli; for example, did he or she respond to questions asked of a roommate (distractible)?
Did the patient show excessive absorption with ordinary objects in the environment; for example, did he or she repetitively fold sheets or examine the IV tube over and over (hypervigilant)?
Did the patient have a recurring thought that prevented him or her from responding appropriately to the environment; for example, did he or she continuously look for shoes that weren't there (persistent thought)?
Did the patient have trouble keeping track of what was being said during the interview; for example, did he or she fail to follow instructions or answer questions one at a time?
Did the patient appear inappropriately startled by stimuli in the environment? Was the patient awake, sleepy, stuporous, or comatose?

INCOHERENT SPEECH*

Was the patient's speech:
Unusually limited or sparse?
Unusually slow or halting?
Unusually slurred?
Unusually fast or pressured?
Unusually loud?
Unusually repetitive (e.g., repeating a phrase over and over)?
Characterized by speech sounds in the wrong place?
Characterized by words or phrases that were disjointed or inappropriate?

(continued)

PSYCHOMOTOR ACTIVITY*

Was there evidence of:
Restlessness (e.g., patient getting in and out of bed)?
Tremors?
Grasping/picking?
Increased speed of motor response (e.g., grabbing for a drinking glass suddenly)?
Wandering?
Lethargy and sluggishness?
Slowness of motor response?
Staring into space?

FLUCTUATING BEHAVIOR*

Did the patient's level of consciousness fluctuate during the interview; for example, did he or she start to respond appropriately and then drift off?
(If present) Did the patient's speech fluctuate during the interview; for example, did the patient speak normally for a while, then speed up?
(If present) Did psychomotor activity fluctuate during the interview; for example, was the patient at first sluggish and then moved very quickly?
Did the patient show emotional lability?

CHAPTER 7

Psychological Testing for Differential Diagnosis and Capacity Evaluations

In Chapter 6 we emphasized the first steps in differential diagnosis: identifying presenting symptoms and problems, obtaining a history of current symptoms and problems, testing for mental status, and what to look for in a medical examination. We now complete that process by examining the uses of psychological and neuropsychological testing for differential diagnosis. We then turn to an issue of increasing importance: capacity evaluations. Just as questions about possible dementia dominate the assessment process, we are often asked to determine whether an older person is capable of performing critical activities—for example, managing his or her money, living alone, or continuing to drive. We look at legal criteria for capacity, as well as the kinds of test data and other clinical information needed for a capacity evaluation.

PSYCHOLOGICAL AND NEUROPSYCHOLOGICAL ASSESSMENT

Psychological testing assesses current functioning in a systematic way and under standardized conditions, yielding findings that can be compared with normative data. These objective results help clarify the more impressionistic findings from a clinical examination. Test performance can also be assessed over time, which is especially important when initial findings are ambiguous. Results from psychological tests have been found to be as accurate as medical evaluations in differentiating dementia from normal aging and other disorders of later life (Tuokko, Kristjansson, & Miller, 1995).

153

Of course, tests should not be used alone in an assessment. Just as a medical evaluation is often incomplete without neuropsychological testing, test results also tell only part of the story. Patients are served best when testing is part of a comprehensive evaluation that includes medical and other relevant assessments.

A full neuropsychological evaluation is expensive and time-consuming, but it need not be conducted in every case. When a client has obvious and significant cognitive deficits, a brief battery, as suggested later in this chapter, can be used to confirm the pattern and severity of deficits. To do more would often be frustrating for the patient without clarifying the situation further. A comprehensive battery should be used when the initial findings from medical workups and the clinical interview are unclear or ambiguous, when a baseline assessment is needed to follow people over time, or when unassailable proof is needed, such as cases in which testing will be used as part of legal proceedings.

Testing plays an indispensable role in differential diagnosis. As we have emphasized, the most frequent question that clinicians will be asked is whether a patient has dementia. Testing provides objective evidence of current performance that can be compared with age norms, as well as individual factors such as education. The evidence from a battery of tests is a more powerful diagnostic indicator than a single score from a mental status test (Ivnik et al., 2001) and provides evidence for differentiation of dementia from other causes of brain damage and from depression.

Using a comprehensive test battery makes it possible to detect early and mild cases of dementia that would not be identified through mental status testing or other clinical procedures. Items on a mental status test sample familiar information that well-educated people can answer easily. Neuropsychological tests include tasks with a range of difficulty. The more difficult or challenging tasks can identify mild deficits in someone with high education. If findings remain ambiguous, however, the results from testing can be used as a baseline and performance then tracked over time. A comprehensive evaluation can also identify specific strengths and weaknesses in cognitive abilities, which is important in planning interventions with the patient, family, or other caregivers. Testing can also differentiate among types of dementia.

Testing Older People

When testing older adults, we need to use special procedures to obtain valid results. Although poor performance is often due to an underlying brain disorder, a number of factors can lead to false positive findings. The tester can exacerbate mild and relatively benign cognitive problems by rushing through an evaluation or conducting it in a noisy or poorly lit setting. Older adults should be tested under optimal conditions in order to minimize the effects of these kinds of noncognitive influences on performance. In structuring the testing situation, clinicians should consider the following points.

Establishing Rapport

As with the clinical interview, clinicians need to begin the testing session by developing rapport with the client. The older person should be relaxed before beginning testing. It is also important to make sure that the client has a comfortable seat and does not have problems such as arthritis that would make sitting for an extended period difficult.

Monitoring Fatigue

Fatigue should be monitored closely among older clients, especially when test sessions are long. Splitting up long assessments into two or more days, taking breaks, and keeping an eye on the client's level of fatigue can address this concern. Giving the client a snack during a long testing session may also help. Sometimes an individual is simply unable to continue because of fatigue. It is advisable to stop testing well before that point is reached in order to ensure that test performance best reflects the client's ability and that the client will agree to return to complete the evaluation.

Time of Day of the Evaluation

Many older people function somewhat better in the morning, although some have difficulty getting up and ready before noon. If the goal is to determine the highest level of functioning, then the assessment should be conducted at a time the patient or family say is optimal. Sometimes the family or some other referral source raises a specific question about whether the client's functioning varies from one part of the day to the next. This question is often raised when concerns exist about the person's capacity to live at home. In that instance, the assessment should be conducted at different times of the day to determine the extent to which fluctuations occur.

Reaction Time and Performance Speed

Reaction time and speed of performance decline with age. Performance suffers if clinicians read the instructions too quickly or do not give clients an adequate amount of time to respond. Clinicians who are used to evaluating younger people need to adopt a completely different pace so as not to rush through tests or press older clients for quick responses in untimed tests. If a clinician hurries through an assessment or tries to do it at the same pace as with younger people, the results will clarify only how an older person responds to time pressure, not what typical functioning might be.

It is useful to allow an older person to complete a timed test even after the allotted time has expired. Although the test should be scored in the standard way, giving no credit for answers made after the allotted time has elapsed, we note that the client was able to complete the task successfully. That allows us to distinguish between people who cannot do a task at all and someone who can perform adequately, albeit very slowly. This finding should be included in the behavioral observation section of the evaluation.

Test Anxiety

Lack of familiarity with testing and test anxiety can interfere with performance. Older people who have not had to perform a structured cognitive task, such as arithmetic or block design, for some time may have difficulty because of lack of familiarity with testing procedures or strategies. Tests that allow for a certain amount of practice can be useful; evidence of improvement over several trials may be a better indication of the older person's functioning than a summary score. Another strategy is to administer tests that use familiar stimuli and tasks that are ecologically valid. For example, recall can be tested by asking people to place familiar objects into the model of an apartment and then to recall each object and where they placed it (Johansson, 1988–1989; Johansson & Zarit, 1991). Money can be used for simple mathematical operations (Johansson & Zarit, 1991). Similar to everyday situations, these tasks can engage people's interest in situations and with stimuli with which they are familiar.

People may also be anxious about what a test will show. Establishing good rapport before starting an assessment and conducting the testing in a supportive and encouraging manner go a long way toward reducing anxiety. Even in the face of obvious deficits, the clinician can be encouraging and positive. One strategy that we have found useful to head off anxiety about making incorrect responses is to begin the session by explaining that the purpose of the tests is to analyze the patterns of errors. We tell clients that although getting everything right might be desirable in other settings, the tests we will give them have been designed so that it is impossible to get everything right.

Sensory Problems

Vision and hearing problems can interfere with test performance in obvious ways. To the extent possible, the assessment should differentiate between decrements in cognition and other areas of functioning due to underlying brain disease and decrements caused by vision and hearing problems. From a functional perspective, a person's cognitive problems can cause difficulties in everyday life whether due to dementia or sensory loss, but people have more opportunities to correct or compensate for sensory deficits. For that reason, assessments should be conducted under optimal conditions. To reduce vision problems, lighting should be adequate and focused on the test materials that the client reads. Clients should be seated so that they are not looking directly into a window or strong light. Glare and low illumination hamper visual functioning. When evaluating a client with hearing loss, talking loudly does not help. Instead, clinicians should speak in a clear and distinct manner, using complete sentences. Background noise should be reduced to a minimum. Testing should be conducted in a room with good acoustics.

Older clients should always be reminded to bring eyeglasses, other vision devices, and hearing aids to the testing session. Before beginning testing, we always check that the client has brought along the appropriate aids. It is better to reschedule an assessment than to try to conduct it when the client does not have eyeglasses or a hearing aid. In addition to determining whether the client has brought sensory aids, the clinician should inquire about everyday visual and hearing function, for instance, difficulty hearing ordinary conversation or hearing what people say on television or difficulty reading newsprint and headlines.

The following example illustrates how sensory loss can complicate an assessment.

The Effect of Sensory Loss on Diagnosis

Frieda, age 84, was brought to an outpatient clinic by her son and daughter-in-law for an evaluation so that they could develop plans to care for her adequately. Frieda had been living in another part of the country until the death of her husband of 50 years. Following his death, she had become deeply depressed and stopped caring for herself. Frieda was hospitalized in an inpatient psychiatric facility for a 2-week period. The staff told her family that she was "hopelessly senile" and recommended that they place her in a nursing home. Following her discharge, her son and daughter-in-law brought her across the country to live with them.

Frieda's son and daughter-in-law began the assessment by reviewing her history. They indicated that Frieda actually functioned quite well in their home and did not have memory problems, but they were concerned that she did not have many activities. Her son was also concerned that her smoking would be harmful to her health. It immediately became apparent in the interview that Frieda was very hard of hearing. She could not respond to even simple mental status questions when administered orally. When the questions were written for her to read, however, she responded quickly and accurately. Frieda performed well on other visual tasks. When discussing her situation, she expressed sadness over her loss and gratitude that her family had taken her in. Rather than managing her "senility," the goal that emerged was to identify activities she would enjoy and to explore ways of minimizing the communication problems caused by her hearing loss.

Additional evidence of Frieda's good cognitive ability came from an incident that took place at the end of the interview. At the beginning of the session, Frieda's daughter-in-law had taken her purse from her and placed it alongside the chair she was sitting in, out of Frieda's line of vision. At the end of the session, the daughter-in-law got up to leave without taking Frieda's purse. Frieda, however, reminded her daughter-in-law that she had put the purse alongside her chair and asked her to pick it up. Consistent with everything else that occurred during the assessment, this type of recall indicated normal cognitive functioning.

The diagnosis of dementia in this case had clearly been erroneous. In retrospect, staff at the psychiatric hospital had probably failed to identify Frieda's profound hearing loss and mistook her lack of responsiveness as dementia rather than sensory loss compounded by depression following the death of her husband. Subsequent follow-up confirmed that Frieda continued to function well.

Test Batteries and Tests

This section describes several test batteries and tests that are useful in the assessment process. Lezak, Howieson, and Loring (2004) provide a comprehensive listing of tests and valuable information on their clinical application and interpretation. Published sources of tests can readily be found on the Web. Most tests can be found at one of two sites: Harcourt Assessment (harcourtassessment.com/) and Psychological Assessment Resources (PAR; www3.parinc.com/). Norms for older people are now generally available, although upper age limits usually do not go beyond 89.

The choice of tests depends on the referral question and the patient's ability. I typically begin with a comprehensive test battery that addresses several relevant neuropsychological functions and then add other tests that help address the referral issue. In effect, I take a middle ground between clinicians who believe that they should administer the same battery to every patient and those who put together a unique combination of tests for each patient. I like the information provided by comprehensive batteries that assess many different functions and allow me to use well-established norms, as well as allowing comparisons with other clients I have evaluated. I also want to supplement the battery with tests that allow me to pursue important questions in a more in-depth way. If it becomes evident that the tests are too difficult and the client is experiencing excessive frustration, I switch to a briefer screening battery (see later in this chapter) that contains easier tasks but still provides information about a range of neuropsychological functions.

This section describes commonly used test batteries and tests and then gives examples of how to put tests together to address specific issues. We want to underscore that choosing tests and interpreting results is a complex process that requires supervised experience. The following material should be helpful to clinicians with a background in testing who are not as familiar with approaches for use with older people. For students, we hope this material provides a framework for learning how to conduct comprehensive assessments.

For clinicians who do not conduct psychological testing as part of their work, we hope this section helps them to know what tests can accomplish and how to use the reports that are provided on test results.

One of the benefits of having experience in testing is learning to use the information that does not go into test scores, such as what clients say about their performance and how they answer questions or solve problems. This nonscorable information is often as important as whether a response is right or wrong. (See Lezak, 1995, for a thorough discussion of qualitative responses.)

Finally, age norms can be very helpful in identifying what is expected with aging and what might be different with dementia (e.g., Kaszniak, 1990). Norms should be interpreted, however, in light of estimates of premorbid levels of functioning. Applying norms is particularly difficult for people at the high and low ends of the spectrum of abilities, because their performance differs more from average performance. As a result, norms may overestimate impairment for someone with a history of poor functioning and underestimate impairment for a person with a high level of intellectual ability.

Years of education can be used in estimating prior performance. Formal education, however, does not tell the whole story for today's cohort of older people. Many older people had only limited opportunities to get a formal education but had work and other life experiences that allowed them to function at a much higher level. Both education and life achievements need to be weighed when evaluating test performance. Some clients may have developed specific abilities to high or expert levels. Decline may occur later in dementia in these well-practiced abilities. An accountant, for example, may still perform at high levels on arithmetic tests, despite early or even moderate levels of dementia. On the other hand, small errors made by a person with a highly developed cognitive skill may indicate a significant decline, even though the same errors would be normal for most people. Reading tests such as the Wechsler Test of Adult Reading (Wechsler, 2001) or the North American Adult Reading Test (Friend & Grattan, 1998) can provide an estimate of premorbid functioning (e.g., Griffin, Mindt, Rankin, Ritchie, & Scott, 2002).

Test Batteries

The Wechsler Adult Intelligence Scale (WAIS; Wechsler, 1997a) remains a popular test, due in no small measure to the extensive literature and adequate age norms (Ivnik et al., 1992b; Ryan, Paolo, & Brungardt, 1990). Recent work has extended these norms to African American samples (Lucas et al., 2005b).

The WAIS-III (Wechsler, 1997a) comprises seven verbal tests and seven performance tests (Table 7.1). It can be used in its entirety, or subscales can be selected to measure specific abilities. Dementia is suggested if the verbal, performance, and total scores are lower than would be expected for a person of a

TABLE 7.1. WAIS-III Subscales and the Abilities They Measure

Subscale	Abilities measured
Verbal	
Information	General knowledge, verbal recall
Comprehension	Reasoning, social judgment
Vocabulary	General mental ability; verbal recall, language fluency
Similarities	Concept formation, abstract reasoning
Arithmetic	Computational skill, short-term memory, concentration
Letter–Number Sequencing	Working memory, attention
Digit Span	Attention, concentration, short-term (working) memory
Performance	
Digit Symbol Coding	Attention, psychomotor performance, response speed
Block Design	Visuospatial organization and construction, conceptualization
Object Assembly	Visuospatial organization
Picture Arrangement	Visuospatial ability, social judgment, reasoning
Picture Completion	Visual reasoning, visual search, recall
Matrix Reasoning	Visual information processing, abstract reasoning
Symbol Search	Visuospatial ability

given age and educational background. Performance scores decline with normal aging (about 12 points by age 65 and 20 points by age 80; see Ryan et al., 1990). This decline occurs in part because many of the performance tests are speeded. They also include more challenging and unfamiliar tasks than the verbal subtests. Low performance scores, but not verbal scores, can reflect normal aging or a disease process that disrupts response speed or visual–spatial functioning (see Kaszniak, 1996, for a review). By contrast, verbal performance is relatively stable until very late life. A lower than expected verbal score can be a very important indicator of cognitive problems.

The Wechsler Memory Scale–III (WMS-III; Wechsler, 1997b) is an updated version of a long-standing battery that provides a comprehensive assessment of memory and attention. The test uses both visual and auditory stimuli and assesses immediate and delayed recall. There are 11 subtests, 6 considered primary and 5 additional, which contribute to scores for the following functions: auditory immediate, visual immediate, immediate memory, auditory delayed, visual delayed, auditory reception delayed, general memory, and working memory. Information and orientation items from typical mental status tests are also included. New tests in this version of the WMS use familiar stimuli that have ecological validity, such as faces and family pictures. Normative data are available (e.g., Ivnik et al., 1992b; Ivnek, Smith, Malec, Kokmen, & Tangalos, 1994), including on older African Americans (Lucas et al., 2005b). The scale has spawned countless research studies comparing different populations of patients with neurological disorders (such as amyotrophic lateral sclerosis, Huntington's chorea, and Korsakoff's psychosis; e.g., Butters et al., 1988).

The entire WMS-III takes about 1½ hours to administer, and it may be frustrating for someone with significant memory impairment. These tests are also fairly challenging for people with low education and occupational attainment. Given these considerations, we sometimes select only those subtests most pertinent to the referral question or use one of the screening batteries described in a later section.

Specific Tests

ATTENTION

Attention is assessed both directly and through observation. Two commonly used tests are digits forward, from the Digit Span task of the WAIS-III, and a letter cancellation task (Lezak, 1995), in which subjects are instructed to cross out particular letters (e.g., all the E's and C's) in a long series. Cancellation tasks can also use geometric figures or pictures. Observations of how the patient focuses on other tasks can also provide good evidence of attention problems (Albert, 1988).

Attention tasks are generally performed well by healthy older people. Impairment in attention is a central feature of delirium. People with early, mild symptoms of dementia do not show attentional deficits, but difficulties develop as the dementia progresses. Patients who are depressed or have other psychiatric disorders may be preoccupied with their own thoughts and show poor attention. Poor attention scores by themselves do not indicate a disorder, but they must be considered in combination with other tests and the overall clinical picture.

EXECUTIVE FUNCTION

Executive function impairment is one of the main indicators of fronto-temporal dementia (FTD), but frontal symptoms can be found in vascular dementia and AD as well, though usually to a lesser degree. Executive functions include flexibility in thinking, abstract thinking, inhibition, planning, and problem solving. The patient with frontal symptoms will generally need more structured and intensive care, and so identification of executive function impairment has both diagnostic and treatment implications.

To assess executive function, we usually use three tests: Trails, Verbal Fluency, and Design Fluency, from the Delis–Kaplan Executive Function System (D-KEFS; see Homack, Lee & Riccio, 2005, for a review). The Trails test in the D-KEFS is improved over the standard version from the Halstead–Reitan Test Battery (Reitan, 1958). The D-KEFS trails are composed of a series of tasks that makes it possible to identify where the patient might be having a problem. The first trails task involves canceling numbers and is a measure of attention. The second task has the client connect numbers in sequence, which tests whether the client is able to sequence the numbers. The third task, a letters sequence, tests whether a client can order letters alphabetically. Finally, the last task, which measures motor speed, makes it possible to differentiate motor slowing from slow intellectual processing.

The Verbal Fluency test also has useful features. It tests fluency for abstract categories (all the words that start with a particular letter) and concrete categories with different degrees of difficulty (animals, boys' or girls' names). Another fluency task involves switching between two categories. Design Fluency adds a nonverbal fluency component.

We also sometimes use the Proverbs test from the D-KEFS (see later in the chapter). The other parts of the D-KEFS are challenging and usually too frustrating for people with dementia or with limited premorbid intellectual skills. They can be useful, however, with well-educated clients when there is a question about suspected frontal lobe involvement.

MEMORY

Memory plays a central role in evaluations for suspected dementia. Memory is not a single function but comprises several different and interrelated processes. Identifying which aspects of memory are impaired is an important part of an assessment. Among the distinctions that testing should make are:

- Differentiating initial acquisition from subsequent recall.
- Identifying rates of acquisition and retention of new information.
- Distinguishing immediate and delayed recall.
- Assessing both verbal (semantic) and nonverbal recall.
- Assessing both recall and recognition.

Memory for old, well-learned information, such as prominent historical events during the person's lifetime, can also be evaluated (e.g., Butters, Salmon, & Butters, 1994).

Tests of short-term memory that involve several learning trials and both immediate and delayed recall are particularly useful in differentiating early dementia from normal aging. In dementia, the rate of learning and retention of new material is poor (e.g., Butters, Salmon, & Butters, 1994; Delis et al., 1991; Johansson & Zarit, 1997; Morris et al., 1991; Welsh, Butters, Hughes, Mohs, & Heyman, 1991). People with dementia perform at lower than expected levels on initial trials and show little or no improvement with repeated presentation of the stimuli. Some healthy older people also demonstrate poor initial recall but show improvement over repeated trials. Delayed recall also helps in differentiating between dementia and normal aging (Welsh et al., 1991). Patients with dementia show a greater dropoff in delayed recall than normal older people. More intrusions during recall, as well as poorer overall delayed recall, can differentiate AD from other dementias, particularly subcortical disorders such as Huntington's disease (Delis et al., 1991) and possibly also vascular dementia (Libon et al., 1997). Intrusions have been found with verbal as well as nonverbal stimuli—for example, recall of geometric designs (Jacobs, Troster, Butters, Salmon, & Cermak, 1990). Improvement in recognition memory will be greater in DLB than in AD (Hamilton et al., 2004).

Depressed patients can be differentiated from those with dementia on many of these indicators. People who are depressed may show lower recall than normal elderly people on initial trials of a memory test, but, in contrast to patients with dementia, they improve with repeated presentations of stimuli. Delayed recall and recognition are also good, compared with those of patients with dementia (Blau & Ober, 1988; Butters et al., 1994; Kaszniak, 1986). Depressed patients also do not typically experience intrusions. Of course, some individuals may have both dementia and depression, which complicates questions of diagnosis.

A well-constructed battery such as the WMS-III tests the different types of memory function. Other tests can supplement or be used in place of the WMS-III. We describe several tests for which good data on older people are available:

• The Rey Auditory Verbal Learning Test (RAVLT; Lezak, 1995) comprises 15 unrelated words that are presented over five trials. Immediate and delayed recall and recognition are scored. Dementia is associated with lower immediate and delayed recall and also with a higher rate of intrusions of words that were not on the original list (Bigler, Rosa, Schultz, Hall, & Harris, 1989). Improvement across trials may help differentiate people with mild cognitive impairment (MCI) who progress to dementia and those who do not (Calero & Navarro, 2004). Extended age norms, including for African American samples, have been reported (Ferman et al., 2005; Harris, Ivnik & Smith, 2002; Ivnik et al., 1992a).

• Some clinicians prefer the California Verbal Learning Test—II (CVLT-II; Butters et al., 1994; Delis, Kramer, Kaplan, & Ober, 1987) because the stimulus words can be organized into semantic categories—for example, types of food that make up a shopping list. The CVLT-II has been found to identify very early, mild changes in people with family histories of AD who subsequently developed the illness (Bondi et al., 1994). Measures of response bias can be computed from the CVLT-II, which can be useful in differentiating dementia from depression (Massman, Delis, Butters, Dupont, & Gillin, 1992). Patients with depression show a more conservative response style, refusing to guess even though they might know the answer, whereas patients with dementia give more incorrect answers.

• The Fuld Object-Memory Test (Fuld, 1978) has been used extensively in research on dementia. This test provides the opportunity to assess rates of learning and recall by selectively reminding patients which items they missed after each trial. Other advantages of this test are its use of familiar objects and the opportunity for the patient to use multiple sensory modalities in learning. Patients are presented with a bag that contains 10 common objects. They are asked first whether they can identify the objects by touch in the bag. If they are not successful, then they are asked to name the objects by sight. Following identification of the objects, they are given a 60-second distraction task. Then patients are asked to recall the objects. Following this trial, patients are reminded of any item they missed, distracted again for 60 seconds, and then tested again for recall. There are a total of five trials of recall, followed by a multiple-choice recognition test. A delayed-recall trial (15 minutes) is also administered. Patients with dementia are able to recall fewer items over the five trials than are normal elderly people or those who are depressed. Delayed recall is also likely to be significantly lower. Norms are included with the test kit (see also Marcopulos & McLain, 2003).

• A related procedure, the Selective Reminding Test (Buschke & Fuld, 1974), has also been found to differentiate normal elderly people from those with dementia (Masur et al., 1989). In contrast to the Fuld test, patients are presented with a series of 12 words. Alternate forms of the test are available.

Finally, we want to note that recall of past information is typically impaired in dementia, though not in normal aging or depression. Some tests of well-known historical events are available (e.g., Butters et al., 1994; Flicker, 1988; Squire, 1974; Wilson, Kaszniak, Bacon, Fox, & Kelly, 1982). One caution about tests of past information is that it is difficult to separate initial exposure and learning from subsequent forgetting. An alternative is to ask people about personal information, such as when they got married or about children and grandchildren. Errors in remembering names of children or grandchildren are highly significant and usually indicate a serious cognitive problem. People who are healthy or who are depressed rarely forget this information. An exception is that someone with a large number of grandchildren may have a bit of trouble recalling all their names and ages but will have no other memory problems. Someone who is severely depressed may refuse to answer or avoid answering. This type of response should be distinguished from being unable to recall the information.

LANGUAGE

Language deficits in dementia can be subtle and not noticeable to the untrained observer. Speech can seem superficially normal because syntax, grammar, and phonology are often preserved until late in the disease (Flicker,

1988). In AD, a particular kind of language deficit, empty language or an overall impoverishment of speech, is often an early symptom. Instead of saying, "Oh, look at the girl," a patient will say, "Oh, look at, um, her." Patients use pronouns instead of nouns and gradually stop using adjectives. Eventually, they use no nouns or adjectives at all. Patients also use a restricted vocabulary and may begin to paraphrase when they cannot recall a word, use an inappropriate word, or misname objects or combine words. Patients may be able to engage in the social process of speech, but the richness of their language declines. As the disease progresses, their speech has little content and contains frequent repetitions.

The vocabulary subscale of the WAIS-III provides information about language functioning. Patients with dementia have increasing difficulty recalling words. Their attempts to define words may be characterized by circumlocutions; they talk around the definition but are not able to produce the specific words needed for an adequate response.

The Boston Naming Test (BNT) is useful for differentiating normal functioning from dementia (Chodosh, Reuben, Albert, & Seeman, 2002; Kaplan, Goodglass, & Weintraub, 1983). The BNT is a confrontation naming test in which patients are shown a series of pictures and asked to give the names. The test starts with a series of easily recognized objects and moves on to harder ones. If the patient does not respond after 20 seconds, the tester gives a phonemic cue, the beginning sound of the word. Not identifying the picture even with a cue is a more serious type of error. Patients with mild dementia have tip-of-the-tongue experiences; that is, they say that they know the word but are not able to recall it. They usually are helped by the phonemic cues. Inability to identify items and misnamings are common with dementia but are relatively rare in normal aging.

The instructions for the BNT specify beginning with item 30 and presenting items 1 through 29 only if 30 is missed. My experience has been that presenting all the items requires no more than 15 minutes and provides important clinical information. Norms are reported by Van Gorp, Satz, Kiersch, and Henry (1986), and by Lucas and colleagues (2005b) for African Americans. Equivalent short forms can be extracted from the full test (Flicker, Ferris, Crook, Bartus, & Reisberg, 1986; Graves, Bezeau, Fogarty, & Blair, 2004).

Another common pattern of language deficit in dementia is in word fluency. As noted, I generally use the fluency tests in the D-KEFS. Patients with dementia who sometimes cannot perform when the stimulus is a letter can respond to semantic categories (Morris et al., 1989). Patients with AD recall fewer items from both letter and semantic categories than normal controls (Ober, Dronkers, Koss, Delis, & Friedland, 1986). In addition, patients with AD make more incorrect responses to the category and have more perseverations and intrusions as severity of dementia increases. People who are depressed may be slowed in their responses but usually perform at adequate levels without intrusions. Fluency tests can be used as the distractors between trials of various memory tasks.

Evaluation of language is more complicated when the client is not a native speaker of English. Someone who has lived in an English-speaking country for 20 years or more can usually manage adequately on these types of tasks. If the person cannot think of an English word, but instead comes up with a word from his or her own language on tests such as the Boston Naming Test, I write it down and then check later to see whether the answer was correct. When a client is not fluent in English, evaluation of language is more difficult. One alternative is to find a translator to work with during testing. Another approach is to tape-record answers in the person's first language and then work with a translator or dictionary to score the test.

VISUOSPATIAL ABILITIES

Visuospatial ability can be assessed with figure drawing. In the Rey–Osterrieth Complex Figure Test (Lezak et al., 2004; Osterrieth, 1944), clients are presented a complex figure and asked to copy it. After a delay, they are asked to reproduce the figure from memory. Both immediate (after 3 minutes) and delayed (approximately 30 minutes) recall are tested. Obvious spatial deficits are apparent in the copying task, whereas the recall task identifies more subtle problems. Rapid decay of the visual icon is typically associated with dementia. Patients with primarily right or left hemispheric damage make characteristic errors. Left-sided lesions are more typically associated with slow organization of the complex details, whereas performance improves with recall. In contrast, right-sided lesions are associated with difficulty in both copying and recall of the figure. Age norms have been reported for this test (D'Elia, Boone, & Mitrushina, 1995; Spreen & Strauss, 1991).

For some individuals, the Rey–Osterrieth figure is too complex. In those cases, a somewhat simpler figure can be substituted from the Repeatable Battery for the Assessment of Neuropsychological Status (R-BANS; see the next section).

Drawing tasks can also reveal deficits. Clients are asked to draw a familiar object such as a house, tree, bicycle, or person (see Lezak, 1995, for a review) or to draw a clock with the hands set to specific times (Johansson, Zarit, & Berg, 1992; Tuokko, Hadjistavropoulos, Miller, & Beattie, 1992; Watson, Arfken, & Birge, 1993). Errors on the clock test are particularly significant because performance does not decline with normal aging (Albert, Wolfe, & Lafleche, 1990; Ferrucci et al., 1996). When drawing a clock, some patients with dementia cannot maintain the shape of the clock face, whereas others are unable to put the numbers inside the shape or to set the time. A step-down procedure is to give patients predrawn clocks and ask them to set the hands to specific times.

CONCEPTUALIZATION

Concept formation can be assessed in several ways. The Similarities subtest of the WAIS-III provides a well-documented approach to concept formation. The Comprehension subtest also assesses conceptual abilities in making social judgments. Block Design assesses concept formation in a nonverbal task. Another test of conceptualization is the Proverbs test in the D-KEFS. Compared with similar measures, this test is useful because it has a step-down option. When clients cannot explain a proverb or when they get an item wrong, they are given a multiple-choice option to determine whether they can recognize the correct answer. There are also age norms, up to age 89, for this task. Sorting tasks, such as the Wisconsin Card Sorting Test, are lengthy and do not adequately differentiate dementia from normal aging (Flicker, 1988). A short version of that test may be more useful (Nelson, 1976).

Screening Batteries

Screening batteries represent an alternative to a full neuropsychological assessment. They should be used when only a limited time is available for an assessment or when a patient is too impaired to complete a full battery without considerable frustration. A screening battery can address diagnostic questions, though without the thoroughness of a complete battery. When using comprehensive batteries, such as the WMS-III, it is possible to administer selected measures as needed, but screening batteries are composed of parts of measures, and so individual components are generally less useful when administered without the rest of the battery.

Three screening batteries are widely used with older people: the Repeatable Battery for the Assessment of Neuropsychological Status (R-BANS; Randolph, Tierney, Mohr & Chase, 1998), the Mattis Dementia Rating Scale (DRS-2; Mattis, 1976, 1989), and the UCLA Screening Battery (Drebing, Van Gorp, Stuck, Mitrushina, & Beck, 1994). Each of these contains a sampling of relevant neuropsychological functions and can be completed in less than an hour. All have established norms for older people.

The R-BANS consists of 12 subtests: List Learning, Story Memory, Figure Copy, Line Orientation, Digit Span, Coding Picture Naming, Semantic Fluency, List Recall, List Recognition, Story Recall, and Figure Recall. Orientation items are included. Scores are computed for five functions: immediate memory, visuospatial/constructional, language, attention, and delayed memory. The figure used as the stimulus for figure copy and recall is less complicated than those in the Rey–Osterrieth Complex Figure Test and can be an informative alternative when the Rey is too difficult.

A major advantage of the R-BANS is the availability of equivalent alternate forms that can be used for retesting. The R-BANS has been able to differentiate mild AD from normal aging. Differences were found mainly on language and delayed memory (Randolph et al., 1998). Norms for people up to age 89 and adjustments for education level are available (Duff et al., 2003; Gontkovsky, Mold, & Beatty, 2002).

The DRS-2 provides a comprehensive assessment of functioning in five domains: attention, initiation/perseveration, construction, conceptualization, and memory. Orientation questions are included. Tasks on the DSR-2 are the least challenging of the three batteries discussed here. It can reliably identify cognitive impairment associated with dementia, but it is less useful in differentiating early, mild symptoms. Like the R-BANS, the DRS-2 provides a profile of the extent of impairment in different functions. As an example, test results may indicate that a patient has poor verbal memory but that visual–spatial functioning is relatively spared. This type of observation is useful in planning interventions that build on the patient's remaining abilities—in this case, using spatial rather than just verbal cues to guide behavior. Because the DRS-2 is generally less demanding than other batteries, it is more useful for tracking changes over time in people with mild and moderate dementia (Salmon, Thal, Butters, & Heindel, 1990). Normative data are available, including on older African Americans (Lucas et al., 1998; Rilling et al., 2005).

The UCLA Screening Battery (Drebing et al., 1994) draws tests from several established measures and includes the WAIS-R Digit Symbol, Trail Making Forms A and B, the RAVLT, the Rey–Osterrieth Complex Figure Test (copy and delayed recall), and the MMSE. The battery is designed for people with functioning ranging from normal to moderate dementia. Cutoff scores are provided that indicate probable cognitive impairment. It can be readministered in 6 months or 1 year to determine whether change has occurred. The scoring system with the UCLA battery, when used in conjunction with other information, leads to clear clinical decisions about diagnosis.

Based on our experience with a large number of patients, the bias of this battery is toward overdiagnosing dementia. That may in part be due to reliance on timed tests. Digit Symbol is a challenging, time-oriented test in which clients have 90 seconds to fill in numbers that match each symbol, as shown in a key. Trail Making is also timed. This weighting toward speeded tests means that people who are depressed or have slowed reactions for other reasons (e.g., PD) do more poorly on the test. There is also no direct assessment of language.

Choosing Tests and Batteries

We want to emphasize again that this discussion of tests is not meant to be exhaustive. Many other tests and batteries have been reported for use with older clients to differentiate dementia from other disorders (e.g., Kaszniak, 1996; Lezak et al., 2004; Parks, Zec, & Wilson, 1993; Tuokko, Kristjansson, & Miller, 1995). The important point is to select a sensible battery, or group of tests, that address the particular question with each client. That can be accomplished in different ways with different sets of tests. It is also critical to know the limitations of the tests that are used.

Qualitative Test Results

Interpreting test findings depends both on objective scores and on qualitative information about how patients responded to tasks or the types of errors they made. Although less research exists to validate these more qualitative aspects of testing, experienced clinicians make use of the nuances and subtle differences in performance. Qualitative features can be of particular help in differentiating depression from dementia. Among the qualitative differences that have been noted: patients who are depressed often are reluctant to guess, whereas patients with dementia make more frequent incorrect answers or intrusions during recall trials; people with depression generally vary more in performance than patients with dementia, who score consistently low on tests except in the earliest stages of their illness; patients with depression can improve with prompts or other cues, whereas those with dementia show little or no improvement; patients with depression are often aware of or exaggerate their deficits, whereas those with dementia typically have less insight into their deficits (Kaszniak & DiTraglia Christenson, 1994). The exception is the highly educated patient with VaD, whose more localized deficits may allow awareness of errors well into the dementing process.

The Use of Repeated Testing

A major challenge for neuropsychological assessment is to differentiate early, mild dementia from normal aging with low rates of false negative and false positive results. This is a difficult task, because cognitive performance can vary for many different reasons besides mild dementia. Norms and cutoff scores represent population averages. An individual who is depressed, has another psychiatric illness, has a poor educational background, or is not a native speaker of English may perform below those levels without having an early dementia. Estimation of likely premorbid performance can reduce but not eliminate these problems. In the final analysis, overlap in neuropsychological functioning will always exist between people with mild symptoms that progress to dementia and those with mild problems that do not progress (Storandt, Botwinick, Danziger, Berg, & Hughes, 1984; Storandt & Hill, 1989).

When we have questions about whether the deficits identified in testing indicate dementia or not, we take a wait-and-see approach. Although there may be benefit for some patients in using the available medications early (see Chapter 12), we believe that the drawbacks of a false positive diagnosis outweigh these potential gains. Diagnosis can be clarified by retesting the client after an appropriate interval (usually a year). Decline in performance over time confirms the presence of dementia, whereas stable or improved performance indicates some other cause of the person's cognitive difficulties. Unfortunately, the current medical standard is to prescribe a cholinesterase inhibitor when a patient complains about memory, thus creating an additional variable to consider in evaluating test results.

The following cases illustrate the use of a test battery as part of an overall evaluation and the decision-making process in clinical assessment.

DETERMINING THE ETIOLOGY OF MILD, ATYPICAL COGNITIVE SYMPTOMS

Ellen was an accomplished 67-year-old woman. She was college educated, had a successful career, and had raised four adopted children. She was in many ways an ideal client. She had a pleasant personality, always showed up for appointments on time, and was always perfectly groomed.

Ellen was referred because of findings of white-matter hyperintensities on an MRI. She had gone to her doctor complaining of fatigue and memory problems. He referred her to a neurologist, who did an evaluation, including the MRI. He then asked for psychological testing to determine whether this was a case of VaD. In the clinical assessment, Ellen was able to tell me about all the specific types of memory problems she was having. Diagnostically, that type of memory complaint with specific recall of incidents points to depression, not dementia. She had a score of 29 out of 30 on the MMSE, her one error being ability to recall only two of the three words after interference. One error, particularly on recall, does not indicate any problem.

Ellen's deceased mother had had AD. As a result, when Ellen forgot something, she worried that it might be a sign of AD. Her worries increased when the neurologist told her about the MRI findings. A complete test battery was administered, including the WAIS-III, WMS-III, and language tests. The WAIS-III indicated that Ellen had high to very high overall intelligence. Scores on the WMS-III revealed an interesting pattern. Her general memory was above average, but her verbal memory was not as good as her visual memory. This pattern is unusual, especially in someone with high education and good verbal skills. Typically, verbal memory scores are higher than visual memory scores. Ellen's lowest scores were in attention and delayed recall. That is a pattern often seen in dementia. Because dementia is a disorder of short-term memory, tests of delayed recall are particularly sensitive to its effects. The language tests were normal.

The test findings confirmed that Ellen was a very bright woman who was generally performing at a level we would expect of someone with her background and history, but she showed a few areas of weakness. Although the tests of attention and delayed recall showed some questionable performance, they were not clearly out of line with her overall functioning. I had, then, evidence of high performance on most tests, a few areas of difficulty, and findings of white-matter hyperintensities on the MRI. What should be done next?

I told Ellen that her test performance did not currently indicate AD or similar problems and that her memory problems could be explained by depression. I told her that depression might be affecting attention so that she was not taking information in efficiently, leading to test scores in that area that were lower than expected. I also explained to Ellen that white-matter hyperintensities have an undetermined significance and prognosis—that is, we do not always know what they mean for functioning, but they did not indicate AD. I proposed testing her at a later time.

Retesting was done a year later. Ellen's WAIS-III scores were the same as before. The WMS-III was also almost identical, but delayed recall was improved. Clinical examination indicated that her mood was also improved. These findings suggest that whatever the white-matter hyperintensities might have meant, they were related neither to obvious cognitive problems nor to progressive impairment. Ellen's stability in performance was good evidence for ruling out AD.

This case had a positive outcome. In some instances, mild findings of impairment in attention and delayed recall may well be the first manifestation of a dementing illness. But very mild deficits can have multiple causes. Because it is often not possible to separate out the effects of depression, as well as other sources of individual differences in test performance, I find it better to wait until I have evidence on the course of symptoms before making a diagnosis. Repeated testing is not necessary when symptoms of dementia are obvious during the first assessment, but it is an essential step in cases with unclear or ambiguous findings.

Another feature of this case is the family history. A history of AD in a parent or in other close relatives increases the risk of developing the disease. Relatives can also become fearful of developing AD and become more vigilant of even minor problems in their memories, as happened in this case. Testing can be a powerful tool for providing reassurance and clarifying the significance of minor problems.

ALZHEIMER'S DISEASE EXACERBATED BY ALCOHOL

History provides valuable information for clarifying diagnosis. In this case, a 66-year-old retired business executive, Robert, was referred for a neuropsychological assessment by a neurologist. The referring physician said he found signs of dementia in his neurological examination but that the MRI was normal.

Robert gave a loose and unreliable history, so much of the information came from his wife. He had been very successful in business, rising to an executive level in a midsize company. Robert had retired 14 years earlier because of hypertension but subsequently took some part-time jobs teaching business classes. He had not been asked to return to his last job. Since 1981, he had had two surgeries on his spine and had become addicted to painkillers. Throughout his life Robert had been a heavy social drinker, though his wife reported some decrease in alcohol consumption in the previous 4 months. His use of pain medication also decreased. His only other current medication was for hypertension.

Robert had no friends or activities, apart from swimming 5 days a week. He spent his days at home alone. His family history revealed that his mother had died 10 years earlier after a long course of AD and that a sister with Down's syndrome was showing AD symptoms. Robert was fearful of having AD.

Current symptoms included significant word-finding and short-term-memory problems. His wife reported that Robert had problems remembering and following recipes (he did the cooking) but that he was able to cook and shop competently. She was concerned about his driving, however, particularly his ability to judge the speed of oncoming traffic. For the previous 4 months, she had stopped serving wine with dinner; this step cut down Robert's alcohol consumption considerably.

Robert was cooperative during the testing, though at times he did not seem to put his whole effort into it. His responses were often impulsive. He frequently had to be redirected to tasks or to have the instructions repeated. He often was frustrated with his performance.

Testing revealed significant problems with memory. Robert scored in the mildly impaired range on the MMSE, mainly because of difficulty recalling the three words and repeating the phrase "No ifs, ands, or buts." On the WMS-III, he scored about 2 standard deviations below normal on most tests of visual and verbal memory, as well as on attention and concentration. Delayed recall was somewhat better. On the WAIS-III, Robert's scores were in the average range, with little difference between verbal and performance scores. There was, however, considerable interscale variability, particularly on the verbal scales. Comprehension was relatively high (scale score = 14), possibly indicating high premorbid reasoning ability. But other scores indicated considerable decline, given his prior occupational functioning. Digit Span and Arithmetic, which are measures of attention and concentration, as well as higher executive function, were among the lowest scores (scale scores of 5). Robert's score on the Boston Naming Test was within normal limits, but he had 11 literal paraphasias, for example, saying "wrath" for "wreath" and "date" for "dart." Word fluency, as measured by the Controlled Oral Word Association Test, was in the high normal range. Scores on Trail Making A and B and on the Rey–Osterrieth Complex Figure Test were low. Recall on the RAVLT also indicated considerable memory impairment.

Although the overall pattern of impairment was consistent with dementia, the history and some features of the test results suggested the possibility that the problems were related to chronic alcoholism, perhaps in combination with pain-killing medications. In particular, the scattering of scores on WAIS subscales, with sparing of some abilities and somewhat better performance on delayed than on immediate recall on the WMS, suggested the effects of chronic alcoholism. It was possible that symptoms were due to a combination of dementia and alcohol use.

To differentiate between these alternatives, I recommended eliminating all alcohol and painkillers to determine whether functioning would stabilize or improve. To reduce his anxiety over AD, Robert was told that his memory problems were due to high blood pressure and his use of alcohol and painkillers. Despite the family history of AD, I was reluctant to make that diagnosis until the alternatives were ruled out.

Unfortunately, a decrease in Robert's drinking did not slow the progression of his symptoms. As it became apparent that Robert had a progressive dementia, his wife decided she did not want to try to control his alcohol intake. Rather, she felt it would be better if their last years together were not filled with conflict.

One year later, a comprehensive medical and neuropsychological examination revealed evidence of continued decline and confirmed a diagnosis of probable AD, though with alcoholism as a secondary cause. Robert's MRI pointed toward AD. In contrast to previous tests, it now showed evidence of brain atrophy. Although an initial finding of atrophy is nonspecific in the absence of pronounced cognitive deficits, longitudinal evidence of changes suggest AD.

In retrospect, Robert's alcoholism probably hastened his decline, but his wife made a decision that preserved his autonomy and, in a way, their relationship. Pressing the issue about his drinking could have had some positive benefits, but his wife's decision to let him live out his life as he preferred had to be respected.

EARLY-ONSET DEMENTIA COMPLICATED BY MEDICATIONS

Donna, a 50-year-old schoolteacher with a master's degree in education, was accompanied to the appointment by her husband, Fred, who provided much of the detail about background and history, as Donna had difficulty giving accurate information. She had a successful career in elementary education that spanned the past 28 years. Donna had had a number of health problems, including severe hypertension and headaches. For more than 2 years, she had been having increasing difficulties with memory and functioning in the classroom. When the problems started, Donna had been referred by her primary care physician to a neurologist for an evaluation of her memory problems and headaches. An MRI revealed tiny zones of increased signal intensity in the midbrain and left periventricular white-matter changes, suggesting the possibility of vascular disease, but the MRI was otherwise considered normal. The results of a brief cognitive screening were also in the normal range (her MMSE score was 28).

Over the following 2 years, Donna's problems in functioning increased, but both her primary care physician and the neurologist still felt there was nothing wrong. Finally, her husband became exasperated by the discrepancy between the doctors' lack of concern and his observation of continuing decline, and he asked for a referral for a neuropsychological evaluation.

Donna was very anxious during an initial testing session but was more comfortable during a second visit. She wanted to perform well and put forth a lot of effort. Her MMSE score was 28, as it had been 2 years earlier. Other tests, however, showed significant impairments. On the WMS-R, her general memory score of 72 was 3 standard deviations below normal. Donna's verbal memory score was much lower than her visual memory score. Her performance on two learning tests, the RAVLT and the CVLT, showed much lower rates of learning and retention (delayed recall) than would be expected. On the RAVLT, for example, she recalled 1, 3, 5, 7, and 9 words (out of 15) over the five trials and then only 3 on delayed recall. The Boston Naming Test was within normal limits (54 out of 60 spontaneously named), but Donna made semantic errors, literal paraphasias, and circumlocutions. These types of errors indicated a problem with language, though she was able to compensate for the most part at this time. The UCLA Screening Battery was consistent with a moderate degree of impairment.

An immediate problem was whether Donna should continue teaching. She had been functioning in the classroom only with the help of two assistants. I encouraged her to take a leave of absence and to reevaluate the situation in the summer. Reports were sent to the neurologist and primary care physician. Although they acknowledged the findings, both of them continued to be unconcerned about Donna's memory problems, at least according to her husband.

In cases such as this one, in which there is some controversy over the diagnosis and in which the implications are significant (in this case, whether Donna could return to work), I like to refer the client for another opinion. Six months after our initial evaluation (a minimum period for seeing changes in functioning in cases of dementia), I referred Donna and her husband to a memory-disorder clinic at a medical center in another town. She was seen there by a neuropsychologist and a geriatrician. The neuropsychologist repeated most of the tests I had done. Donna now scored only 23 on the MMSE, a drop of 5 points in 6 months. As in the previous testing, she had a great deal of difficulty learning and retaining new information. This problem was more pronounced on verbal tests but was also found on nonverbal tasks. Other tests were stable or showed a mild decline from the previous testing. Given her functioning, the neuropsychologist reached the same conclusion that I had, that Donna was no longer capable of continuing in her old job.

A diagnosis was given of VaD or possibly mixed VaD and AD. The medical findings, a history of hypertension, and the MRI abnormalities pointed toward a VaD. AD, however, could not be ruled out from Donna's test performance. In fact, all three clinicians involved, the two psychologists and the geriatrician, felt that Donna seemed in behavior, appearance, and test performance more like a patient with AD, a clinical sense based on having evaluated many patients with dementia.

The geriatrician who saw Donna recommended several changes in medications. She suggested changing the two antihypertensives Donna was taking because they had more cognitive side effects than other available drugs, discontinuing two common over-the-counter antacids that can affect cognition, and discontinuing a pain medication (Ultram) that also has cognitive side effects. After making these changes, Donna's husband reported an immediate improvement in her functioning. Her memory was a bit better, and she asked fewer repetitive questions. She generally seemed more alert. Although it was clear that Donna still had dementia, the medications had obviously been contributing to her problems.

This case shows how dementia can affect someone relatively early in life. Early-onset cases are often difficult for everyone involved, because the illness seems premature. Whereas someone who is over 65 has a number of safety nets, such as Medicare and Social Security, a person under 65 must deal with early retirement and disability. The financial consequences can be catastrophic if the person does not have sufficient resources. Patients often encounter obstacles in trying to qualify for disability payments and Medicare. It takes a lot of determination and usually an appeal to get disability insurance, so unless the patient has a family member who is an effective advocate, the patient's resources can easily be depleted before he or she is approved.

The other noteworthy feature of this case is that the patient's cognitive functioning and behavior improved following changes in medication. This improvement illustrates that there can be treatable components in cases of dementia, a fact that is often overlooked because of the pessimism associated with the diagnosis.

EVALUATIONS OF DECISION-MAKING CAPACITY

Clinicians are increasingly called on to make complex judgments about the decision-making capacity of older adults in five main areas: (1) daily living activities, including living alone, (2) finances, (3) contracts, (4) wills, and (5) medical treatment, including ability to refuse treatment. Capacity for driving may also be assessed, though by somewhat different procedures and criteria. These evaluations may be part of a legal process to determine diminished capacity or competence, or they may occur in hospitals, nursing homes, or other service settings whose staffs have to make decisions about where a person can live and what kind of help is needed.

Capacity evaluations pose many challenging ethical dilemmas and can literally have life-and-death implications. Clinicians must be able to conduct objective and sophisticated assessments that carefully weigh the evidence from multiple sources and to write reports that address the pertinent legal criteria for competence. The well-trained geriatric specialist can provide an informed opinion that helps resolve an often tangled or conflicted situation in an optimal way. The American Bar Association and the American Psychological

Association (2005) have prepared a joint publication, *Assessment of Older Adults with Diminished Capacity*, that provides a useful summary of the legal issues, assessment strategies, and suggestions on how to organize capacity reports. This book is available through both organizations and can also be downloaded at the American Bar Association website (www.abanet.org/aging).

Defining Competence and Capacity

The terms "competence" and "capacity" have evolved over time in efforts to establish equitable legal processes for identifying people unable to make adequate decisions about their own health, safety, or self-care. "Competence" and "incompetence" are legal terms and are decided by a judge who has weighed all the evidence. "Capacity" refers to the assessment of decision-making ability in specific areas, such as managing one's money, used in making judgments about competence. A psychologist who conducts an assessment would comment on the person's capacities, whereas a judge would decide on competence. The use of these terms, however, is not uniform, and sometimes "capacity" or "diminished capacity" is used to describe the outcome of the legal process and "ability" is used to refer to the assessment of a specific domain.

The specific legal definitions and procedures for determining competence and capacity vary from one country to another, and within the United States from one state to another. Clinicians must familiarize themselves with the laws where they practice. We describe some common features in the United States. Although legal proceedings are likely to be different in other countries, the assessment approach described here should have some relevance.

Legal statutes regarding capacity typically address four key points. First, competence and capacity are presumed, until a court decides otherwise. Determination of incompetence involves due process, that is, a court proceeding in which the "defendant" has the right to representation and to contest the proceeding. Some states now require the person to be present during the proceedings. Historically, absence of due process in competence decisions led to occasional abuse. A person with a history of mental illness or who was old could be ruled incompetent without any presentation of evidence or without being able to challenge the proceeding. Unscrupulous relatives or other individuals would try to get control of an older person's assets this way. That still can happen, but now more legal safeguards regulate competence decisions.

Second, capacity and competence are now generally regarded as specific to a task. In the past, legal definitions of incompetence and related terms were global, and so a competence evaluation involved an all-or-none decision. A person found to be incompetent in one area (e.g., managing money) was considered so for all types of decision making. Under current statutes, capacity is evaluated for specific abilities. A person can be found to lack decision-making capacity for a single ability but could be considered capable of carrying out all other activities. The finding that someone does not have the capacity for managing finances, for example, does not presume an inability to take care of personal needs or to make decisions about where to live.

Third, capacity comprises multiple components. Current legal definitions of incapacity usually include four components: presence of a disabling condition, cognitive impairment, functional impairment, and the need for another party to intervene in order to prevent harm or other adverse consequences to the individual (American Bar Association & American Psychological Association, 2005). In the past, a medical diagnosis of a disabling condition such as dementia alone was sufficient for determination of incompetence (Willis, 1996). Over time, however, courts recognized that presence of a disease did not necessarily compromise functioning. Legal criteria now emphasize functioning—specifically, how the person performs the ability in question and his or her reasoning about it. Some states have even omitted diagnosis from their definitions of incompetence (Sabatino, 1996). With the evolution of these definitions, the courts have also become more accepting of non-physicians as experts who can provide evidence about capacities. In fact, training in testing may provide the best background for conducting the kind of objective evaluation needed for this situation.

Fourth, incapacity involves more than just eccentricity or engaging in risky behavior. To be found incompetent, a person has to be unable to recognize the implications of decisions or to understand the information used in reaching a decision.

The goal of an evaluation is to determine whether a substitute decision maker needs to be appointed to act in an individual's best interests. When a court evaluation finds that a person is incapacitated, the court assigns a guardian as a substitute decision maker to act in his or her best interests. Guardianship orders can be global or limited to the specific realms in which the person has been found to lack capacity. In some states, a conservator will be appointed specifically to manage finances.

The legal procedure for obtaining guardianship is expensive and can often be avoided. Many people already have assigned a durable power of attorney to a trusted family member or friend. This mechanism becomes effective when a person becomes incapacitated. The person named as having durable power of attorney can act as a substitute decision maker for financial and/or medical decisions. In addition, people can complete an advance medical directive that indicates preferences about medical care in end-of-life situations (see Chapter 15). Usually, durable power of attorney and advance directives are implemented automatically and without controversy when the person cannot make his or her own decisions. The only reasons for a capacity evaluation in these situations are that a third party contests the actions of the person holding power of attorney or that the older individual asks to take back decision-making power. It is also possible to contest the person's capacity to grant power of attorney.

The court oversees guardianship and conservatorship, and reports are due on a regular basis to protect against abuse, such as improper use of the person's financial assets. This precaution, unfortunately, does not prevent all abuses, and some legal disputes revolve around the question of whether the guardian is acting in ways consistent with the individual's values and preferences. By contrast, there is no formal supervision of the actions of someone with power of attorney. Most families act in the patient's best interests and do not abuse their power of attorney, but sometimes other family members will raise questions about the decisions being made.

Adult Protective Services may take on responsibility for living arrangements and other matters affecting older adults. The procedures that Adult Protective Services uses to determine need may be different from legal requirements for capacity. When making an evaluation for Adult Protective Services, however, the clinician should apply the usual standards for capacity.

Capacity Evaluations

Capacity is assessed through interviews with the person and with relevant informants, such as family members and staff in an institution, through direct assessment of behavior and decision making relating to the capacity or capacities in question and through psychological testing that assesses the capacity for decision making in specific domains (American Bar Association & American Psychological Association, 2005; Grisso, 1994, 2003; Kapp, 1996; Willis, 1996).

A capacity evaluation should be constructed around the type of question being asked. Questions of capacity may address different situations: the ability to make a will, to enter into a contract (including marriage), to make a donation, to live independently and take adequate care of oneself, to make medical decisions, and to drive. Legal criteria for capacity in these areas are summarized in *Assessment of Older Adults with Diminished Capacity* (American Bar Association & American Psychological Association, 2005). Sometimes lawyers will request an evaluation but will not be specific about the reasons. In those instances, the clinician should clarify what areas of capacity are being questioned.

Except when the evaluation is ordered by the court, the clinician needs to obtain consent to perform the assessment and to gather information from other people or from medical records. If someone is already serving as guardian or exercising power of attorney for the individual, that person should also provide consent.

The specific elements that we examine in an evaluation are the presence of an illness or disabling condition; cognitive impairment; and the person's functional capacity and decision making, including the person's values and preferences (American Bar Association & American Psychological Association, 2005; Grisso, 2003).

Illness or Disabling Condition

A capacity assessment may yield information that clarifies diagnosis and prognosis, for example, the likelihood that the person's condition will improve, deteriorate, or fluctuate. The clinician obtains relevant information about history and diagnosis from all possible sources, including the person being evaluated, informants, and medical records.

Medications may be involved in evaluations of capacity in two different ways. First, medication, especially pain medications, may either render patients incapable or contribute to their incapacity. In a recent case, a gentleman was clearly incapable of making decisions for himself; cognitive impairment, psychiatric illness, and pain medications each contributed equally to his incapacity. He was seen after spending 30 days in a nursing facility to ensure that he had not been abusing the pain medications. The evaluation showed him to be incapable of making decisions, although it was not possible to partial out the exact contribution of each of the three contributing factors. Second, an individual may not take his or her medication optimally at home, but after admission to a nursing facility and receiving correct doses, he or she becomes capable of making informed decisions. An example of this situation appears later in the chapter.

Cognitive Impairment

A major part of a capacity evaluation is to determine whether the person has the cognitive ability to understand and make decisions. Two things can lead to cognitive impairment: (1) deficits in neuropsychological functions such as attention, learning, and memory, expressing information, reasoning, and other areas that are relevant to decision making and (2) distorted thought processes due to psychiatric problems such as psychosis or severe depression (American Bar Association & American Psychological Association, 2005; Grisso, 2003).

In conducting an evaluation of capacity, I select tests from among the batteries and tests discussed earlier. I usually begin with a brief screening test, such as the MMSE (Folstein et al., 1975), to obtain a gross estimate of the degree of cognitive impairment. If testing reveals severe dementia, it does not usually make sense to put the person through a whole battery of tests. In that case, I do fewer tests or administer a screening battery such as the R-BANS so as not to frustrate either the patient or the tester.

Tests should assess the abilities that are most directly related to those in question. It is generally important to know whether a person can attend to, process, and retain information in an adequate way. For that reason, I include a test of attention (usually the Digit Span subtest from the WAIS) and tests of verbal memory and language. I am also interested in judgment and reasoning and use the Comprehension and Similarities subtests of the WAIS. If there is a question about the person's ability to manage finances, I use the arithmetic subscale of the WAIS, which assesses ability to do simple computations involving spending money and making change. These tests constitute a minimum battery, provided the person does not have severe dementia.

The amount of testing beyond that minimum depends on the person and the question that is being asked. It is not necessary or desirable to have everyone complete a long and comprehensive test battery. Many tests do not bear directly on the question of competence. A comprehensive battery of tests (e.g., a complete WAIS and WMS) is useful, however, when capacity issues are complex, when results from a short battery of tests reveal ambiguous findings, or when the case is highly contested. For other suggestions of tests that are useful in capacity evaluations see the American Bar Association and American Psychological Association (2005) and Grisso (2003).

In addition to focusing on test scores, the clinician needs to examine the quality of reasoning and judgment the person reveals in responding to test items (Kapp, 1996). Often I ask the person to explain answers or to discuss the reasoning used in giving a response. As with testing for differential diagnosis, I assess factors such as fatigue and sensory impairment that can interfere with test performance.

In addition to testing, I interview the person to evaluate mood and the possibility of psychotic thought processes that could be affecting decision making. A depression scale can be used to document severe depression.

Functional Capacity and Decision Making

Functional assessment focuses specifically on the type or types of capacity in question. To assess capacity, I ask the person specific questions about the function. I want to learn whether he or she understands information about a given situation and about the consequences of the choice he or she is making. I also want to learn about the person's values and preferences. When a person makes choices that are not congruent with his or her preferences, it is necessary to explore why he or she might be doing so. I would also want to get the perspective of relevant informants about the person's decision-making capacity. Finally, I review documents such as medical records, advance directives, or any statements made by the person that bear on the situation.

Kapp (1996) suggests examining five specific and two general factors that reflect capacity. The specific factors are:

1. Can the individual make or express choices about life situations?
2. Can the person offer reasons for these choices?

3. Is the reasoning process that underlies these choices rational, that is, based on facts rather than delusions?
4. Can the person understand the implications of these choices?
5. Are the choices consistent with the person's values and preferences, or do they represent a departure that might be due to illness or excessive influence by another person?

The two general factors that reflect the capacity for making decisions are:

1. Can the person take in factual information?
2. Can the person understand his or her own situation as it relates to the facts?

Of course, it is important to be aware that one or more relatives or friends may be trying to influence the person who is being evaluated for their own self-interests. In some cases, the person does not have the capacity to make reasoned decisions and so becomes easily manipulated. In other cases, the person being evaluated can formulate reasoned decisions but will do what this other person wants, even though it is not consistent with his or her preferences.

Questions about functioning should be specific and should reveal understanding of the situation, decision-making capacity, and the ability to carry out plans effectively. When the focus is financial management, the clinician should determine whether individuals know what and where their assets are and whether they have a plan for managing the assets. The clinician can also assess the client's ability to manage a variety of everyday tasks that are relevant to financial management, such as making simple purchases, making change, understanding a checkbook or bank statement, and paying bills. Tools are available for assessing financial capacity (e.g., Griffith et al., 2003). The person's ability to resist the influence of people who might defraud him or her can also be evaluated.

For assessment of *testamentary* capacity, the clinician should determine whether the person understands what making a will involves, has knowledge about his or her assets, recognizes those individuals who would be considered the natural heirs (e.g., a spouse, children), understands the scheme in the proposed will for dividing assets, and indicates that the plan is consistent with his or her intentions and values. For *contractual* capacity, the person needs to show an understanding of the provisions of the contract and its effects. In a sale, for instance, the seller should understand that he or she is selling property to the buyer, as well as the purchase price involved, the fairness of the price, and any fees that are paid as part of the transaction. For *donative* capacity, the person needs to understand how the gift affects his or her financial situation and what might remain in an estate for natural heirs (American Bar Association and American Psychological Association, 2005).

In evaluating capacity for medical decision making, the starting point is determining whether the individual understands information about the illness and the consequences of choosing one treatment or course of action compared with another. The person's preferences and values should also be determined. Preferences and values are particularly relevant if the evaluation concerns a request to terminate a treatment. In that case, it is essential to find out whether or not prolonging life is what the person wants. When a person is not able to provide this information, we would rely on informants, as well as any written statements, such as an advance directive (see Chapter 15).

Capacity to remain at home has become an increasing focus for evaluations. Two standards that are used in some states for evaluating capacity to remain at home are "essential needs"—which is sometimes called "endangerment"—and "least restrictive environment." Essential needs refers to whether the person is able to provide for his or her own basic requirements, such as food and housing, or whether his or her efforts to do so are so poor as to cause endangerment. The assessment of essential needs takes into consideration whether supporting people are available to give the assistance that the person needs. The legal standard of living in the least restrictive environment recognizes that there are advantages to remaining at home that can offset risk, particularly if remaining at home is what the person wants and if he or she understands the risks involved. The implication of this standard is that risks associated with remaining at home need to be balanced against the benefits as well as risks associated with moving to a protected setting. The goal of least restrictive environment frequently conflicts with the preference of families and some judges to avoid any possible risk of harm to an older person. The person's own understanding of the risk involved in remaining at home is often critical in these circumstances.

In assessing the capacity to remain at home, the clinician can ask questions that probe the individual's judgment in making decisions in key situations, his or her ability to provide for self-care and safety, his or her understanding of the implications of decisions, and the person's values and preferences regarding staying at home. The person's ability to carry out the activities of daily living (ADL) necessary to sustaining life can also be evaluated. ADLs are evaluated by asking the individual and relevant informants directly about difficulties in performing activities. I would ask about basic or personal activities, such as dressing, bathing, and using the toilet, and about instrumental activities, including using public transportation, using the telephone, or managing finances (Lawton & Brody, 1969). I would also ask about any other activity or function relevant to this particular case, for example, whether the person had been reported to leave the house at all hours of the day or night.

A problem with ADL assessment is that people with dementia may underestimate their problems and some caregivers may overestimate problems. As an alternative to standard self-report measures, several instruments are now available that conduct direct assessments of specific functions. These measures include the Community Competence Scale (Loeb, 1983), the Direct Assessment of Functional Status Scale (Lowenstein et al., 1989, 1995), the Structured Assessment of Independent Living Skills (Mahurin, DeBettignies, & Pirozzolo, 1991) and the Everyday Problems Test (Marsiske & Willis, 1995). These tests use specific tasks to assess functional abilities, for example, telling time or being able to understand the information on a prescription drug label. Table 7.2 gives examples of sample tasks.

As with psychometric tests, however, these performance tests may not bear directly on the question of capacity. For example, someone might not be capable of making decisions about different health insurance plans but may still be able to handle daily expenses. There is also no agreement on what critical tasks might adequately assess domains such as financial management or being able to live independently (see Willis, 1996, for a review of these issues).

For those reasons, visiting the person at home can often provide the best information about how he or she functions in the setting. Home visits are recommended by the American Bar Association as part of capacity evaluations whenever possible (Kapp, 1996). In a home visit, it is possible to observe the person's performance directly and to get a firsthand look at possible safety hazards. The following example shows how a home assessment revealed supports in place that enabled a person with memory impairment to function safely at home.

TABLE 7.2. Examples of Tasks That Assess Instrumental Activities of Daily Living

Domain	Exemplar task
Managing medications	• Determining how many doses of cough medicine can be taken in a 24-hour period • Completing a patient medical history form
Shopping for necessities	• Ordering merchandise from a catalog • Comparison of brands of a product
Managing finances	• Comparison of Medigap insurance plans • Completing income tax return form
Using transportation	• Computing taxi rates • Interpreting driver's right-of-way laws
Maintaining household	• Following instructions for operating a household appliance
Meal preparation and nutrition	• Evaluating nutritional information on food label

Note. From Willis (1996). Copyright 1996 by Springer Publishing Company, Inc. Reprinted by permission.

Home Visit to Evaluate Competence

Thelma, a 96-year-old woman, lived alone in a house in the country. The court asked me to evaluate her ability to live safely at home. The case had gone to court because of a dispute between Thelma's daughters. One daughter felt that she was not safe at home and wanted her to be placed in a nursing home. The other daughter believed that her mother was better off remaining at home and that it was safe for her to do so. Testing revealed a significant deficit in short-term memory, but no other obvious cognitive deficits. Thelma's memory problems may have been an early manifestation of dementia, but in the absence of other obvious cognitive problems, it was not sufficient for diagnosis of dementia.

The main question posed in the evaluation was Thelma's safety at home, so I visited her there. The home was small but neat and clean. We talked about food preparation, and I had Thelma show me how she went about preparing her meals. I also questioned her about what she might do in an emergency situation, such as a fall. Thelma told me she had a neighbor who checked in on her regularly. The neighbor made sure she was safe and also gave her reminders, for example, that it was time to prepare dinner. With her permission, I talked to her neighbor, who confirmed that she checked on Thelma regularly and indicated that she was willing to continue doing so. From the information I obtained, I concluded that Thelma was competent to remain in her home.

These types of supportive arrangements can come into play with other capacities. A person no longer able to manage finances may have set up arrangements for one person to manage the estate. As long as that person is carrying out the intentions of the agreement, there would be no need for a guardianship or other court action.

The Capacity Report

In a report, the clinician reviews and integrates findings and makes a recommendation about the capacities that were in question. This should be done in a succinct way, free from jargon. A sample report would include the following (American Bar Association & American Psychological Association, 2005):

1. Reason for the request.
2. Informed consent.
3. Presenting problem and history.
4. Collateral interviews.
5. Test results.
6. Functional evaluation.
7. Summary and conclusions.

The court's decision will weigh this information in light of specific statutes. The decision then leads to legal action or to clinical interventions (e.g., instituting or withholding a medical treatment).

Evaluation of Driving

One of the most difficult decisions for older people is giving up driving. Some people restrict their driving or give it up altogether, but others (mostly men) continue to drive long past the point at which their families consider them to be safe (Kaszniak, Keyl, & Albert, 1991). Families, however, are often unable or reluctant to take the car away from these unsafe drivers.

Not surprisingly, patients with dementia are the most at risk of getting into accidents (Dobbs, Heller, & Schopflocher, 1998; Kaszniak et al., 1991; Sims, McGwin, Allman, Ball, & Owsley, 2000; Tuokko, Tallman, Beattie, Cooper, & Weir, 1995). Even people with mild dementia make more serious errors while driving than do other older people (Hunt, Morris, Edwards, & Wilson, 1993; Uc, Rizzo, Anderson, Shi, & Dawson, 2004). Individuals who suffer from other mental disorders or vision loss or who take medications that interfere with attention and reaction time also can have higher rates of traffic accidents than age-matched controls (Tuokko et al., 1995).

Cognitive deficits are strongly related to increased accident rates and decreased performance on a test course and in traffic (Dobbs et al., 1998; Hunt et al., 1993; Odenheimer et al., 1994; Reger et al., 2004; Sims et al., 2000). Visual–spatial skills, which contribute to positioning a car in a traffic lane or judging the distance of oncoming traffic, are among the strongest predictors of performance. Considerable work has been done on useful field of view, a composite measure of selective and divided attention and speed of processing of visual stimuli. This function has been consistently found to be related to increased crashes and other driving problems (Ball & Owsley, 2003; Myers, Ball, Kalina, Roth, & Goode, 2000; Owsley et al., 1998).

As with other capacities, a medical diagnosis of dementia is not sufficient to take away a driver's license. Some states now mandate reporting people with dementia to the motor vehicles department, but they do not lose driving privileges unless they cannot pass a driving test.

Clinicians are increasingly asked to evaluate driving capacity. Neuropsychological tests, including evaluation of functions, such as useful field of view, that are directly related to driving, provide evidence of impairment likely to be related to driving ability. In cases of extensive impairment, neuropsychological findings are probably sufficient evidence to restrict driving. In other circumstances, on-the-road tests yield the most definitive evidence. Driving simulators are also used, but many people without driving problems have difficulty with them.

A promising assessment approach is DriveABLE, which is widely available in Canada and in some parts of the United States (Dobbs et al., 1998; www.driveable.com). Developed specifically to identify unsafe older drivers, DriveABLE involves a two-part assessment. First, clients are assessed on a computer-based test involving driving situations that depend on memory, judgment, decision making, attention, and motor speed. Second, clients are taken for an on-the-road test drive by a trained driving evaluator using a car with dual brakes. The driving evaluator rates the number and type of errors that the driver makes. Hazardous or potentially catastrophic errors or many less serious errors, such as overcautious driving or poor positioning of the car, indicate impaired capacity for driving.

The following cases illustrate several issues discussed in this chapter that a clinician may face when asked to perform capacity evaluations.

Tailoring the Capacity Evaluation to Specific Abilities

Marvin, age 68, became depressed when his wife discovered he had been having a long-standing affair. He took a gun and shot himself through the head. The bullet entered and exited through the frontal region of the brain but did not kill him. Marvin's wife subsequently divorced him, so he was living on his own and in charge of his finances. He had a daughter and a son, and he gave power of attorney to his daughter. She promptly spent about $100,000 of his money on herself and her family. His son went to an attorney to protect the father's assets out of concern that Marvin would run out of money if his sister continued spending his assets. The attorney referred Marvin for an evaluation of his ability to make decisions about his finances.

Testing in this case proved to be a challenge. Marvin had frontal lobe damage and was hard to manage. In the middle of testing, he would lose track of what he was doing. For example, he would suddenly stand up during the testing and start to walk around or get ready to leave. These interruptions did not reflect resistance or hostility; he was simply forgetting what he was doing.

I performed a thorough evaluation that included the WAIS, the WMS, and language testing. Because the main question was Marvin's capacity to make decisions about finances, I focused particularly on tests of comprehension and ability to abstract. Could he think logically and develop and implement a plan? Based on the test findings and on discussions with Marvin, it became apparent that he was highly suggestible. If someone presented a scheme to him, he would turn over some money. But the situation was complicated because he was also capable of making logical plans. Testing revealed that comprehension and reasoning were adequate. When I asked Marvin specifically what he wanted to do with his money, he could give a logical answer.

The assessment, then, indicated that Marvin was capable of logical decisions but had difficulty implementing them. Because he was very distractible, it was possible to confuse him and take his money from him. Based on these findings, the judge put safeguards in place to prevent Marvin's daughter from continuing to spend his assets on her own needs.

Marvin was not capable of decision making because of his suggestibility, and therefore he needed protection from one of his daughters.

CAPACITY ISSUES IN REFUSING TREATMENT

Julia, age 78, was living in a nursing home but wanted to move back to her own home. She had been placed in the nursing home by her sister, who felt that she was not making good decisions about her care at home. On a couple of occasions, Julia had returned home on a trial basis but would not take her medications properly. As a result, she would become sicker, and her family would put her back in the nursing home. Julia would then get very depressed and say she did not want to go on living.

Julia's attorney requested an evaluation to determine whether she was competent to decide to go home, even if it might compromise her care. The key to the evaluation was talking with her in depth to determine whether she really understood what the implications of going home would be. I asked her specifically whether she understood that if she went home, the likelihood was that she would die sooner. She replied, "I know I am sick and am going to die soon, and I'd rather die at home." Given that that was her wish and that she was cognitively able to make that decision, the judge ordered that she be permitted to go home. She went home and lived there for about 3 months before she died.

This case illustrates that people can competently make decisions that put them in potential danger. Julia understood the implications of going home and therefore was competent to make that decision.

As in both of these cases, it is often family conflict over the decisions that bring these cases into the legal system.

Examples of other end-of-life decisions and the use of advance directives are found in Chapter 15.

CONCLUSIONS

In this chapter, we discussed the uses of psychological testing in differential diagnosis and capacity evaluations. Testing provides a structured assessment that yields data that can be compared with age norms, thereby helping to clarify the significance of presenting symptoms or problems. When there is a question of possible dementia, a thorough neuropsychological evaluation can confirm the presence of a degenerative process or suggest other possible causes of symptoms.

Just as dementia is the focal point for differential diagnosis of older adults, cognitive functioning is a major issue in evaluations of capacity. Capacity evaluations require integration of interview, testing, and observational data with an understanding of individual and family issues out of which the concerns about capacity arose. At the heart of these evaluations is the broader issue of how to balance respect for individual rights with protecting an older person with impaired judgment and the surrounding community from harm. With the continued growth of the older population, we expect these questions to become even more common and more complicated.

CHAPTER 8

Foundations of Treatment

The previous chapters laid a foundation for conducting psychotherapy with older adults by describing the normal processes of aging, common mental health problems of elderly people, and assessment. We now strengthen that foundation by discussing the fundamentals of treatment. This chapter begins with a discussion of the application of psychotherapeutic skills and the adaptations that need to be made when working with older clients. The focus then turns to some "hot button" issues that can arise when treating older adults and concludes with case examples that illustrate treatment issues and skills.

We do not believe in a single or unique type of psychotherapy to be used with every older client. Rather, therapists working with older people apply varied psychotherapy skills as needed to meet the special circumstances and qualities older clients bring into treatment. Treatment also requires specialized knowledge of problems and issues that change with aging, such as the more frequent interaction of medical and psychological problems and the differences in how older people respond to medications. In subsequent chapters, we extend this framework and apply it to common disorders, problems, and settings.

At the most basic—and often most rewarding—level, psychotherapy can address older people's problems and help restore them to fulfilling and productive lives, as the following case example illustrates.

FINDING NEW MEANING IN RETIREMENT

Vernon, age 68, had recently retired and was trying to decide what to do with the rest of his life. His initial plan was to leave the town where he had spent his life. Vernon associated the town with his work, and he was bitter toward his former employer for not giving him the recognition he believed he deserved and toward his colleagues, who, he believed, had prevented him from being promoted to senior management.

Like many professionals, Vernon derived much of his sense of identity from his job. His work had been his main interest, and the few friends he had made were colleagues. When Vernon retired, his relationships with them ended. I focused treatment on coming to grips with his bitterness toward his former employer and on finding an interest that would be an outlet for his talents. He was able to give up the hope of receiving recognition from his former employer and to explore activities he had always wanted to pursue but had not had the time to do because of work. Instead of ruminating about the past or running away from his problem by moving, Vernon got involved in a new activity, painting with water-colors, which provided him with a sense of accomplishment. Vernon's success in resolving his retirement issues made it easier for him to return to therapy years later when his health began to fail and he became depressed.

Treatment in this case was fairly typical. It focused on an age-related transi-tion, retirement, as well as the client's long-standing beliefs and problems. Timely psychological intervention can improve functioning and may even be cost effective, for example, in reducing unneeded physician visits or improving rehabilitation following an illness or injury. Furthermore, psychotherapy with older people is effective, perhaps as much so as with younger clients (Gallagher-Thompson & Thompson, 1996; Gatz et al., 1998; Scogin & McElreath, 1994; Smyer, Zarit, & Qualls, 1990).

PLANNING AND INITIATING TREATMENT WITH OLDER CLIENTS

Successful treatment of older adults involves a combination of sound basic skills in psychotherapy and specialized knowledge of the issues and problems likely to arise when treating older adults. We emphasize those issues that are most important when working with older clients. Practice of what we might call a *geriatric-focused psychotherapy* includes attention to the following: (1) the critical role of assessment, (2) the influence of treatment setting, (3) pre-paring the client for psychotherapy, (4) goals of treatment, (5) establishing a healthy therapeutic alliance; (6) the role of the family, and (7) the role of medical conditions and medications.

Assessment

The starting point for good treatment is good assessment (see Chapters 6 and 7). Knowing the likely diagnosis is critical to treatment planning. There are times, however, when we begin treatment with only a tentative or provisional diagnosis; for example, we think someone is suffering from depression, but we have not conclusively been able to rule out the possibility of early dementia. In that situation, we continue gathering information to clarify diagnosis. It may also take a few sessions to determine whether a personality disorder exists, which would lead to more circumscribed treatment goals and strategies.

Treatment Setting

Treatment of older people can take place in a variety of settings. The therapist needs to decide at the outset where treatment will take place and what the implications of the location will be. Most older clients can either drive themselves or arrange for transportation to a therapist's office. In many locales, special transportation is available that can bring older people to an appointment. For people who do not get out often, a trip to the therapist's office can be helpful in itself and can contribute to discussions about increasing activities outside the home. Information on transportation services is available from local Area Agencies on Aging.

There are, however, times when it is important to make home visits—for instance, to establish rapport with a reluctant client or to see a disabled client who cannot get to the therapist's office. When older clients live in a nursing home or other residential setting, it is often more practical to treat them there rather than in the office. Residents in those settings, however, have very little privacy. It is absolutely essential to be able to hold therapy sessions in a private place where you will not be interrupted by staff members or other residents. We return to the issue of treatment in institutional settings in Chapter 14.

Preparing the Client for Psychotherapy

Psychotherapy has changed greatly during the lives of our older clients, both in terms of how it is practiced and how it is viewed by the general public. When today's older people were young, the predominant treatment was psychoanalysis, and only people who were "crazy" took medications. It is useful to find out the client's ideas and expectations for therapy. I explain to clients how therapy works and how they can benefit from it. Explanations about how the clinician will conduct treatment can clear up misconceptions and also allow clients to be more active in their own treatment. This type of socialization for treatment has been found helpful in many different types of psychotherapy (e.g., Lewinsohn, Muñoz, Youngren, & Zeiss, 1992; Orne & Wender, 1968) and results in improved outcomes.

Therapists should also find out about a client's past treatment experiences. Some older clients have a great deal of knowledge and sophistication about psychotherapy. They may have been in and out of therapy throughout their lives and can recount the whole history of psychotherapy in the United

States. Over the years, I have encountered people who were treated by some of the most famous therapists from earlier generations: Rogers, Perls, Minuchin, Ellis. Although clients with a history of prior treatment are more sophisticated about therapy, I still discuss with them how I plan to proceed. In particular, these clients often have been passive in their past treatment, whereas I work with them in more collaborative ways. Although I use contemporary treatment approaches, I do try to build on what may have been helpful in past therapies.

Older clients sometimes have had bad experiences in therapy when they were younger. These incidents were often due to practices that are now outmoded or theories that have been discredited. As an example, a 68-year-old gay man who sought treatment had spent his young adulthood in and out of treatment with therapists who had tried to "cure" him of his homosexuality. Rather than helping the problem, the therapists only made him feel more guilty and confused, contributing to two psychiatric hospitalizations. Given this history, it was essential for me to convey acceptance of his homosexuality at the outset and to assure him that treatment would focus on the issue he was most concerned about—feelings of anxiety and depression that had increased since he retired.

Goals of Treatment

Given the diversity of the older population, goals of treatment necessarily vary considerably, depending on clients and their circumstances. Goals should be developed collaboratively as part of the interaction between client and therapist. The expectations clinicians have about what goals might be realistic can have a powerful impact on clients. If a therapist believes that not much can be accomplished, little will be attempted. On the other hand, therapists who hold unrealistically positive expectations will be frustrated when treatment does not yield the good outcomes they hoped for.

How much can older people change? When working with younger clients, therapists often believe that far-reaching changes in behavior and personality structure are possible. Our colleagues have expressed wonderment that we would work with older people, who they believe have a more limited capacity for change than the young clients they see. In fact, older clients' maturity and experience is often an asset in therapy. They possess knowledge and abilities that can be brought to bear on their current problems. In the example of Vernon, the retired man embittered about his job, the treatment goal was to decide whether or not he should move, which was related to coming to terms with retirement. This discussion led Vernon to uncover interests and abilities he had not pursued when he was employed. By comparison, our college-age clients often do not have the basic life skills for finding and keeping a job or a relationship and have difficulty making major life decisions or even managing their daily lives. Although some possibilities may be more limited with older clients, therapists can find strengths to build on.

Although goals depend on the unique features of every case, two general principles should guide their selection: identifying treatable aspects of the situation and supporting autonomy. Many older clients have problems that seem at first to be intractable. They may be suffering from chronic and degenerative illnesses. Or they may have longstanding psychological problems that have not responded to treatment in the past. In instances such as these, some aspects of the problem may still be modifiable. Consider an "untreatable" disorder—AD. Early on, people with AD might benefit from counseling that helps them come to terms with their illness and make plans for their future while they are still able to consider the alternatives (Zarit, Femia, Watson, Rice-Oeschger, & Kakos, 2004). As their illness progresses and they can no longer engage in a therapy process, their family members can benefit from counseling that will help them manage the many challenges they face in providing care (see Chapter 13). Even in the late stages, when patients may be living in a nursing home, it is often possible to improve quality of life by working with staff or family members (see Chapter 14). Similar treatable components can be found in other chronic physical or mental health conditions. When a complete recovery is not possible, treatment of some features of the situation may result in significant improvements for the patient and/or the patient's family.

MANAGING ANXIETY AND A HUSBAND'S GROWING DISABILITY

Lisa, age 61, originally sought treatment from her physician for her failing memory. She was referred for neuropsychological testing, and it was determined that although her memory was within normal limits, she had lifelong anxiety and perfectionist beliefs. Further inquiry revealed that Lisa's husband, who had been diagnosed with PD 10 years earlier, was becoming increasingly disabled. The couple had enjoyed an active social life, including entertaining at home and ballroom dancing, but these activities were becoming much more difficult and stressful. Treatment was focused on helping Lisa adjust her expectations for herself and her husband, preserving the activities that they could both still enjoy but letting go of or simplifying other activities. Lisa's anxiety decreased, and so did her memory complaints.

Sometimes an appropriate goal is maintenance, not treatment. This is especially the case with people who have an Axis II disorder (American Psychiatric Association, 1994) or other chronic problem. Although maintenance is frowned on in this era of time-limited treatment and managed care, the goal for individuals with particular types of problems may be to prevent the situation from getting worse. In the end, that approach may cost less money than no intervention at all. Often, patients with borderline personality disorder go from doctor to doctor, getting tests and treatments that they do not need and as a result sometimes experiencing adverse side effects or complications. Therapists try to interrupt this cycle so that clients can get the care that they need and not unnecessary treatment that can make their situations worse.

MAINTENANCE AS A GOAL

Theresa, age 64, had a long history that suggested borderline personality disorder and multiple medical problems. Suffering from chronic health problems that required ongoing care, she would repeatedly get mad at and fire her doctors. Theresa's present physician was providing excellent treatment for her medical problems and so far had been able to tolerate her emotional flare-ups. I sensed, however, that Theresa was getting frustrated with him and that a major outburst might be in the works. I empathized over her frustrations with the doctor but also worked with her to understand the need to tolerate him during her appointments. Although I did not in any sense "treat" Theresa's borderline characteristics, I was able with this and other interventions to prevent her situation from getting worse.

The second overarching principle in treatment of the elderly is supporting autonomy. Many older clients face immediate or potential threats to their autonomy. The biggest is moving from home to an institution. Weighing the advantages and disadvantages of a move like that can be complex. Placement becomes an issue when older people have chronic health problems that make it difficult for them to continue living independently. Their families may be concerned about their ability to stay alone safely or to get needed medical care. Moving them to a protected setting where supervision is available would reduce these concerns. But the potential gains of relocation have to be weighed against the risks associated with taking away someone's autonomy and independence. Older people often function better in familiar settings and maintain their mobility and self-care activities longer at home. Furthermore, they may prefer to stay in their own homes, and unless their competency is compromised, they have the right to make that decision. In general, we try to support autonomy as long as it is feasible, even for people with dementia, and to encourage placement only after all the ways of supporting someone at home have been explored.

The pioneering geropsychologist Robert L. Kahn (1975) proposed that treatment decisions for older clients should be guided by the "principle of minimum intervention." Minimum intervention means choosing a treatment that is the least disruptive to clients' usual functioning. Although this principle could apply to people of any age, minimum intervention is especially relevant for older adults, who maintain a fragile balance between independence and dependence. Minimum intervention means supporting continued independence whenever possible, because that expands the choices older clients have and ensures that they have the opportunity to make decisions about how they live that are consistent with their own values.

Kahn (1975) contrasts minimum intervention with the usual approach to treatment of older people, which he characterizes as "custodialism." Custodial approaches emphasize an older person's dependency while failing to identify or support remaining areas of competence. Much of our long-term-care system is custodial in nature, stressing security over independence, maintenance over rehabilitation. By contrast, treatment guided by the principle of minimum intervention identifies strengths of the client or situation, as well as resources that can be drawn on to reduce the risks or problems.

Minimum intervention applies to many different types of treatment decisions. A basic principle of geriatric medicine is that the more one does, the more potential exists for adverse or unintended effects. Adding more medications is not necessarily better because of the risk of side effects or drug–drug interactions. It is also better not to make changes in medications when a person is doing all right on his or her current regimen. Tests or surgeries should also be considered carefully, weighing the potential gains against possible losses and complications. As one geriatrician we worked with always emphasized, a fundamental principle in geriatrics is "if it isn't broken, don't fix it."

It is important to take a similar approach in mental health practice. The therapist should not set goals that clients do not agree with. It is always easy to see what has to be done to improve clients' situations, but that does not mean it will be therapeutic in the long run to impose our values on them. To the extent possible, therapists need to avoid upsetting a client's usual way of doing things or undermining their remaining areas of competency. That includes supporting people so that they can live at home as long as possible. Although there may be a lot of pressure from family and/or physicians to institutionalize an older person, it is important to weigh the perceived advantages of placement against the disadvantages.

Trading autonomy for security introduces new problems. The move can be stressful and adjustment difficult. Older people who move to an institution may experience a loss of functioning, or what Kahn (1975) called "excess disabilities." Excess disabilities result when institutions limit independent behavior, for example, by insisting on dressing a resident because she takes too long to dress herself or by not allowing a resident to walk independently because of a fear that he might fall. There has long been a concern about the risk of excess mortality in nursing homes. Although people go to nursing homes because of health problems, their mortality rates are higher than those of individuals with comparable health problems who remain in the community (Aneshensel, Pearlin, Levy-Storms, & Schuler, 2000). In the end, placement may become the best option, but that conclusion should be reached only after exploring all the alternatives.

As an example, an older woman living alone might be prone to dizziness and falls. Because she lives alone, she could potentially injure herself and not be able to get help. One solution would be to place her in special housing, such as an assisted living facility, a board-and-care home, or even a nursing home, where there would be someone to check on her. That would be a reasonable solution if she preferred it and there were no other alternatives. Some individuals readily move to assisted living because it makes them feel more secure to have watchful helpers around. But along with addressing the risk of falls, a move would place restrictions on this woman that have nothing to do with her problem. Depending on the facility, she might have to give up her furnishings and live with a roommate not of her choosing. She might not be familiar enough with the neighborhood to go out for walks or shopping. Or the facility might be reluctant to let their clients go out, for instance, if the neighborhood is unsafe or if they are concerned that clients might wander off, fall, or get into other difficulties. Although it addresses one problem—the risk of falling—the move to a protected setting could set off a chain of other changes that would restrict the client, compromise her independence, and possibly set a downward course in physical and/or emotional functioning.

Alternatives to moving this woman would be to provide her with an emergency call system, which she could use to get help, or to find a neighbor or volunteer who could check on her at regular intervals. These approaches are consistent with minimum intervention; they address the main problem or concern, the risk of falling, but do not compromise the woman's independence in other ways. We return to these issues in Chapters 12 and 13.

Establishing a Healthy Therapeutic Alliance

The client–therapist relationship is at the core of all psychotherapy. Many of the steps for building this relationship with older clients are the same as with people of other ages, but these procedures sometimes have a different twist or emphasis.

Empathy plays a central role in successful therapeutic relationships. Introduced originally by Rogers (1951), empathy involves being able to understand the client's feelings and behavior from his or her own perspective and to convey that understanding. In other words, the clinician must try to see the world through their clients' eyes. Empathy is especially important when marked differences in background separate client and counselor. Because there is usually an age difference between older client and therapist, as well as cultural and social differences, empathy is critical.

Empathy has two functions in the therapeutic relationship. First, empathy provides a check for the therapist against accepting biases or stereotypes about clients. By communicating empathy, clinicians push themselves beyond social stereotypes and view clients in a more individuated way. They gain a sense of what the client thinks and feels. Second, empathy conveys to clients the feeling of being understood. This feeling can bridge the differences that may exist between therapist and client in social class, education, or ethnic background.

Using Empathy to Bridge a Generation Gap

Sandra, age 73, was depressed and lonely. Her counselor was a student trainee in her mid-20s who looked even younger. During the first session, Sandra was reviewing her problems but then stopped and said to the counselor, "You haven't been through what I have been. You're not old. You can't possibly understand." The counselor had been trained to use a medical analogy to respond to this complaint by stating that a doctor did not need to have had chicken pox in order to know how to treat it. That statement did not seem right to her, and, instead, she responded spontaneously, "I'm not old, but I have been lonely, too." This response identified Sandra's core feeling of loneliness and conveyed understanding through self-disclosure. This brief exchange was crucial in establishing an effective therapeutic relationship between Sandra and her young counselor, which subsequently contributed to a successful treatment outcome.

Rogers (1951) emphasized two other core qualities in the therapeutic relationship: warmth and genuineness. As with other clients, therapists should be warm and accepting toward older clients and not hide behind the role of "expert" or "doctor."

Some older clients may express racist, sexist, or political beliefs that are offensive to the therapist and that make it difficult to convey empathy or warmth. It is important for therapists to recognize that some of these attitudes were more socially acceptable in the past and so not overreact to them. The therapist needs to remain focused on the client's psychological issues and not be distracted by opinions that are not relevant to treatment.

A particular issue with older clients is touching. Therapists should *not* touch clients routinely, because touching can easily lead to misunderstandings. Occasionally, however, touching is appropriate, such as when a client is retelling a very painful story. Therapists need to overcome the culturally induced apprehensions about touching an older person so that they can convey comfort in the same way they would with a younger client. In fact, it may be more helpful to touch an older client than a younger one because some are rarely touched by another person. But although touching has therapeutic potential, it needs to be used on a limited basis. Because of the improprieties taken by some therapists with their clients, companies that provide malpractice insurance now mandate that physical contact be restricted to touching a client's hand.

The Role of the Family

A major difference in treating older adults compared with younger ones is that key family members are more likely to become involved in an older person's treatment, at least for a brief time. Few older people enter treatment for family therapy or have goals that involve making fundamental changes in their families. The more typical pattern consists of brief involvement of the family that is focused on particular issues. As discussed, families may initiate contact with the therapist and provide useful information that contributes to diagnosis. They also may contact the therapist during the course of treatment. With the client's permission, it is possible to talk with family members over the phone or bring them in for a session with the client. The perspective that they offer is valuable in moving treatment forward. It gives a view of clients that goes beyond how they present themselves in sessions and may reveal information about critical incidents that clients are unable or unwilling to provide.

A FAMILY SESSION HELPS CLARIFY TREATMENT GOALS

Bill, age 59, had been coming to therapy for several months in an effort to resolve his grief. His wife had died suddenly 2 years ago, and he was still unable to focus on anything else. Concerned friends urged Bill to go into therapy. Every week he had a new stack of articles about his wife's illness that he wanted to discuss. There was a strong obsessive–compulsive quality to Bill's presentation. I allowed him to educate me about his wife's illness in order to build empathy. When it became clear that trust had been established, I asked about the effects of his wife's death on their children, who were in their 20s. We agreed that the children would meet with me. Bill remained in the waiting room while they talked with me. What they described was a classic, lifelong obsessive–compulsive pack rat. Bill had not only filled their home with "things too good to throw away" and "things he might need again," but he had also filled his parents' home and two storage spaces. This information from the children helped me readjust my expectations and focus treatment in a more realistic way. Bill's unresolved "grief" was part of his long-standing obsessive–compulsive behavior that held on to everything. Without this information, I might have proceeded too aggressively or might have become frustrated by the slow progress that Bill was able to make.

When an older person is unwilling or unable to benefit from treatment, family members may become our clients. Parents with long-standing personality disorders, for example, may begin making excessive demands on their children's time. Their children may initiate contact with the clinician in order to get help for their parent, but their parent may not agree to participate in anything more than an assessment and, indeed, may see nothing wrong with his or her own behavior. In this type of situation, the therapist can redefine the problem as the child learning to cope with and set limits with his or her parent.

Medical Conditions and Medications

One of the biggest differences in treatment of older people is the amount of time we spend coordinating psychotherapy with medical care. Most older people suffer from one or more chronic illnesses, and these problems can influence their moods and cognitive abilities. Their medications can have similar effects. In treatment, it is necessary to continue monitoring health issues for changes that might affect psychological functioning. As an example, a client's fatigue caused by a new medication may overlap with anergia resulting from depression. Sometimes just identifying the possible physical cause of a symptom helps a client cope. If clients know that a beta blocker can make them feel tired until they get used to it, they will not attribute their tiredness to psychological causes. It is also important to be able to differentiate between irreversible limitations and those medical problems that may respond to treatment. In that way, therapists can help their patients adjust to losses or encourage them to pursue further medical treatment or rehabilitation.

When working with older clients, it is critical to keep abreast of new developments in medical treatment for common diseases. If a client has an illness or takes a medication the therapist is not familiar with, the therapist should read up on it and, with the client's permission, consult with his or her physician. That way it is possible to get a better idea about what might be realistic goals and how psychotherapy can contribute to the situation. There are many resources for obtaining this information. Morrison (1997) provides a comprehensive summary of psychological symptoms associated with medical disorders. Resources on the Web can provide updated information about causes and treatment of medical problems, though we caution readers to stick to reputable websites. The U.S. National Institutes of Health (www.nih.gov) provides comprehensive information on illnesses and on current clinical trials. Many advocacy organizations such as the Alzheimer's Association (www.Alz.org) maintain up-to-date sites that feature current research and treatment.

Therapists also need to become familiar with commonly used medications and particularly with their side effects and potential interactions with other drugs. It is not necessary to know about every medication in use today, but you should know enough to ask the right questions. Pharmacists can be a valuable resource when you have questions about medications.

EFFECTS OF HORMONE IMBALANCE ON MOOD

Vivian, age 67, had taken care of her husband through a long course of Alzheimer's dementia. She was in her early 60s when he died. Two years after his death she began a relationship with a man who was unable to fully commit to her. Vivian became severely depressed and made a serious suicide attempt. She was given antidepressants, mood stabilizers, and atypical neuroleptics, but her suicidal ideation and an intense, irrational anger persisted. Finally, during a therapy session, I happened to ask her about her dosage of an estrogen replacement medication. Vivian replied that she had run out and that her physician did not want her to take it because of research findings on the risks of hormone replacement. Her discontinuation of estrogen coincided with the suicide attempt. I was aware that estrogen is known to be a factor in maintaining a stable mood, whereas progesterone can produce angry feelings. The abrupt discontinuation of estrogen would lead to a relative imbalance of progesterone. Vivian consulted with her gynecologist, who agreed to prescribe a low dose of estrogen, with yearly endometrial biopsies to detect any precancerous changes in the uterine lining. As she resumed taking estrogen, Vivian was able to reduce the psychotropic medications she was taking, and her anger disappeared.

Older people may respond differently than younger people to any medication, whether for psychiatric symptoms or medical problems. As discussed in Chapter 3, physiological changes in the older body increase the risk of adverse effects, especially when a patient is taking multiple medications. It is also more difficult to identify a therapeutic window in dosage with older patients. There may not be guidelines about how much of a medication to give to an older person. With psychotropic medications, geriatric specialists often follow the precept, "Start low, and go slow"—that is, begin treatment with a lower dosage than would be given to younger patients and then increase gradually as needed. There will, however, be wide individual variations in dosages that are effective and tolerated.

Given the multiple interactions possible among illness, medications, and mental health, a critical role for clinicians is learning how to consult with physicians and other health care providers. In a typical outpatient practice with younger adults, the need to consult with a client's physicians rarely arises. When it does, the discussion almost always focuses on psychotropic medications. With older clients, consultation is a frequent and often a key part of treatment. Consultations can clarify the significance of current somatic complaints and lead to coordination of treatment efforts. They can also address issues such as identifying the therapeutic dosage of common psychotropic medications or changing medications to reduce side effects or improve the therapeutic response.

Physicians are often very busy and may not understand or appreciate the contributions to treatment that can be made by mental health practitioners. I have found, however, that it is possible to build collaborative relationships with physicians through several means. First, it is important for the mental health professional to be familiar with common illnesses and medications. That is the physician's area of expertise, but it helps in discussions of clients' problems if the mental health professional understands common terms and issues.

Second, information should be presented to physicians in a succinct way, free from psychological jargon. (Of course, any release of information should be done only with a client's written consent.) Third, the therapist's own treatment plan should be presented briefly and clearly. When physicians understand that therapists can actually help their patients, they welcome collaboration and, indeed, often become a source of new referrals.

I consult with a physician for several reasons. First, I talk with a physician in order to understand a client's situation. Second, I call a physician before a client's scheduled appointment if I think it is necessary to explain what is going on with the client. Clients can find it difficult to communicate their psychological symptoms in a succinct way when they are under the time pressures of a physician office visit. A quick call to alert the physician to specific symptoms can assure prompt implementation of an appropriate treatment.

INTERVENING WITH THE PHYSICIAN

Charlie, age 74, went to his physician three times about his anxiety without getting an appropriate response. After I discussed these interactions with him, it became apparent that he was telling the doctor about his sleep problems and fatigue, that is, telling how he felt, but not using the word "anxiety." In response, the doctor had ordered a sleep test and blood tests. Until I called and focused on the psychological symptoms of anxiety, the doctor was not able to put the pieces of the puzzle together.

When physicians call with questions about the client's functioning and treatment, it is imperative to respond promptly, which helps build their confidence in you. It is also important to have appropriate signed consent from the client before initiating these contacts.

The biggest asset of mental health specialists who treat older adults is that they are likely to be the only professionals who spend a significant amount of time with the client. As a result, they usually have the most complete picture of the client's functioning. They are also more likely to become aware of new symptoms, as well as problems associated with medications. They can consult with physicians when problems arise and encourage clients to see doctors when new or significant symptoms appear. In some cases, they may note symptoms that the physician has overlooked and then either talk with the physician directly or send the client back for another visit.

OVERLOOKED SYMPTOMS

Conrad had seen his primary care physician earlier in the week, complaining about fatigue and light-headedness. He felt that the physician had been less than thorough but that he would have noticed anything major. However, in our session, Conrad was short of breath and unable to focus his attention on the therapy. I called Conrad's doctor's office, alerting the office staff to the problems Conrad was having, and then his wife was able to get an urgent appointment there later in the day. Blood work revealed a severe anemia that required intravenous treatment.

Later in the chapter, we turn to the issues that arise in psychotherapy concerning medical illnesses.

BASIC SKILLS IN TREATMENT OF OLDER PEOPLE

Psychotherapy with older adults involves incorporating the knowledge and skills of geropsychology with a solid foundation of psychotherapy technique. Many different psychotherapy approaches have been used successfully with older clients (see Gatz et al., 1998, for a review). We have chosen to highlight the strategies that have formed the core of our approach over the years. We noted previously the central role of empathy in the therapeutic relationship. We also draw on concepts and techniques primarily from three other traditions: (1) behavioral therapy, (2) cognitive-behavioral therapy, and (3) family systems.

Behavioral Approaches

Behavioral approaches, such as relaxation, desensitization, and shaping new responses, have many potential applications with elderly persons (Zeiss & Steffen, 1996). Behavioral treatments are effective with insomnia, depression, and anxiety and in helping families manage problems related to dementia and other chronic medical and mental illnesses (Bootzin, Engle-Friedman, & Hazelwood, 1983; Burgio & Burgio, 1991; Gallagher et al., 1981; Green, Linsk, & Pinkson, 1986; Haley, 1983; Hussian, 1986; Hussian & Davis, 1985; Lewinsohn, Antonuccio, Steinmetz, & Teri, 1984; Lewinsohn et al., 1992; Pinkston & Linsk, 1984; Rusin & Lawson, 2001; Scogin, Rickard, Keith, Wilson, & McElreath, 1992; Smith et al, 2002; Teri, Logsdon, Uomoto, & McCurry, 1997; Teri et al., 2003; Wisocki, 1991). Many behavioral interventions have been conducted in institutional settings. The targets of these programs have included increasing social participation, increasing exercise, improving self-care activities, managing incontinence, training social skills, and, particularly, controlling problems such as wandering and agitation (see Carstensen & Fisher, 1991; Hussian & Davis, 1985).

Behavioral therapy is valuable with older clients as much for its basic concepts and approaches as for specific techniques. The overriding emphasis in behavioral therapy is on observation—observing the specific behaviors, thoughts, or feelings that are problematic for a client, their frequency (or absence), and the circumstances in which problems occur. This direct approach to problems appeals to the practical side of many older people. As with the use of empathy, careful observation challenges therapists to go beyond cultural stereotypes about aging. The focus on overt behavior in particular also helps therapists and clients alike get beyond incorrect attributions of problems. Clients, for example, may mislabel problems. They may describe a problem as occurring more or less often than it actually does. Similarly, they may fail to note antecedents and consequences of their problems, that is, the events that trigger and reinforce behaviors or feelings. By obtaining the specific details of what the problem is and when and how it occurs, the clinician gains valuable information for planning treatment.

The next example illustrates how observation can change the attributions both the therapist and the client make about a problem.

BEHAVIOR MONITORING AND ATTRIBUTIONS

Sonia, age 53, was caring for her mother, who had dementia. She reported that one of her biggest problems was that her mother would ask the same question over and over again; "When is your husband coming home?" Sonia reported that this constant questioning was driving her crazy. I undertook a behavioral assessment to determine how frequently and when the repetitive questioning was occurring. Sonia's task was to record on a log sheet each time her mother asked the question. Reviewing this record a week later, it was immediately obvious to me, but more important, to Sonia, that her mother was not asking the question often. Rather, Sonia realized that she became annoyed with her mother on the occasions that she did ask the question. Sonia interpreted the question as a criticism of her marriage—that if she were a better wife, her husband would be home already. By getting the specifics of what happened and when, it was possible to change the formulation of this problem from an excessive rate of verbal behavior by a patient with dementia to Sonia's own appraisal of her mother's comment. Careful observation clarified in an important way the characteristics of the problem and led to an appropriate treatment.

Behavioral therapy provides a simple framework for helping clients understand and learn to handle their problems. Through discussion of findings from behavioral assessments, such as the one in the case example, therapists demonstrate the A–B–C (antecedent–behavior–consequence) model of behavior (Teri et al., 1997). Behaviors have antecedents, that is, specific events that trigger them, as well as consequences or events that appear to reinforce the problem. This approach helps clients understand that problems do not emerge out of the blue and that they have some control over what is happening to them. This type of concrete framework works well with clients who are not well educated and for whom more cognitively demanding approaches might be problematic.

Another approach that is especially useful with older clients is to emphasize implementing new behavior in specific, graduated steps. Rather than instructing a client to carry out a complex set of behaviors, the therapist breaks down tasks into steps or components that are easy to master and remember. In many instances, clients agree to carry out new behaviors but delay or put off actually doing anything new. Behavioral approaches address this problem with schedules for specific behaviors and reinforcements for carrying them out. The detailed, concrete steps involved in planning and scheduling new behaviors are often critical in helping depressed or dependent clients break out of a cycle of passiveness and inaction. In a broader sense, behavioral approaches encourage clients to take an active role in treatment, which is especially useful for older clients who feel helpless or overwhelmed. The strong educational component helps clients understand why they are having problems and how new behaviors can help them overcome those problems.

Probably the most useful feature of a behavioral orientation is its emphasis on evaluating the outcome of treatment. Health care professionals, family members, and older clients themselves often are pessimistic about the possibilities for change. An effective way to counter this skepticism about the value of treatment is to demonstrate that there have been measurable improvements. A detailed assessment, which is the first step in behavioral treatment, provides a clear baseline against which outcomes can be evaluated. By obtaining concrete evidence of progress, clinicians can reassure clients about their capacity to improve or to benefit from psychotherapy.

Cognitive-Behavioral Treatment

What older people believe about themselves and their experiences and how they typically appraise events in their lives is a major focus of treatment. Cognitive-behavioral approaches (e.g., Beck, 1995; Beck et al., 1979; Gallagher-Thompson & Thompson, 1996; Zeiss & Steffen, 1996) provide a systematic framework for identifying and modifying thoughts that lead to maladaptive behaviors and emotions. In a sense, cognitive-behavioral therapy addresses many of the same issues as traditional psychodynamic approaches, but it uses a structured framework to bring thoughts out in the open more quickly and to treat them in a direct manner. Clients become aware of how they distort or misinterpret the events in their lives and how these distortions relate to negative concepts about themselves.

Several features of cognitive-behavioral therapy make it well suited for work with older people. First, as with behavioral approaches, there is a strong psychoeducational component. Clients learn about how their thought processes affect behavior and emotions, as well as learning to identify the thoughts they are having that trigger emotions. As in behavior therapy, the techniques are applied to everyday situations. The detailed process of planning and scheduling intervention helps overcome a client's passivity. Other features that cognitive approaches have in common with behavior therapy are the emphasis on identifying when, how often, and in what context problems occur and on evaluating the outcomes of specific interventions.

The heart of cognitive therapy is identifying what people think about themselves and their circumstances. There are so many negative stereotypes about elderly people that clients readily incorporate these stereotypical beliefs into their self-concepts. The issues older people raise often have a basis in reality but are also somewhat exaggerated. One of the most complex issues for therapists is differentiating realistic implications of losses from exaggerated beliefs. Cognitive-behavioral techniques provide tools for therapists to explore the difference between a reasonable sense of sadness or grief over loss and an overgeneralized and excessive preoccupation. Clients who have experienced losses often believe that life is not worth living or that they cannot be happy anymore because of a particular problem or loss. The cognitive-behavioral therapist can discuss the appropriateness of being sad over a loss while challenging the exaggerated belief that the client will never again be happy.

When therapists use cognitive-behavioral approaches with younger clients, they can readily identify which beliefs are excessive or exaggerated. If a college student proclaims that her life is over because her boyfriend has broken up with her, the therapist recognizes the exaggeration right away. He or she knows that the client will have more and probably better relationships in her life and so feels secure in challenging this negative belief. When an older client makes a similar generalization following the death of a spouse, clinicians may accept it uncritically. The death of a spouse is, of course, more serious than breaking up with a boyfriend or girlfriend, and a period of grieving is normal. But when grief persists long after the spouse's death, it is usually due to exaggerated beliefs that make the loss worse than it needs to be.

In order to differentiate the realistic and reasonable consequences of loss from exaggeration, the therapist engages clients in a gentle process of questioning and challenging beliefs. Clients learn to identify overgeneralizations or other distortions in their appraisals of themselves and the events in their lives and to activate more realistic appraisals of themselves. This questioning process always must be embedded within empathy. It should never become harsh or argumentative, even when the therapist is directing clients to examine critically the assumptions they have been making.

Family Systems Perspective

As we have stressed, family members are frequently involved in treatment of older adults. The substance of treatment frequently involves family issues as well. Therapists must make complex judgments about what actually may be going on within a family and when to bring in other family members for the purpose of gathering information or to involve them in treatment. Treatment usually does not involve family therapy in a traditional sense; that is not what older people or their families seek, nor is it usually necessary in addressing the presenting problems. Rather, we apply a family systems perspective to understand how the family functions and then focus on those features that are most relevant to the stability of the system.

Families of older people come in all different shapes and sizes. There is no single "dynamic" of an older family or of children's relationships with their elderly parents, such as role reversal, that influences interactions. Rather, the variations in family structure and relationships are considerable. Each family has its own history, structure, and rules, many of which are implicit. Shared memories and unresolved grievances color how family members deal with one another. Interactions from childhood may continue to affect relationships in the present between parents and children and among siblings, but so may the ongoing exchanges that have taken place since children reached adulthood. Many parents provide considerable emotional and tangible support to children well into their adult years, whereas others may use their resources to manipulate children or may place demands on children for attention. From the children's perspective, some learn to appreciate and relate to parents as adults, whereas others persist in psychological struggles that were laid down in childhood—for example, to gain recognition or acceptance from a withholding parent. The clinician must encounter each family with an open mind about what the psychological issues might be in order to intervene effectively.

Working with families demands a different perspective and set of skills than are used with individual clients. One of the biggest mistakes that inexperienced therapists make is to assume that family members can easily get down to business to address a current problem in a rational and straightforward way. A family systems perspective goes beyond a focus on the individual and instead looks at patterns of interactions among family members and the roles that each person has within the family (e.g., Haley, 1976; Herr & Weakland, 1979). This perspective helps guide the therapist in thinking about when and how to intervene.

The starting point is gathering information about how a particular family functions. It is important to consider who is influential or powerful within the family, who makes decisions, who is viewed positively by other people, and who is seen as weak, needy, or problematic. How family members communicate with each other is also relevant. Building on these observations, it is possible to conceptualize problems as caused by interactions rather than by the behavior of one person or another. Viewing problems in this way opens up more possibilities for intervention. When working with a couple or a family, formulating problems as interactions can help break the cycle of accusations and help them try out new ways of relating with one another. In many of the situations that involve families—such as when someone is suffering from dementia or chronic psychiatric problems—the "patient" cannot change. Nevertheless, it is possible to change the interactions others have with that person and with one another, thereby lessening strain on the family as a whole.

One of the most important elements of a family systems approach is that the therapist does not take sides, assign blame, or support one person against another. Clinicians are often caught up in tense family situations rife with disagreement about what is best for an older client. The issue of whether an older person should move to an institutional setting is likely to produce disagreements. We have often seen therapists in this situation reflexively taking sides with the family member they most identify with. Sometimes, that might be the older person, sometimes his or her spouse, sometimes one of the children. Whoever that might be, that person has a role in the family and elicits certain reactions from everyone else. By taking that person's side in the discussion, the therapist will either produce the same reactions from other family members that this person usually provokes or will fail to bring the family together on a course of action.

Families are not always involved in treatment, nor should they always be involved. But when the older client wants their involvement or is dependent on them, they need to be included, at least to some extent. Even when the family is not included in treatment, a systems perspective is useful for understanding an older client's relationships with them.

HOW THE PROCESS OF THERAPY CAN DIFFER WITH OLDER CLIENTS

We now discuss some of the ways that conducting therapy can differ with older compared with younger clients. We view psychotherapy with older adults as involving application of the usual skills but with some subtle and not-so-subtle variations in style that make treatment work better for many older clients. Treatment also requires being comfortable with discussions of issues that do not arise frequently with younger people. It is not necessary to make all these adjustments with every older person. In fact, the similarities in treating older versus younger people usually outweigh the differences (Miller & Silberman, 1996). Rather, therapists need to be ready to modify their basic approach some of the time in order to improve the effectiveness of treatment.

Addressing the Youthfulness of the Therapist

One of us (JMZ) referred a client to another member of our practice. When I told the client that she would be seeing Dr. Young, the client responded by asking, "Is she?" The answer was "Yes," which was a concern for this client.

Most therapists who work with older adults are younger than their clients. Although age differences are usually not a barrier, they may become an issue in treatment. The geriatric specialist learns to recognize and address problems associated with age differences that might arise during treatment. In the example, the client was concerned not about the therapist's youth per se but about her experience. In other instances, clients feel that a young person cannot understand what they are going through. I have found that explaining my training in geropsychology in a nondefensive way usually is sufficient. The development of a therapeutic relationship quickly allays most of these concerns.

I start a relationship with an older person with the assumption that although I am "one up" on my client in my role as therapist, I am "one down" in terms of age and experience. I always treat clients with respect. One of the reasons I initially allow older clients more leeway in getting to the point is that it is not respectful to interrupt. As the relationship evolves, it becomes more collaborative.

Accommodating Sensory Problems

Just as sensory loss can affect assessment (Chapter 6), it can also be a problem in therapy. When working with older clients, I have trained myself to talk louder (though not too loud), slower, and at a lower pitch. If someone hears better in one ear, I make sure to sit on that side.

Being Patient with the Pace of Treatment

The biggest change therapists have to make when working with older clients is to be patient with the pace of treatment. Older people move at a slower pace, and change comes in smaller increments (e.g., Zeiss & Steffen, 1996). In part, this slower pace is due to differences in communication style. Older clients frequently take longer to get to the point. They may digress, telling anecdotes or recounting events that seem unrelated to the issue we are discussing. Some clients feel they have to tell the therapist everything about an issue or problem or about their lives in order to be understood.

I allow older clients as much time as they need to say what they have to say. Allowing them to take the time they need is helpful in building a therapeutic relationship. They may not have many people in their lives who take the time to listen to them. When few people value or pay attention to what they have to say, they may adopt the strategy of holding onto someone's attention for as long as they can—and then feel that doctors and other professionals are rushing them. A therapist needs to build a different kind of relationship and should not be in a hurry. I often remind myself that I may be the only one who gives this older client my undivided attention, and that helps me be more tolerant of the slower pace.

The balance between directing conversations too much and allowing too many digressions is always delicate. Early in treatment I allow more digressions. Sometimes I learn something important during a digression. As I get to know clients better, I can redirect them when a digression seems to be a distraction.

Treatment with older clients involves more repetitions, both of things they say to me and what I say to them. We sometimes go over a point several times. Although this process may feel repetitious to the therapist, it does not to the client.

The slow pace and repetitions may partly reflect the learning process for some older clients. Older people generally learn more slowly and thus benefit more from repetitions and a slower pace. They may also make decisions more cautiously, which may contribute to the slower pace (see Chapter 2). Clients who are not sophisticated about how to use therapy also may make slower progress.

A counterforce is sometimes at work: Older clients are frequently more goal oriented in their treatment than younger people. They want to work on some specific problem or issue and then move on with their lives. Of course, older people who are excessively dependent or for whom the therapist is their main social outlet prolong therapy as long as possible. But many older clients are comfortable with time-limited and goal-oriented treatment.

The slower pace of treatment with older people runs counter to the emphasis on managed care and controlling costs that dominates health care in the United States. Up to now, Medicare has allowed unlimited numbers of weekly sessions, but older people who have enrolled in a managed care plan may experience some restrictions. If health care for older people moves more in the direction of managed care, there are likely to be more restrictions on the number of sessions the therapist can offer. We should also note that the session limits that have been adopted by managed care plans are based on the expectations of how quickly younger clients might respond to treatment—and even then, the number of sessions is often unrealistically low. Guidelines for older people need to reflect the fact that the pace of treatment is slower. In the end, providing an adequate amount of treatment in the first place is the best approach because it saves costs later on.

Using Written Records

Because therapy places a considerable load on a client's short-term memory, some therapists recommend approaches that help older people compensate for deficiencies in memory (e.g., Zeiss & Steffen, 1996). Using written notes, summaries, reminders, and similar approaches can reduce the load on a client's memory. Forms for recording events, behaviors, or feelings between sessions can also compensate for memory problems. Sometimes, though, the issue is not memory but difficulty initiating and accepting change.

Giving Clients Control

For many older clients, actual or perceived threats to their independence is an important issue. As part of how I deal with these threats, I allow clients to take control of some therapy issues, for example, sometimes allowing clients to control how frequently they see me. After an initial period of weekly visits that allows us to make progress on the presenting problems, the client may decide to come biweekly or just once a month. There are several reasons why they may want to reduce the frequency of visits. In some instances, they may not want to overuse their resources. Medicare covers only 50% of their costs, and the copayments they make can strain their budgets. In other cases, it has seemed that clients did not want to indulge themselves by coming too frequently. Rather, they space out contacts and, paradoxically, may place more value on the sessions than if they came weekly.

These intermittent clients use their sessions productively. They get clarification of what has been going on in their lives, or they get help sorting out medical or other problems they may have been having. They also know that they can come more often in the event that they face pressing issues.

Coordination of Treatment with Community Services

Many older clients need help or assistance to remain safely at home. When families cannot provide this help, community services can sometimes fill the gap.

Therapists need to know what type of help is available and where to find it. In some countries that have national health care and social service systems, such as Sweden and France, linking people to community services is a relatively easy task. A coordinating agency carries out this task, and government financing helps make services affordable. The United States, by contrast, has a piecework system of public and private services that varies to some extent from state to state and even from community to community. However, several sources of information can be helpful. Every community is served by an Area Agency on Aging, which can provide information on the types of programs for older people and their costs and what types of assistance may be available to help pay for them. Some Area Agencies also provide care management. They conduct an assessment of the person's functional needs and then identify appropriate services. Care management is also available from some service agencies and from independent providers. We have frequently worked with a private care manager who helps older people and their families identify appropriate services to bring into the home.

Another valuable source of information about local services is voluntary organizations, such as the Alzheimer's Association or similar groups that focus on a specific problem or illness. Local chapters of voluntary organiza-

TABLE 8.1. Community Services for Frail Older People

- Care management
- Lunch programs (often located in senior citizen centers)
- Home-delivered meals (e.g., "Meals on Wheels")
- Transportation (usually for doctor's visits, but sometimes for shopping and other special needs)
- Home health (nursing care for medical problems)
- Home care (nurse's aides providing help with activities of daily living)
- Adult day service programs
- In-home respite care
- Overnight respite care
- Home modification and repair (usually arranged through the Area Agency on Aging)
- Caregiver programs

tions frequently maintain lists of agencies that provide assistance and may even be helpful in identifying physicians or other professionals who work well with people suffering from a particular disorder.

The types of services that may be available to support someone at home are shown in Table 8.1. For healthy older persons, there are opportunities for activities with other older people, such as in senior centers or through volunteer programs.

Duration of Treatment

Most treatment with older adults is problem focused and has a relatively brief duration of between 4 and 6 months. Sometimes, the pattern is more episodic. The initial problem-focused treatment lasts for a few months, and then the client returns at periodic intervals to address changes in his or her situation.

TREATMENT AT PERIODIC INTERVALS

Melissa, age 70, was caring for her husband of more than 40 years, who had a VaD. Melissa came to therapy regularly for about 6 months, then she felt that her needs had been met, so we terminated. Perhaps a year would go by, and then a new problem would bring her back for a few months. This pattern has now gone on for more than 15 years. When her husband was placed in a nursing home, I did some consultation with the staff on his behalf. Three of Melissa's children married, her husband died, and several grandchildren were born. Her most recent return to therapy was precipitated by depression in reaction to a hip fracture that required surgery and a long, slow rehabilitation period.

I see a small number of older clients on a long-term basis. These clients often have chronic physical and mental health problems and have either no family at all or relatives who live at some distance. Therapy serves as a sounding board for relatively isolated individuals. It helps them address problems and concerns and probably reduces their inappropriate use of medical services for their psychological complaints. I often see these clients monthly, or as needed when problems develop. The role that these long-term clients often place me in is that of the valued child who is supportive and accessible. I can accept this role while keeping in place appropriate boundaries on my time and involvement.

Long-Term Clients

Occasionally, clients work their way into our hearts. One such was Morris. We introduced Morris and his wife Sally in Chapter 6, when Sally came for an evaluation of dementia symptoms. Morris began treatment by being very defensive about "needing" therapy, and with his anxiety and obsessive–compulsive tendencies, he needed to control the therapy in the beginning. As I met and passed his many tests and was able to treat him respectfully and honestly, he became more open about his problems. After about 4 years of weekly meetings in the office, where Morris would berate himself for not paying his bills, he agreed to allow me to visit him and his wife at home, and then he would write the bills as he talked with me. One of the major barriers that had to be crossed was allowing someone into his home, which had literally not been cleaned in a decade, and where there were impressive piles and collections of everything from recordings to newsletters to junk mail and, everywhere, books. For the next 5 years, I made weekly home visits, which spanned the period from Sally's decline into her dementia to her placement in a nursing home and subsequent death to a surgery and recuperation that Morris had and then to his bypass surgery, which led to his final months in a nursing home. In all, our weekly contacts spanned about 14 years. His daughter, who lives about 4 hours away, became an adjunct to treatment as his health declined and still maintains occasional contact.

Frequent Themes in Therapy

The topics and themes that are likely to emerge in therapy with older clients are sometimes different from those with younger clients (Knight, 1996). Four themes that are not typically encountered with younger people or that take a different form with older clients are (1) medical issues, (2) dealing with "what if" questions, (3) death and dying, and (4) relationship issues and sexuality.

Medical Issues

The focus of treatment with older clients is often on medical problems. Just as I take medical issues into account when conducting an assessment and coordinating treatment with physicians, I also spend time understanding and interpreting the ongoing medical problems and experiences clients have.

Emphasis on medical problems takes different forms. I spend a lot of time gathering information, explaining, and clarifying. Sometimes I help the physician understand the symptoms the client is presenting; sometimes I help the client understand what the physician is recommending. I often play a consulting role with clients, going over with them what the physician has recommended and examining their choices. If a client is confused about what the doctor said, I offer to consult with the physician and get a copy of the medical records so that I can go over them with the client. I do not supplant the physician, but I have the time to help clients understand their medical problems and treatment alternatives.

Generally, older clients present themselves to physicians in the same way they do to therapists, that is, they have trouble getting to the point and identifying which complaints are important. As a result, physicians sometimes stop paying attention and may fail to identify important new symptoms. To deal with this problem, I teach clients a set of strategies for communicating with their doctors. I developed this approach based on conversations with physicians about how they evaluate and respond to patients' symptoms. Physicians have been trained to listen for certain kinds of information. When they do not hear that information or get distracted by too many complaints or digressions, they become frustrated and even lose interest. I teach clients how to phrase their complaints so that physicians are likely to pay attention. It could be argued that physicians should be skilled enough at interviewing patients to draw out the information they need, and some certainly are. Nonetheless, it is more practical to instruct patients how to present their problems effectively than to wait for physicians to change how they practice.

The starting point for effective communication with a physician is to plan an agenda for each visit. The agenda should be limited to one or two problems. Physicians often stop listening when the patient brings a long list of complaints, dismissing the patient in their minds as a hypochondriac or complainer. The problems should be relatively recent, typically originating within the preceding 3 months. Physicians tend to lose interest in a problem that has become chronic, believing that there is less they can do to treat it. I help clients to be as specific as possible when presenting symptoms, for example, stating "I have had a sticking pain in my left shoulder" rather than "I have had lots of pain recently." Clients should also plan the questions they want to ask the doctor. Some clients may need to work on their listening skills so that they can process what the doctor says.

I also talk with my clients about the implicit rules that physicians have about how the interaction with a patient should go. Even though the doctor may start the conversation by asking "How are you feeling?" he or she is really interested in finding out what the patient's main concern is. Getting to the point and being specific helps the interaction. Patients, however, should let the physician ask the first question rather than launching into a list of complaints.

Besides these specific suggestions, I help clients understand the time pressures modern physicians face and that they cannot expect the more leisurely and personalized care they received in the past. These procedures help people present information to a physician in a clear and organized manner. That creates a favorable impression and also gives doctors the information they need to make a diagnosis and develop a treatment plan. With the immense financial pressures on medical practice, the physician's time is at a premium. The more efficiently patients can present their concerns, the better the process will work.

Whether illness contributes in a primary or a secondary way to psychological distress, psychotherapy can be an effective component of treatment. I address both the emotional consequences of illness and the limitations that the illness has placed on daily life. Sometimes depression is a barrier to seeking treatment or rehabilitation opportunities that may be helpful. When a problem is not reversible or is life threatening, therapists can help clients sort through the variety of practical decisions they are facing and come to terms with the situation.

Medical problems come into play in a direct way in many cases. Clients with whom I work for any length of time invariably experience an unexpected illness, such as a heart attack or stroke. Their therapists need to be able to deal with clients' health changes, conveying support during the acute phase of their illnesses and then helping them maximize their potential for recovery. Therapists working with older people need to be comfortable talking about illness and disability and dealing with problems that sometimes cannot be changed.

Some clients talk excessively about somatic symptoms. I have heard more about digestive problems and bowel movements from older clients than I ever wanted to know in a lifetime. It is important to listen to these complaints, however, to find out whether something psychological is leading a client to be so focused on a somatic symptom or whether there might be a real medical problem. Interestingly, many somaticizing older clients do not think of themselves as frail or vulnerable. Rather, they are not good at identifying which complaints are important.

When treating older clients with serious illnesses or disabilities, clinicians sometimes focus on how they would feel in that kind of situation. They may identify the situation as hopeless or overwhelming and so might fail to recognize what the client might be feeling or whether there are realistic alternatives to managing the problem. Learning about the illness and the treatment possibilities, however, can contribute to effective psychotherapeutic interventions.

One of us (SHZ) developed a psychological services program for a comprehensive rehabilitation center for people with vision problems. At the beginning, I did not know much about vision loss and rehabilitation, and I found myself at a loss for words when clients were depressed over their deficits. When they said things such as that their lives were no longer worth living because they could not see, part of me thought that they could possibly be right. As I gained more knowledge about the problem, however, I became familiar with the many ways people can compensate for vision loss and engage in satisfying and meaningful activities. I came to recognize that thoughts of hopelessness and helplessness, though having a basis in reality, also reflected the kinds of exaggerated negative appraisals typical of depression. My role became helping clients overcome their sense of loss and depression so that they could explore the full range of options available.

Dealing with "What Ifs"

Another difference with older clients is the amount of time they dwell on possible risks, or "what ifs." This preoccupation is often found when people do not have many activities or a lot of other things that they are thinking about. They focus on one event far in the future and worry about all the possible things that can go wrong along the way leading up to that event. As an example, an older woman is planning to move from her house to a condominium because it will be easier for her to manage. Although she wants to make the move, she is spinning a series of "what ifs," in which everything starts to go wrong; for example, her house does not sell soon enough or sells too soon or she will have difficulty getting movers to deliver her things when she needs them. As a result, she dwells on the thought that the move will turn out badly.

Cognitive interventions for "what ifs" are generally possible. Continuing with the example of moving, the therapist can begin by suggesting that it is not possible to solve hypothetical problems that might arise in the future. There are too many unknowns that will come up—for example, when the client's house will sell—before the situation reaches the bad outcome that she is imagining. Instead, the therapist would encourage her to focus on the next steps (e.g., getting the house ready to show to prospective buyers) and not worry about a hypothetical outcome. Taking care of the next steps will create a feeling of being in control and make a positive outcome more likely. In other words, it is possible to help people differentiate between immediate risks that they need to do something about now and far-off risks that are hard to plan for because many other things have to happen along the way to reach that point.

Many older people are concerned about what would happen to them if they fell or needed help for other types of emergencies. People who already have lost some functioning are particularly concerned about what will happen to them if they decline further. Probably the biggest "what if" is the fear of going into a nursing home. I work with these clients to develop scenarios that they are comfortable with about the type of help they can use should they need it. Finding ways of controlling what might happen reduces feelings of helplessness.

Death and Dying

Older clients, even healthy ones, are often concerned about their own deaths or about the deaths of people close to them. As Knight (1996) points out, much of the literature on this topic is based on case studies of younger people with illnesses that have predictable trajectories, such as cancer. Older people can have more varied courses of decline. They also may have different ways of dealing with death. Some older people may feel fear and anxiety about death, but these feelings do not seem as common as among younger individuals. Although not afraid of dying, they are often concerned about the circumstances of their deaths. They do not want to endure painful or unnecessary medical procedures and may want to pass away at home rather than in the hospital. They may question why they have been left behind when others have died or believe they cannot go on with their lives. People may also have unfinished emotional business with their families or issues that they want to resolve before they die. These issues can be value laden for both therapist and client. The most desirable therapeutic stance is one of neutrality, allowing the individual the freedom to express his or her own beliefs and explore the possibilities.

Therapists need to be comfortable talking about death and dying and letting clients know they can talk about these issues. Someone who is uncomfortable talking about death and dying will convey that discomfort to clients. Therapists also have to know where they stand personally on end-of-life issues. They need to come to terms with their own beliefs and feelings so that they do not distort or misinterpret what clients say or feel and do not let their own beliefs interfere with clients' making their own decisions.

It is also possible to be too focused on issues of death and dying. One of us (SHZ) once supervised a doctoral student who had a great deal of interest in death and dying. When the student's first client began focusing on these issues, it seemed to be a happy coincidence that the client's concerns matched the therapist's interests. When her subsequent clients also began dwelling on death and dying instead of on their presenting problems, however, it became apparent that the therapist was shaping their responses to what she believed was the main issue, rather than letting them define their concerns in their own way.

Therapists also have to be prepared to lose clients. One of the consequences of empathy is that we get attached to our clients. Seeing people who are declining and who will ultimately die is not easy and raises complex feelings in us. These losses can feel like the death of a good friend. We come to know clients well and are very involved in their lives. But with our older clients, death is not just a loss but can be the culmination of a process that ends suffering or frees them from a life they would not want to live.

A very important part of our work as therapists is helping clients negotiate this last transition. We are there to be supportive and to help clients deal with the medical system and any family issues that might arise. In this role, it is very important to stay focused on the quality of life. Most clients do not want their lives artificially prolonged. They reach a point at which they are ready to let go, and our role is to be an advocate for them. To do that, we have to be comfortable talking with them and the people around them about death and with the decision to let them go when it is time.

Letting Go When a Client Dies

There are many textures to death. The hardest death of a client that I experienced was a 21-year-old woman who died in an automobile accident. That death was sudden, unexpected, and off-time in the life span. That does not describe my older clients. For them, death is often a relief; they are ready to go.

I was driving to visit a long-standing client, Eve, who had moved to a nursing home in the previous month because of multiple health problems that made it impossible for her to manage on her own. Her health was declining rapidly, and this proud woman could now do very little by herself and had to receive help for most of her daily needs. As I drove, I thought to myself that this was this last time I would make this trip. It was a feeling that the end was near. I felt sad but also relieved for her, because she was ready to die. Eve passed away within the week, before my next visit.

When appropriate, I attend clients' funerals, both for myself and to respect my client and his or her family. We return to this issue in Chapter 15 when we discuss advance directives.

Relationship Issues and Sexuality

Though old age is often a time of losses, it is also a period in life when important relationships continue and even when new relationships form. Older clients may be concerned about working out problems in a long-standing relationship or developing new relationships. They may want to address conflict with a spouse or child, or they may seek help for family strains that have emerged as the result of recent life changes.

Sexuality and sexual feelings are not frequently part of treatment, but therapists need to be aware that they can emerge as an important issue. Clinicians can be helpful in a number of ways. They need to convey acceptance of a discussion of sexual feelings. Because of stereotypes about sexuality and aging, some older people believe that they should not have these feelings or should not talk about them. Several years ago, one of us (SHZ) conducted an initial assessment with an older woman who was concerned that she might have a sexually transmitted disease. She had previously raised this issue with her doctor, who dismissed her concern, saying that that was impossible for someone her age. In the history she gave me, however, she said she had recently had unprotected sex with someone she did not know well, and so there was a foundation for her concern. Although this is an extreme example of stereotypical thinking about aging and sex, it underscores the importance of recognizing that older people have sexual feelings and sexual activity. As therapists, we need to help them feel comfortable talking about these issues. We also need to be aware of generational differences in sexual beliefs and practices and the degree of comfort different people have in talking about their sexuality.

As with other problems of aging, sexual difficulties may have their origins in illnesses and/or medications, as well as in the normal processes of aging (see Agronin, 2004, for a review). The starting point for treatment is a careful medical assessment to determine the extent to which illness and medication may contribute to sexual difficulties. When obvious physiological factors do not play a major role in sexual difficulties, sex therapy techniques that have proven effective with younger clients can be used with older people (Whitlatch & Zarit, 1988). These techniques include the use of specific procedures and exercises to improve functioning, as well as helping clients recognize and adjust to changes that occur with aging, such as more time needed to become aroused. Although newer medications have shown promise in treatment of erectile dysfunction in men, reports of adverse effects suggest that these medications should be used with caution.

The Client–Therapist Relationship

Many of the issues presented in preceding sections have to do with not letting one's own biases enter the therapy situation. When working with older people, issues such as illness, death and dying, or sexuality, as well as age and generational factors, can kindle a therapist's own fears or prejudices (Knight, 1996). Therapists can also have idiosyncratic reactions toward clients based on relationship issues or conflicts they have in their personal lives. When undetected, such responses interfere with treatment.

Therapists can also develop a positive bias toward a client. In that situation, the therapist may overlook or minimize the client's problems or join the client in denying evidence of possible deficits in functioning. Sometimes new or inexperienced counselors see every negative attribution as part of the negative bias and stereotypes about old age. But as with any other group, the elderly include people who are not likable or who engage in self-defeating or otherwise aggravating patterns of behavior. An overly positive counselor will not recognize these behaviors or how they are contributing to the client's life problems.

Conversely, all therapists sometimes experience negative reactions to clients. These feelings are important because they can help identify ways in which the client is having trouble in other relationships. But therapists must be able to differentiate between reactions to the client's behavior and reactions that occur because the client in some way reminds the therapist of someone in his or her life. Therapists are obligated to work these issues out on their own or through consultation or supervision.

Clients, of course, can have a distorted view of the therapist (Knight, 1996). Therapists must learn to monitor how clients are responding to them and how to recognize and use distortions in treatment. Sometimes distortions reveal how clients approach other relationships in their lives. Rather than pointing out distortions to clients, which would not do any good, I develop strategies for using them. When clients view me in an exaggeratedly positive way, I build on that to encourage new behaviors. It is also possible to use negative reactions creatively. As an example, an older woman who is angry with her children may regard a therapist who is the same age as her children as taking their side or failing to understand her needs. Empathizing with this client, that is, agreeing that the therapist cannot really know or understand what the woman has gone through, can paradoxically provide understanding and build the basis of a therapeutic alliance.

Working with Couples

Most of the work I do with couples involves caregiving situations, but sometimes I do see them in therapy for other reasons. I may bring a husband or wife into treatment for strategic purposes for a few sessions. The reasons for doing so would be to gather more information about the client, to see how the couple interacts together, or to work on a specific and manageable problem (e.g., a husband helping his wife in one area).

Older couples do not frequently seek out marital therapy. Many conflicted couples have divorced long before later life. Others have accepted the limitations and even the ongoing conflict in their marriages. Many older people, of course, are happily married.

As with other problems in later life, one of the key questions is how long a couple's marriage has been troubled. Couples with long-standing marriages who seek treatment often have problems that go back many years. They fall into a pattern that might be called the "stable incompatible" marriage. What characterizes them is the predictable course of their communications and the certainty that they will not leave the marriage. They are still trying to win the old battles with each other after all these years. They carry around a list of grievances that may go back to the start of their relationship. Whenever one of them discusses a current problem, one or both of them will identify instances in the past that show how his or her spouse has been wrong all along. Each of them tries to engage the therapist into taking his or her side in these long-standing arguments. Therapists need to avoid getting drawn into alliances with one or the other person and should mainly comment empathically on these conflicts. The potential for change may be limited, because each person is too invested in his or her version of past wrongs to make a commitment to change. The best outcome often is a resolution of any current issues, for example, concerning medical problems or relationships with children, but without the expectation that this could now become a happily married couple.

One of the issues that may arise with older couples is whether forgiveness is possible. A spouse may still be angry because of a past affair or for a host of small grievances that were never resolved. Because the events that produced this anger were often far in the past, it is clear that whatever the other person had tried to do to gain forgiveness did not work. Exploring with the couple what it would take to forgive each other for past behavior can sometimes be helpful.

Some couples can make progress. Often, these are couples who were recently married. They often are struggling with adjustments to being married after a period of living single. Sexual difficulties can also be part of the picture. These couples are typically motivated and learn new skills readily.

As with younger clients who are seen in marital therapy, it is important to begin by finding out from each person individually whether there are secrets in the relationship, either past or present. Even though the couple is older, the possibility that one of them is currently having an extramarital affair should not be dismissed. Of course, in a couple that has been married for many years, there may be many secrets, though it can turn out that the other person knew the secret all along.

Treatment involves a combination of problem solving and enhancing communication skills. It is possible to improve communication with one another when both people are committed to doing so. Couples can learn to listen and respond in empathic and nonjudgmental ways. Improving listening skills and helping each understand his or her spouse's feelings can go a long way to improving the relationship.

WORKING WITH A STABLE INCOMPATIBLE COUPLE

Vernon (who was introduced earlier in this chapter) and his wife, Marcia, are a perfect example of the "stable incompatible" pattern. They married when Vernon was 27 and Marcia was 20. He was finishing graduate school and beginning his first professional job, and she had not finished her undergraduate degree. They began having children, and much later Marcia finished her degree and found her own career. One of their chronic problems was that Marcia had felt that Vernon had "stolen her youth." Whenever he would hear her say that, he would feel guilty, and when she said it, she felt angry. These two emotions characterized many of their interactions when they were alone. Curiously, they were both charming, intelligent people and could entertain beautifully and function at a very high level in their work and socially. They saved their unpleasant interactions for their most intimate moments.

When this type of interaction is uncovered, it is wise to set limited and achievable goals. It is possible to uncover the motivations for the interaction, but one or both individuals may not be able to let go of the strategies that they have employed in the relationship for so many years. However, it may be possible to utilize their strengths to help them meet the challenges that they will face with aging, specifically changes in health and dependency. In this case, Vernon became ill in his early 70s. Marcia was not a natural caregiver, but she found herself forced into that role. His role had been to be the provider and the authority figure, and he became depressed and anxious as he lost the ability to fulfill that role. Both were able to benefit from therapy, learning to respond differently to the present situation, without ever resolving or changing the underlying dynamic of their relationship.

Working with Difficult Clients

Over the years I have worked with many challenging and difficult older clients. Many of these individuals have personality disorders or other complex and chronic problems that are difficult to treat. They may have poor boundaries, may be emotionally demanding, or may verbally attack me during sessions. Or they may be so passive that no strategies seem able to get them to work on their problems. Of course, each therapist will find a different set of behaviors difficult. (See Chapter 5 for more details on personality disorders.)

These clients become an emotional drain on therapists, which can easily lead to feelings of burnout that spill over into work with other clients and into our personal lives. Although we do not have solutions that eliminate the stress of working with difficult clients, we have developed survival strategies that usually keep the strain within manageable limits.

The beginning point is having patience and realistic expectations for these individuals. They have spent a lifetime perfecting their maladaptive approaches and are not likely to change significantly. As noted earlier, our role is often to prevent their problems from getting worse, rather than achieving significant improvement. We need to be patient with the slow rate of change and the persistence of maladaptive behaviors.

Another important consideration is setting boundaries. Many of these patients become an emotional drain by making excessive time demands. I limit the length of sessions, the number of sessions (no more than once a week, and sometimes less often), and, particularly, the number of phone calls between sessions.

We can set boundaries successfully when we are fully engaged during sessions and provide a safe environment that focuses on the client's needs. Many of these clients sense when the therapist is not paying attention, which increases their anger and demands. It is also important not to convey rejection through verbal or nonverbal communications. These clients have usually experienced considerable rejection in their lives, and the perception of rejection from the therapist will make the sessions much more difficult.

It is also important to intervene cautiously with these clients. Changes can be difficult to make and may upset a precarious balance for someone who already has considerable problems with everyday life.

LEARNING FROM DIFFICULT CLIENTS

As difficult as clients with personality disorders can be, they can also teach us a great deal about ourselves as therapists and as people. They will challenge you to become a better listener and a more honest person and to stay educated in your interventions. When Pat started therapy she had been "fired" by many previous therapists. She demanded to know what theoretical orientation I was going to use and argued against anything that I offered. She fully expected to be rejected again and continuously challenged me as a therapist, devaluing my services and pointing out how unhelpful cognitive therapy was to her. At the outset, I let her know that I would not be "firing" her and that it would be Pat's decision as to when to leave therapy. There were times when Pat angrily stormed out of sessions early, and, when a session had been going well, at the very end she would announce that I had completely missed what was bothering her (again). Over the 12 years that she has been in therapy, these episodes have diminished, and the pattern of bringing her anger at the outside world into the session and directing it at me has diminished. She has taught me a great deal about how clients perceive their therapists, because she is so sensitive to the slightest change in my affect. She will comment on changes in the furniture, in dress, or in office staff, and those comments are often valid. It has been a challenge not to be defensive in the face of such direct critical comments, but I have to say that on balance, I have learned at least as much from her as she has from me.

As this example suggests, as therapists we need to know ourselves and our own limitations. There are certain clients that we do not do well with, and it is best not take them on in the first place. When we do take on a difficult client, we need to separate our reactions from their problems. Clients with boundary problems will push those boundaries with us. They will often distort what we say. Sometimes we can tell that something went wrong only when the client starts to berate us in a session or because the client cancels the next appointment. We need to be able to approach these encounters in a nondefensive way, knowing what we said and how we conveyed what we said. It does not help to be drawn into the client's dramas, because these behaviors have not been adaptive. Rather than letting clients push us away with their anger, we need to be patient with them and, when there is sufficient trust, use these examples to help build up more adaptive responses.

Finally, I try both to limit the number of difficult clients I am seeing at any one time and the number I see on any given day. That is easier to say, of course, than to implement. People suffering from chronic and severe problems tend to stay in treatment, whereas those with good adaptive skills and who are enjoyable to work with get better quickly and leave. After a while, anyone in practice with adults will find him- or herself with a caseload weighted toward difficult clients. When I find myself reaching that point, I am especially careful about which new cases I take. I know in the end that I have to set these limits in order to continue to provide good treatment to everyone I am seeing.

Developing Empirically Based Treatments for Older Adults

There has been an emphasis in recent years on using empirically validated treatments. Toward that goal, the Division of Clinical Psychology of the American Psychological Association developed criteria for empirically validated treatments (Chambless et al., 1996). Using these criteria, Gatz and her colleagues (1998) reviewed the literature on treatment of older people. Although there have been far fewer controlled outcome studies of older adults than of younger adults, many approaches met the standard for effective treatment (see also Gallagher-Thompson & Thompson, 1995; Scogin & McElreath, 1994).

We support this effort to develop a more rational, research-based body of knowledge for making treatment decisions. Much still has to be learned, however, about treatment of older people. As we review the empirical literature, there are three obvious limitations. First, most of the outcome studies have been conducted on people with a limited range of disorders, mainly depression. Second, treatment trials usually select participants who do not have other complications, particularly comorbidities with other psychiatric or medical disorders. Our experience tells us that these treatment protocols need to be modified when working with someone who has, for example, a comorbidity between depression and an Axis II disorder or when the client has significant medical problems. Third, there are individual differences in treatment response. Some people do not respond to the empirically validated treatment but may improve with other approaches. Thus, although it is a positive step to emphasize the use of empirically validated treatment, it would be premature to limit practice to only those treatments. That approach would stunt development of clinical practice by preventing therapists from taking new and creative directions in their work. It would also greatly limit the number of older people who could receive treatment to those who fall within diagnostic categories that have been investigated to date or who present without any complicating factors.

A responsible approach to treatment is to begin with an empirically validated treatment when appropriate for the presenting problem and person. If that treatment is not sufficient, then the therapist can proceed to another approach that has at least some evidence of efficacy. Each case can be viewed as a single-participant experiment. In other words, the therapist can monitor how the targeted symptoms respond to the treatment. That way it is possible to know whether the treatment is helping, and, if it is not, the therapist can try something else.

With the growth of managed care and other pressures to reduce the cost of treatment, we expect efforts to restrict psychotherapy with older adults. We believe in practicing responsibly, that is, not running up costs with unnecessary assessment or treatment and not prolonging treatment. By practicing responsibly, therapists can contribute valuable clinical findings on the uses of psychotherapy with older adults that justify the cost and point to the benefits that their clients receive.

The following two examples illustrate some of the unique features that form the foundation for treating older clients.

Helping a Client Maintain Control and Manage Medical Problems

This case illustrates the role medical problems play in treatment and how therapists can help their clients make decisions about their medical care. Roberta was previously introduced in Chapter 6. She had suffered a delirium when a physician changed a blood pressure medication she had been taking. She was referred for treatment to get help in her recovery from the delirium and to deal with the consequences of her health problems.

Roberta, age 76, suffered from multiple health problems. In her 60s she developed emphysema, and more recently, she had had heart bypass surgery. She suffered from hypertension and diabetes, and diabetic retinopathy was affecting her vision. Despite Roberta's health problems, she was completely independent, living in her own apartment in the community. One factor contributing to Roberta's good functioning was that she kept exact records of her health. In a notebook, she wrote down her vital signs, when she took each medication, and every calorie she ate. As a result, her diabetes was in very good control.

The initial plan was for short-term treatment to get Roberta back on an even keel. After making gradual progress over the course of several sessions, Roberta took control of the frequency of visits, setting appointments about 1 month apart. I could have insisted that a younger client come every week. But I believed that Roberta needed to feel in control of her life, so I let her set the frequency.

The focus of sessions initially was her anxiety that the delirium would return. Roberta had been greatly unnerved by feeling out of control during the delirium. It took her a year to feel competent again and not embarrassed over what she had said and done during the delirium. Gradually, the focus of treatment shifted to consultation on her medical problems. During the year I treated Roberta, all her medical doctors changed. Her therapist was the one constant for her during this time. Changing physicians is another frequent issue older clients face when their doctors retire or, as in this case, move out of the area. The readjustment to new physicians is often associated with anxiety, especially for someone whose medical condition is fragile. I helped Roberta understand the plans developed by her new doctors. For example, she went for the first time to see an optometrist about the vision problems caused by her diabetic retinopathy. After that visit, with her permission, I had the optometrist send over a copy of her records so that I could review them with her. I played a similar role with Roberta's other doctors. Although her problems were mainly medical, she had a component of anxiety that potentially could have made her condition worse. The monthly therapy visits, however, had a calming effect.

Other concerns arose as well. Winter driving worried Roberta. She did not want to drive in icy or snowy conditions but feared being completely cut off, unable to shop or get to the doctor. To deal with this concern, I introduced Roberta to a geriatric care manager, who could arrange help if she needed it. That winter turned out to be relatively mild, and she did not need a driver, but it relieved her anxiety to know she had someone to call.

Roberta's emphysema steadily worsened as time passed. She began using helpers, first to take her to the grocery store and later to buy food and bring it home to prepare meals for her. Finally, one day, during a home visit, she asked to have an ambulance called because she could not get her breath. She went from the hospital to a nursing home, where she died 2 months later. Until the end, Roberta directed her own care and determined how much help she wanted.

This case illustrates several typical features about treatment of an older person. First and foremost was the focus on the client's medical problems and my role in clarifying and helping her interpret what her doctors were doing, thereby lowering her overall anxiety. This case also shows that an older person can take control of the frequency of visits and other aspects of her treatment. Third, I linked Roberta to a community service, in this case, to a care manager who could arrange for a driver. Finally, I felt the loss with her death, as I do when I have become emotionally engaged with clients.

A LACK OF FOLLOW-THROUGH COMPLICATES THE COURSE OF A DISORDER

Myra, age 68, had become progressively anxious and depressed, though there was no clear precipitating event. Seeking treatment for the symptoms, Myra's family took her to a psychiatrist, who wrote a prescription and then went on vacation. When Myra's symptoms worsened on the medication and she could not get hold of the psychiatrist, the family had her hospitalized. After a brief examination by a hospital psychiatrist, Myra was given a major tranquilizer and a drug for a bipolar disorder. (There was no apparent history of manic depression, and the reason for prescribing these medications was not clear.) Her condition worsened on these medications, and she gradually withdrew and became inactive. Discharged from the hospital, Myra came under the care of a third psychiatrist, who changed the medications once again, this time to an antidepressant, a tranquilizer, and a sleeping pill. At this point, Myra's daughter contacted me for an assessment and treatment.

The initial session was conducted in Myra's home. Myra lived with her husband. Both of them had been very active in community organizations until her depression. I found her to be very depressed, but she gave no indication of cognitive impairment. She was spending most of her time in bed and was not engaging in self-care activities. Myra's husband was continuing his activities while providing assistance to her.

The treatment plan was psychotherapy for depression. I consulted with Myra's most recent psychiatrist, who decided to continue the current medications for a while (the change had been made quite recently) to determine whether they were having any effect. He did make one change, however, advising that Myra wean herself off the sleeping pill she was taking, as sleeping medications are most effective for short-term treatment of insomnia and could now be making her situation worse.

Treatment involved building an empathic relationship and utilizing behavioral and cognitive-behavioral strategies to reduce depression. A major goal of these approaches was to encourage Myra to resume activities that she had previously enjoyed and valued and to address negative beliefs that prevented her from increasing her level of activity. Because her husband was involved in helping her with self-care activities and in encouraging her to resume some of her former activities, I decided to hold one session a week with both of them and one session with Myra alone. In this manner, her husband could work with Myra in encouraging specific activities or in supporting the steps she was taking in treatment. Leaving him out would have left open the possibility that he would work at cross purposes with me or that Myra would resist his suggestions to become more active and therefore also resist my efforts. By holding a joint session, I could pursue a strategic approach that enlisted both husband and wife in agreed-on assignments. Myra showed gradual but steady improvement and was able to resume her normal activities.

___

This case incorporated several common features of therapy with older clients. A critical first step was coordinating psychotherapy with the use of psychotropic medications. A basic approach to psychotherapy for depression was initiated that used a family approach, as well as individual treatment. The complexity of this case is by no means typical, but it does indicate the types of knowledge and skill therapists must draw on when working with older clients.

CONCLUSIONS

In this chapter, we have presented a foundation for psychological treatment of older people. Is psychotherapy with older people different from treatment with younger age groups? In many instances, treatment proceeds in similar ways and is equally effective. But there are subtle and not so subtle differences. The psychotherapist needs to draw on a wider range of skills when working with older clients. Medical comorbidities are likely to be of far greater importance with older clients, as is an understanding of the client's family system. Goals may be more focused and limited, and treatment may proceed more slowly than with younger clients. More needs to be learned about the efficacy of various treatments and the conditions under which treatment response can be maximized. Nonetheless, a growing body of clinical studies and controlled research is emerging that indicates that psychotherapy is an effective treatment with older people. In subsequent chapters, we explore how psychotherapy approaches have been adapted for treatment of specific problems.

CHAPTER 9

Treatment of Depression

A growing body of evidence indicates that treatment of older depressed people is effective, whether with medications, psychotherapy, or a combination of the two. Despite these optimistic findings, older people frequently do not receive optimal treatment, or any treatment at all. In this chapter we examine treatment for depression, with particular attention to features of treatment that are unique or different when working with older people. We begin with a discussion of psychotherapy for depression, focusing on three empirically validated treatments: behavioral therapy, cognitive-behavioral therapy, and interpersonal psychotherapy. Next we turn to how therapy and medication can be used in combination for positive results. We then focus on other treatment considerations, including comorbidity of medical problems, involvement of the family, and use of electroconvulsive therapy (ECT). We end with case studies that demonstrate how treatment is implemented.

PSYCHOTHERAPY AS A TREATMENT FOR DEPRESSION

There is now considerable evidence that psychotherapy is an effective treatment for depressive disorders in later life. Although the literature on treatment of depression among older people is limited, Scogin and McElreath (1994) reviewed 17 studies that used a control group and found that psychotherapy was reliably associated with decreases in depression. In fact, the effect size (a statistical estimate of the amount of improvement, expressed in standard deviation units) was somewhat greater in the studies of older clients than that reported for younger clients. Older clients receiving psychotherapy improved, on average, three-quarters of a standard deviation on depression measures. Gatz and colleagues (1998) also found consistent evidence that different types of psychotherapy were effective with older clients.

Psychotherapy also has been found to be as effective as antidepressant medication in treatment of depression, with some indication that combined therapy may be slightly more effective than either approach by itself (e.g., Arean & Cook, 2002; DeRubeis, Gelfand, Tang, & Simons, 1999; Elkin et al., 1989; Hirschfeld et al., 2002; Reynolds et al., 1992; Thompson, Coon, Gallagher-Thompson, Sommer, & Koin, 2001). Combined treatment may be particularly useful in preventing relapses in older people with a history of recurrent depression (Reynolds et al., 1999).

We focus on three psychotherapy approaches that show considerable empirical evidence of efficacy: behavioral therapy for depression, developed by Peter Lewinsohn and his associates (Lewinsohn et al., 1992); cognitive-behavioral treatment, developed by Aaron Beck and colleagues (1979); and interpersonal psychotherapy (IPT), developed by Gerald Klerman and associates (1984). Although they draw on somewhat different theoretical traditions, these three treatments for depression share many points of similarity, suggesting that some techniques may be an essential part of any intervention with depressed clients. The therapist plays an active role in structuring sessions and building a collaborative relationship with clients to confront symptoms in a direct way. The focus is generally on the here and now, that is, the immediate events and beliefs associated with feelings of depression. All have a strong psychoeducational component, teaching clients how their own actions affect their moods and how they can change their moods. Clients are helped to break out of the cycle of depression by changing behaviors in their daily lives and thinking differently about themselves and other people. To do that, clients are assigned tasks to perform between sessions as a way of either gathering data for treatment or implementing new actions. This convergence of techniques in the three approaches suggests that the method of treatment—direct, structured, focused on the here and now—may be as important to positive outcomes as the specific theoretical orientation.

As discussed in Chapter 8, a somewhat slower pace of treatment, the use of written assignments and other aids to offset memory problems, and the careful handling of the therapeutic relationship are all helpful when treating older clients. Depending on the client, a therapist can focus on increasing or decreasing specific behaviors, on automatic thoughts, or on social relationships. As in any situation, therapists should monitor a client's progress closely to ensure that treatment is having a positive effect on depressive symptoms.

All the treatments are also time limited, between 12 and 20 sessions, although additional sessions are sometimes needed. The time-limited nature of the treatment is welcomed by some older clients who may be concerned about the cost of treatment. For those clients who want to use therapy as a substitute for relationships, each treatment has ways of redirecting them to people in their lives.

Behavioral Therapy for Depression

Building on the work of Peter Lewinsohn (Lewinsohn et al., 1992), a behavioral therapy for depression has been developed that has had good outcome results with both younger and older adults (Gallagher-Thompson & Thompson, 1995; Scogin & McElreath, 1994). The starting point for this approach is observation of what depressed people do and don't do. As Lewinsohn and his associates detailed in a series of studies, depressed people engage in fewer behaviors than do nondepressed people, particularly pleasant or reinforcing behaviors—what Lewinsohn calls "pleasant events" (PE). This low rate of output of behaviors that are reinforced or reinforcing leads to a vicious cycle in which mood is lowered, further decreasing the output of behavior, and so on. Given this association between mood and pleasant events, the most parsimonious approach to treatment of depression is to increase the frequency with which clients engage in behaviors they find enjoyable.

As experienced clinicians know, just telling clients to change their behavior is usually not successful. Lewinsohn and his colleagues (1992) have developed a sophisticated approach that goes beyond simple advice and facilitates change. Seven features of treatment are particularly relevant to treatment of older, depressed patients:

Involving Clients as Active Participants in Treatment

Clients are actively involved in the treatment process. Lewinsohn's model includes a strong psychoeducational component, which instructs clients about behavioral causes of depressive symptoms and about the process of change. Treatment begins with an explanation of the rationale of the approach, in effect instructing clients how they can use therapy to get better. The therapist explains that the client's mood is related to everyday activities. Engaging in more pleasant or rewarding activities will improve mood, whereas engaging in fewer of those activities worsens mood. Depression is viewed as the result of a vicious cycle in which a person may feel sad because of events in his life, then decrease pleasant activities, feel worse as a result, and then decrease activities further. Treatment involves breaking out of this vicious cycle. As treatment proceeds, clients become increasingly active, completing various assignments and tasks. This approach contributes directly to reducing depression because it breaks the cycle of passivity and withdrawal. It may also foster skills to improve coping or self-efficacy, thereby reducing the probability of a recurrence of depression.

Contracting with Clients

Of course, encouraging depressed patients to be more active and their actually doing so are two different matters. A key part of the treatment is developing a contract with clients through which they agree to perform certain tasks. In the context of an empathic and accepting relationship, the therapist can work with clients to develop specific plans for action and to gain their agreement to try out these steps. Although behavioral therapy can sometimes be presented in didactic ways, we have found it better to use a collaborative approach with clients, an approach that is more likely to gain compliance and lead to clients taking more responsibility for their own behavior.

One of the specific challenges when working with older adults is differentiating between the real and perceived limitations associated with old age and disability. Older clients often make a convincing case that they cannot do more than they are currently doing. This is where the therapist's knowledge of various medical conditions and the prospects for rehabilitation are essential. A naïve therapist can be persuaded that an older person *cannot* really do more, because of illness or disability, when there are opportunities for intervention. With experience, it becomes possible to identify when feelings of helplessness and hopelessness are exaggerated responses to disability. Almost all cases present opportunities to increase the level of pleasant activities. One way to engage reluctant clients is to frame treatment as an experiment to find out how much they can do, making sure to proceed in small steps. Throughout this process, therapists have to perform a balancing act—maintaining empathy yet understanding that the client can do more. Without empathy, therapists will come across as harsh or punitive; without goals, clients will remain mired in their depressive beliefs. We return to this issue later in the chapter.

Developing Graded and Specific Tasks

A major feature that contributes to the success of behavioral approaches is breaking clients' goals into a series of graded tasks. Initial tasks need to be planned carefully, with the dual purposes of gaining compliance and producing some initial, albeit small, success. Once clients successfully complete a task, it becomes easier to implement the next part of the treatment plan. Tasks in a treatment plan should be graded; that is, they should proceed from simple steps that are likely to be successful to more complex and challenging behaviors. Initial tasks should not be difficult or complex to perform and should have a high probability of success. For example, a depressed older person might be asked to exercise for 5 minutes a day. Although the client might have exercised previously for longer periods of time, the client and the therapist might decide that 5 minutes is an amount that the client can manage right now. In addition to keeping initial tasks simple, they also need to be specific (e.g., what type of exercise) and scheduled for a definite time and place.

Clients may maintain that doing such simple tasks cannot help them with such a large problem as depression. They may also compare their performance to what they previously could do. In these instances, the therapist can explain that these tasks are building blocks, the first steps that need to be taken in treatment, and that they will make it possible to address more serious problems.

The main problem an inexperienced therapist encounters is not spending enough time working out the details of assignments. A poorly specified task that does not include when, where, and how often the task is to be performed leaves an opening for the client to fail. Depressed clients avoid or postpone plans that are overly ambitious or vague.

Monitoring Mood and Behavior

Clients learn to monitor their own moods and activities and to observe connections between what they do and how they are feeling. These steps are essential for treatment. They enable clients to take more control over their moods and to become active in the treatment of their depression.

Clients monitor their moods by providing a summary score each day of how they are feeling. Depression scales can be used during office visits to provide additional information on the course of symptoms. Clients also record specific behaviors, including pleasant and aversive events. Working with these records, the therapist can demonstrate how mood varies in relation to activities.

Increasing Pleasant Events

The central element of treatment is to increase the frequency with which clients engage in pleasant activities. As a first step, the clinician works with the client to identify what events or activities are potentially reinforcing, that is, events the client experiences as pleasant. Pleasant events differ from simply telling someone to get more active or choosing a set of activities for them. They are activities that reflect the client's own preferences, not those of the therapist or anyone else who might have an opinion about what is best for the client.

Lewinsohn and his colleagues (Lewinsohn & Libet, 1972; Lewinsohn & MacPhillamy, 1974) developed the Pleasant Events Schedule, a list of more than 300 activities that people experience as pleasant. Clients respond to each activity by indicating how frequently they have engaged in it recently and how enjoyable they find it. A shorter form has been developed specifically for use with older clients (Teri & Lewinsohn, 1982).

The second step is to obtain a baseline of the frequency with which clients engage in activities they find pleasurable. Usually the rate is quite low for depressed clients. Sometimes variations appear during the baseline period. The therapist may be able to use the records to point out that small increases in pleasant activities are associated with improved mood.

After establishing the baseline, therapist and client develop a plan to increase the number of pleasant activities. As noted, this plan must start with simple and manageable tasks and be specific. Written schedules and assignments are used as reminders for clients of any age and may be particularly helpful for older clients (Zeiss & Steffen, 1996). Schedules serve as a concrete way for clients and therapists alike to monitor the progress of treatment.

As clients increase the frequency of pleasant activities, their moods generally begin to improve. This is often a critical point in therapy. Clients may come back after doing a behavioral assignment and say that they do not feel better, yet they look better and rate their mood as improved compared with prior ratings. What they are telling the therapist is that they do not yet feel as they used to. Client and therapist review together the records of mood and pleasant activities to confirm the association between what the client is doing and what he or she is feeling. The therapist may reframe what clients are saying to reflect the fact that they are still in the early stages of treatment. By pointing out that his or her mood has improved, the therapist can assure a client that he or she is on the right track and that continuing in this direction will lead to further improvement.

Once their moods begin improving, clients can go on to other tasks that may be more difficult, including addressing aversive events in their lives, dealing with problems in social relationships, and treating cognitive features of depression, such as negative thoughts.

Decreasing Aversive Events

In a comparable way to pleasant events, Lewinsohn and associates (1992) assess which activities or events clients find unpleasant. Events are defined as aversive based on clients' perceptions, not on an arbitrary classification system. An activity such as housecleaning can be experienced differently by different clients. Some find it pleasant to clean the house, whereas others experience it as aversive. An instrument similar to the Pleasant Events Schedule has been developed for assessing aversive events (Lewinsohn et al., 1992). The therapist focuses on reducing unpleasant or aversive events once a client's mood has begun to improve.

Again, it is important to begin with problems that can be managed readily or problems over which clients have some control. For example, a client may want to have fewer arguments with her daughter. That is a goal that may require the client to change her behavior in complex ways, and it may be partly out of her control, as her daughter must also respond differently to her. As a result, it might be better to start with a simpler task over which the client has more control (e.g., limiting the amount of time she cleans the house so that she has more time for other activities).

Developing Cognitive and Social Skills

The behavioral model of treating depression also focuses on changing beliefs or cognitions that contribute to depression and on improving social skills, such as becoming more assertive or learning how to communicate more effectively with other people. These features are dealt with extensively in the other two treatment approaches, discussed later.

Applications of Behavioral Treatment for Older People

Zeiss and Steffen (1996) summarize the advantages of the behavioral approach for treatment of older people. The therapist is a collaborator with clients, developing a supportive relationship and encouraging them to be actively involved. The therapist brings one type of expertise into the relationship concerning treatment methods, but clients are the experts in their own experiences and skills. This approach is very useful with older people who are not psychologically minded. Behavioral treatment contains a large element of common sense and an absence of psychological jargon, which appeals to many clients. For older clients, record keeping and scheduling can reduce concerns about failing memory. Finally, treatment is time limited, which reduces the trepidation many older people have about the cost of treatment and counters the common stereotype of psychotherapy as open-ended and always long term.

Cognitive-Behavioral Therapy for Depression

Although it shares many elements with behavioral therapy, cognitive-behavioral therapy differs by giving primacy to the role of cognitions in the development of mood problems. (See Chapter 8 for a brief overview of CBT with older patients.)

Cognitive-behavioral therapy deals with a process that is central to later life: how people respond to setbacks and losses in their lives. Bad things *will* have happened to one's older clients, and so it will seem natural to an inexperienced therapist that they are depressed. From a cognitive perspective, however, it is important to distinguish between feeling sad, which is appropriate after a loss, and depression, which depends on exaggerated or distorted interpretations of the events in one's life. The strength of a cognitive-behavioral approach is that the therapist has strategies that encourage clients to tackle their practical problems while using that process to help them understand how their interpretations of events have contributed to their depression.

Beginning Steps in Cognitive-Behavioral Therapy

As in behavioral therapy, the therapist begins with an explanation of how cognitive therapy works. The therapist explains that people's interpretations of events affect how they feel.

Also as in behavioral therapy, the focus is on daily behaviors and activities. Focusing on an activity is a good way to produce some immediate relief from depression, giving clients more energy to work on cognitive dimensions of depression. Working on activities also generates examples of the client's typical thought patterns or ways of interpreting events.

The cognitive therapist uses graded task assignments. After clients agree to a task, the therapist can have them cognitively rehearse the steps involved in carrying it out to identify potential obstacles (Beck et al., 1979). The obstacles that are identified in this way may be practical or cognitive. The therapist and client worked together on these obstacles so that the assignment is eventually carried out.

Cognitive Dysfunctions

The main emphasis in treatment is on identifying characteristic thought patterns, that is, how clients typically appraise the events in their lives. People with depression have thought patterns that are marked by logical errors that lead to incorrect attributions about experiences and, consequently, to feelings of depression. For example, an older woman had interviewed for a job and had not heard from the company. She concluded that she had not gotten the job, that companies preferred hiring only younger women, and that she would never get a job. That is certainly a possibility, but the client did not know whether that was the reason the company had failed to call back. The therapist encouraged her to test her inferences by calling the company. It turned out that they had been trying to call her back for another interview. Her incorrect inferences (that she had not gotten the job) led to exaggerated or catastrophic interpretations and to intense feelings of depression.

In cognitive-behavioral therapy, clients are taught to recognize and then record these "automatic" thoughts. By writing these thoughts down as close to the occurrence of an event as possible, clients learn to recognize thought processes that trigger depressed feelings. Once dysfunctional thought patterns are identified, therapist and client work collaboratively to test the beliefs behind them.

The following dialogue illustrates the process of treatment with cognitive-behavioral therapy.

> CLIENT: I feel all alone in the world. My husband is dead, and since we never had children, I don't have anyone to look after me.
>
> THERAPIST: Who do you see on a day-to-day basis?
>
> CLIENT: Well, my neighbors in the apartment building, but they have enough problems of their own.
>
> THERAPIST: Do you see any of your relatives?
>
> CLIENT: I talk to my brothers every week and my niece comes by to take me out nearly every week. But they have their own families.

THERAPIST: Do you do anything in the community?

CLIENT: I want to go to Senior Citizens, but I haven't gotten there yet. When the weather is good, I go to church.

THERAPIST: So it sounds as if you really are lonely for your husband, but when you look at your day-to-day life, there are a number of people you are in contact with.

CLIENT: I guess I'm not completely alone, but I am lonely.

By examining the evidence, the therapist shows that the client's extreme statement that she is all alone in the world is not accurate. Extreme statements result in strong feelings of sadness and hopelessness. Being lonely is associated with negative feelings, but these feelings are not as strong or immobilizing as they were when the client viewed herself as being all alone in the world. This example also illustrates that the therapist does not dispute with the client but instead uses questions to gather information and then summarizes the information in a way that gently reframes the conclusions the client has drawn about herself.

The next example illustrates the use of alternative explanations:

CLIENT: My son and his family don't care about me. That's why they didn't invite me along when they drove up to Massachusetts to pick up my grandson.

THERAPIST: I wonder if you can think of any other reason they might not have asked you?

CLIENT: No, I think they don't want to spend time with me.

THERAPIST: Could they have thought that such a long ride would be uncomfortable for you? Or might they have been looking forward to the drive to have some time alone to talk together?

CLIENT: I never thought about that. They *might* have some other reason.

When working with older clients, therapists need to be able to differentiate exaggerated or negative thoughts from social stereotypes about aging (Blazer, 2002). A client may claim that she is too old to change or that her problems are due to a lack of good alternatives available to her because she is old. These types of beliefs may seem especially compelling if they are linked with physical disabilities or the death of a spouse or other close relative. Examination of these types of thoughts reveals that they represent overgeneralizations and that clients have alternatives they are overlooking. We return to this point later in the chapter.

The relationship between client and therapist should be supportive and collaborative. As the focus of treatment turns to clients' beliefs, therapists should avoid turning these discussions into arguments. They should also avoid fostering excessive dependencies.

Concluding Treatment

During the final session, cognitive therapists usually review the therapy, summarize the problems presented and the techniques that were most effective, and predict certain anticipated problem areas in the future. Closing sessions can be used to prepare clients for the possibility of relapses and how to deal with them. The therapist can make a booster session available should something unexpected occur. Sometimes just knowing that this is possible eases the anxiety the client might have about termination. Because of the tendency for depressed people to exaggerate negative events, it is also important at termination to remind clients that relapses are minor and expected events rather than evidence that the therapy has failed and that they have the skills to manage these setbacks.

Interpersonal Psychotherapy for Depression

Interpersonal psychotherapy (IPT) focuses on interpersonal problems in the patient's life as the major source of depression. Developed by Klerman and associates (1984), IPT has been found to be an effective treatment both with younger individuals (e.g., Elkin et al., 1989; Frank et al., 1990) and with older clients (Miller & Silberman, 1996), including those who are also medically ill (Mossey, Knott, Higgins, & Talerico, 1996).

Characteristics of Interpersonal Psychotherapy

IPT focuses on relationship issues, which are a common complaint among depressed older adults. Clients may have problems in their relationships with husbands or wives or with children or friends. They may also complain of difficulties in meeting new people and forming friendships. Some older clients say they are lonely, yet they may behave in ways that drive people away. Interpersonal psychotherapy explicitly examines these relationship problems and what older clients can do to improve them.

Treatment begins with an assessment to identify depressive symptoms and their sources. The assessment includes a review of the client's past and current relationships. The therapist identifies people who are or have been important in the person's life, which interactions are conflicted or problematic, and which relationships are associated with the current episode of depression or with prior episodes. As with behavioral therapy and cognitive-behavioral therapy, IPT emphasizes establishing rapport with clients and explaining how treatment works.

The interpersonal therapist focuses on four areas that are considered critical in the development of depression: (1) grief, (2) interpersonal disputes, (3) role transitions, and (4) interpersonal deficits (Klerman et al., 1984; Miller & Silberman, 1996). Each of these issues is likely to be relevant for older clients. The initial assessment is used to determine which areas are involved. The therapist then encourages clients to develop more adaptive behavior to overcome these problems. With grief, for example, the therapist supports the mourning process and then works with clients to identify ways to replace or compensate for the loss. The therapist is active throughout treatment, offering reassurance and support.

A major focus of treatment is helping clients improve their communication with other people. Although past relationships are acknowledged for their influence on the present, clients are encouraged to work on their current situations.

Modifications of Interpersonal Psychotherapy for Older Clients

As with the other depression treatments, IPT is modified somewhat for use with older clients (Miller & Silberman, 1996). One such modification is the use of shorter sessions if an older client cannot tolerate a full-length therapy session. Older clients may have more limited options for replacing problem relationships, so the therapist is more likely to encourage working out these problems rather than discarding relationships. The therapist may also need to role-play with the client to develop new interpersonal skills.

Other Types of Psychotherapy for Depressed Older Adults

The principles used in these treatments for depression can be implemented in other formats besides traditional one-on-one psychotherapy. A group therapy protocol for cognitive-behavioral therapy has been found to be effective (Beutler et al., 1987). Lewinsohn and his colleagues (1992) have developed a class called "Control Your Depression," which has had promising results. Thompson, Gallagher, Nies, and Epstein (1983) have modified this approach specifically for older adults and report that participation in the classes has resulted in reduced depressive symptoms, improvement in life satisfaction, and decreased negative thinking.

Group treatment, whether in a therapy group or a psychoeducational class, presents opportunities for intervention not available in one-to-one therapy. Groups may be particularly helpful when people share a common problem or concern and can use the group to share information and build mutual support. An example is a group for people with the same illness or disability. In a group setting, it is also possible to assess and build relationship skills in a more direct way. Groups also offer the potential for clients to learn from one another. Clients are more likely to be able to make changes in their lives when changes are suggested by other members of a group rather than by the therapist. Psychoeducational groups and classes have the additional advantage of not having the stigma that is associated with traditional mental health treatment. These approaches can be used as part of a primary prevention program and to reach out to nontraditional clients who might not come for psychotherapy but who are willing to attend classes about mental health issues.

We recommend screening clients before enrolling them in a therapy group or psychoeducational intervention. Some older clients do not do well in groups or have strong negative feelings about being in group treatment. Indications that group treatment should not be undertaken include (1) hearing loss that is severe enough to interfere with understanding conversation in a group setting, (2) evidence of personality disorder, (3) severe depressive symptoms, and (4) a prior history of poor response to group treatment. When a class is offered, it may not be possible to screen clients in advance, so the therapist/instructor needs to be proactive in dealing with participants who are disruptive or who derail the discussions.

Combined Treatment with Psychotherapy and Medications in Late-Life Depression

Many older clients we see are treated with a combination of psychotherapy and medications. They have often sought help first from their primary care physicians, who prescribed an antidepressant, and then were referred by the physicians or came on their own for psychotherapy. Sometimes we bring up the possibility of medication with clients and then with their physicians. Clients who previously responded well to an antidepressant or whose symptoms are fairly severe are likely to respond best to a combined treatment. Consultation with a psychiatrist can be helpful in complicated cases or when patients have not done well on a standard medication protocol.

Therapists must weigh the advantages of combined treatment against the potential drawbacks. Clients may get an immediate boost from the antidepressant, either real or placebo, which then helps the therapist work with psychological material. It is also easier to keep depressed clients engaged in treatment when they begin to see benefits sooner. The main disadvantage of combined treatment is that the antidepressant medications may have side effects that clients have difficulty tolerating. Because of the amount of time we spend with clients, however, we are more likely to hear about side effects and other concerns that would otherwise lead a client to discontinue medication and to work with them and their physicians to resolve these problems.

To conduct combined treatment effectively, therapists need to be familiar with antidepressant medications, their main effects and side effects, and how to manage those effects. Next we review the most commonly used antidepressant medications and then discuss the therapist's role in conducting combined treatment. When referring to drugs, the scientific literature uses generic names, whereas physicians and patients typically mention the brand name. We provide both the generic and brand name of a medication when it is first presented, then refer to it subsequently by the brand name.

The Antidepressant Medications

Antidepressant medications block the reuptake by brain neurons of neurotransmitters that are associated with depression, particularly serotonin, norepinephrine, and dopamine. As a result of the medication's actions, the amount of one or more of these neurotransmitters that is available at neuronal synapses is increased. The main types of antidepressants and the neurotransmitters they target are shown in Table 9.1.

The choice of an antidepressant depends on the presenting symptoms, as well as medical conditions and other medications that might potentially interact with certain drugs. Most drug trials have determined the efficacy of antidepressants with people suffering from a major depressive disorder, but there

TABLE 9.1. Types of Antidepressant Medications and Their Mechanisms

Medications (generic and brand names)	Primary targets
Selective serotonin reuptake inhibitors (SSRIs)	
• Citalopram (Celexa) • Escitalopram (Lexapro) • Fluoxetine (Prozac) • Fluvoxamine (Luvox) • Paroxetine (Paxil) • Sertraline (Zoloft)	SE
Selective serotonin and norepinephrine reuptake inhibitors (SSNRIs)	
• Venlafaxine (Effexor) • Trazodone (Desyrel) • Duloxetine hydrochloride (Cymbalta)	SE, NE
Tetracyclics	
• Mirtazapine (Remeron)	SE, NE
Atypical antidepressants	
• Bupropion (Wellbutrin)	NA, DA
Tricyclic tertiary amines	
• Amitriptyline (Elavil, Endep) • Imipramine (Tofranil) • Doxepin (Adapin, Sinequan) • Clomipramine (Anafranil) • Nortriptyline (Aventyl, Pamelor) • Protriptyline (Vivactil) • Trimipramine (Surmontil)	NE, weak impact on SE
Monoamine oxidase inhibitors (MAOIs)	
• Tranylcypromine (Parnate)	NE, SE, DA

Note. NE, norepinephrine; SE, serotonin; DA, dopamine; NA, increased noradrenergic activity. Data from Alexopoulos (1994), Blazer (2002), De Leo and Diekstra (1990), and Swartz (2005).

is some evidence that antidepressants are effective in other depressive syndromes (Kocsis et al., 1997). Useful overviews of the antidepressants can be found in Jacobson and colleagues (2002), Preston, O'Neal, and Talaga (2002), and Swartz (2005). These texts discuss differences among various antidepressants, potential interactions with other medications, and contraindications for the use of medications with people suffering from particular illnesses. Current information about treatment of depression can be found at the National Institute of Mental Health website at www.nimh.nih.gov/healthinformation/depressionmenu.cfm.

The selective serotonin reuptake inhibitors (SSRIs) are generally considered the first choice in treatment of depression unless there are specific medical contraindications or a prior history of a good response to another antidepressant (Jacobson et al., 2002; Swartz, 2005). These medications have three principal advantages over other medications. First, they mainly target one neurotransmitter, serotonin. As a result, it is possible to determine whether altering levels of serotonin alone is sufficient to alleviate depression. If not, medications that affect the other neurotransmitters associated with depression can be used. Second, the SSRIs have fewer side effects than most of the alternatives and can be tolerated more easily by most older people (Salzman, 1994). Third, patients feel symptom relief relatively quickly, typically from a few days to 2 weeks. Contrary to popular opinion, the SSRIs do not have a greater impact on depression than the drugs they largely replaced, the tricyclics, or other antidepressants (Jacobson et al., 2002; Schneider & Olin, 1995). Their main advantage is having fewer side effects, thus allowing more people to reach a therapeutic level of the medication.

Among the SSRIs, the most likely side effects are serotonergic (see Table 9.2). Clients complain of difficulty falling asleep, poor appetite with weight loss (not always a problem!), a feeling of "jitteriness," and sometimes headaches. Although most of these problems disappear within a few weeks, people often need support to wait them out. Once the side effects disappear, they feel "better than good." More significant side effects of SSRIs may also occur. Some people develop diarrhea to such an extent that the medication has to be discontinued. People with a history of irritable bowel syndrome or other gastrointestinal problems will do better on some SSRIs than others. Another problem is that some older patients become drowsy and hypersomnic on SSRIs, particularly if they are also taking antihypertensives. Patients may com-

TABLE 9.2. Serotonergic Side Effects

• Headaches	• Insomnia
• Nausea	• Sexual dysfunction
• Gastrointestinal problems	• Weakness
• Nervousness	• Dizziness
• Anxiety	• Increased sweating
• Tremors	

plain of loss of libido and other sexual problems. Weight gain can be a problem for people who already are overweight and for whom the additional weight may affect other health conditions, such as diabetes or arthritis. Finally, parkinsonian symptoms have been reported in rare instances and require immediate attention (Swartz, 2005).

Some antidepressants, called selective serotonin and norepinephrine reuptake inhibitors (SSNRIs), act on both of those neurotransmitters. These medications are generally tried when a patient does not respond to an SSRI. One such medication is venlafaxine (Effexor). An SSNRI is generally tolerated well by older patients, though not as well as the SSRIs. Bupropion (Wellbutrin), which is considered an atypical antidepressant, primarily blocks reuptake of dopamine. This medication has been found to be effective with older adults (e.g., Branconnier et al., 1983; Weihs et al., 2000).

Prior to the introduction of the SSRIs in the late 1980s, the tricyclic antidepressants (TCAs), such as amitriptyline (Elavil) and imipramine (Tofranil), were the most widely used antidepressants. These drugs block the reuptake of norepinephrine and, to a lesser extent, serotonin and have both antidepressant and sedative effects. There is considerable evidence that these medications reduce depression, and they may be more effective for severe depression than the SSRIs (Jacobson et al., 2002).

TCAs, however, are rarely used today as the first medication prescribed because of high rates of side effects. In particular, the TCAs have high anticholinergic effects, resulting in such symptoms as dry mouth, blurred vision, urinary retention, and constipation. Another anticholinergic effect is memory loss, which is particularly a problem in older patients because symptoms can resemble dementia. Another possible side effect is orthostatic hypotension, which can lead to falls and serious injuries (Swartz, 2005). Other severe reactions can include psychotic thinking, hyperthermia, worsening of glaucoma, and cardiac problems (Jacobson et al., 2002). TCAs are not recommended for patients with ischemic heart disease. Patients may also experience weight gain, motor tremor, liver toxicity, decreased sexual interest, or impaired sexual functioning and seizures (Blazer, 2002).

The sedating feature of the TCAs can be an advantage when treating a patient with depression who has anxiety and/or sleep problems, but it is sometimes difficult to achieve the proper balance of antidepressant and sedating effects. Some clients may not be able to tolerate the sedation. Nortriptyline (Pamelor) and desipramine (Norpramine) are more frequently used with older adults because they have fewer anticholinergic and sedating side effects (Blazer, 2002; Jacobson et al., 2002). As with other TCAs, however, they may have adverse cardiac effects.

Monoamine oxidase inhibitors (MAOIs), such as tranylcypromine (Parnate), have a broad effect, increasing the availability of norepinephrine, serotonin, and dopamine (Shuchter et al., 1996). MAOIs have often been used for depression that does not respond to other treatments. These medications are more difficult to administer because clients must avoid many common foods, such as cheeses and wines, that have a high amount of the amino acid tyramine. Interaction of an MAOI with tyramine can lead to a hypertensive crisis or a stroke. MAOIs also have adverse interactions with many common medications. MAOIs have been reported to worsen cognitive functioning and to result in symptoms such as agitation and paranoid thinking, especially in people with evidence of prior cognitive deficits (Blazer, 2002). They can cause orthostatic hypotension and, more rarely, hypertension (Salzman, 1993). These medications are generally no longer used with older adults because of their higher risk of side effects and lack of therapeutic advantages over other available drugs (Salzman, 1993; Swartz, 2005).

Mood stabilizers are used in bipolar disorders and can be tolerated by older patients (Blazer, 2002; De Leo & Diekstra, 1990). Concern about long-term side effects of lithium in the elderly have led to recommendations for use of valproate instead (Jacobson et al., 2002). Mood stabilizers must be monitored carefully because of the risk of toxic side effects, cardiac problems, and a variety of other adverse symptoms.

Finally, some stimulants (e.g., methylphenidate and D-amphetamine) have been used with older depressed and medically ill patients. The rationale for this use is that these medications have fewer cardiovascular side effects than TCAs and work quickly. Controlled studies, however, suggest that stimulants are not effective as antidepressants (Schneider & Olin, 1995).

Some people turn to natural substances for treatment of depression. St. John's wort (*hypericum*) has been very popular among advocates of alternative medicine. Although initial evidence suggested that St. John's wort had antidepressant properties, more rigorous trials found little support for its efficacy for major depression (Hypericum Depression Trial Study Group, 2002; Shelton et al., 2001). Though it may have some benefit for mild depression, there is also evidence of possible adverse effects with long-term use, as well as toxic interactions with other medications (Swartz, 2005). There have not as yet been conclusive tests of another supplement with possible antidepressant effects, SAM-e.

Some individuals do not respond initially to medications. It is estimated that between 18 and 40% of older depressed patients do not respond to standard medication protocols (Bonner & Howard, 1995). When the initial response to a medication is poor, the prescribing physician usually tries one of the alternatives. Differences among the SSRI medications result in somewhat different benefits. Responses to a medication are not always predictable, as a great deal of individual variability can exist in effects. In clinical practice, a certain amount of experimentation with medications is done to identify which drugs are more likely to be effective for a patient and at what dosages. This approach can work. The main problem we have observed is continuing treatments that are not effective or that are having significant side effects. On the other hand, switching rapidly from one medication to another without careful evaluation of the response can overwhelm the depressed individual and lead to resistance to the use of *any* treatment. When a client has not responded well initially to medications and continues to be depressed, a consultation with a geriatric psychiatrist or another specialist who is knowledgeable about treatment of older adults should be considered.

Sometimes patients display a combination of anxiety and depressive symptoms or experience an increase in anxiety as a result of the antidepressant medication they are taking. Insomnia is also another common symptom associated with depression. In Chapter 10, we look at medications that can be useful for anxiety and sleeping problems.

The Therapist's Role in Combined Treatment

It is helpful to spend time with clients discussing the side effects of medications they are taking and also helping them recognize the positive benefits. Particularly with the SSRIs, some side effects are transitory. When clients understand this and that it takes a while to experience the therapeutic benefits of medications, they are often more compliant and give the medication a chance. When side effects are serious, it is important to work with patients to contact the physician about a possible change. Usually there is another medication in the same class that has fewer of the particular side effects in question. For example, people with a history of irritable bowel syndrome tend to develop significant gastrointestinal symptoms on SSRIs. This response appears to be idiosyncratic rather than due to a particular SSRI. The best approach is to discontinue the offending medication and wait for symptoms to clear before starting a different SSRI. It is usually possible to find an SSRI that can be tolerated.

Patients may want to discontinue an SSRI because they begin to feel detached and less concerned about the things that bothered them. Although this change can be viewed as improvement, some clients become concerned that they will lose the intensity of feelings that they had in the past. We assure them that in time they will recapture the ability to experience positive feelings, but without also having strong negative emotions.

Collaborating with Physicians

Nonphysicians need to work collaboratively with physicians to coordinate use of antidepressant and other psychoactive medications. Therapists are in an ideal position to monitor effectiveness, compliance, and side effects of medications. They see patients often and listen in depth to their experiences. Thus they can provide valuable feedback to physicians on the effectiveness of a medication. They can also discuss with physicians the experiences that other patients had with certain medications. In a successful collaboration, information flows freely between physician and therapist, so that the patient perceives a united effort in treatment. We strongly recommend that mental health professionals who work with older clients be trained in psychopharmacology to give them a thorough understanding of the uses of medication. Excellent programs sponsored by the American Psychological Association and the National Institute of Mental Health, among others, provide the latest research on the uses of psychotropic medications.

OTHER ISSUES IN TREATMENT WITH DEPRESSED OLDER PEOPLE

In treating older depressed patients, therapists also need to be aware of: (1) the possibility of using electroconvulsive therapy (ECT), (2) the need to address the family's role in the client's depression, (3) comorbidities of health problems and depression, and (4) comorbidity of personality disorders.

Electroconvulsive Therapy with Older Depressed Patients

ECT remains controversial, but it is widely used with depressed patients, including those who are older. Given the controversy surrounding ECT, the American Psychiatric Association (2001) has proposed guidelines for its use. ECT is recommended for severely depressed and suicidal patients, with whom an immediate treatment response is needed, and with patients whose medical conditions preclude use of antidepressants. Patients who do not respond to antidepressant medication may also be considered for ECT. It may also be used if a patient responded well previously to ECT and requests it for treatment of a new depressive episode.

Many strong advocates of ECT argue that recovery rates are high, perhaps higher than with medications, and that improvement is rapid. Some evidence suggests that older patients have an even better response to ECT than younger ones (O'Connor et al., 2001).

Critics, however, cite adverse effects associated with ECT and argue that it should be used rarely, if at all. Although ECT is usually considered medically safe with older patients, several potential problems exist. The greatest medical risks involve cardiovascular problems and falls (Sackheim, 1994). Blazer (2002) estimates that one-third of older patients are likely to experience some adverse effects (falls, cardiovascular symptoms, confusion) following ECT. Other side effects are headaches, nausea, and muscle pain. The oldest old (75 and over) are most likely to have medical complications and increased mortality (Cattan et al., 1990).

The most troubling problem associated with the use of ECT with older patients is its effects on cognitive functioning. ECT results in some short-term memory loss immediately following treatment. Memory problems include both anterograde and retrograde amnesia. Patients have trouble remembering some events from prior to the ECT and have difficulty with new learning. These problems usually clear up within a month, but some patients have been found to have more persistent deficits (Sackeim, 1992). We have encountered people in our practice whose cognitive difficulties apparently originated with or were intensified by ECT.

There are competing explanations for these long-term effects. One possibility is that ECT may cause permanent brain damage, which results in deficits in cognition. That can happen if the ECT is administered improperly. An alternative explanation is that the patient's memory problems are associated with other pathologies or even with normal aging rather than with ECT. Some depressed older people are at risk of developing dementia, especially if they have cognitive symptoms at the time of the depressive episodes (Alexopoulos, Meyers, Young, Mattis, & Kakuma, 1993). In that situation, the emergence of dementia symptoms would be inevitable and unrelated to ECT. The effects of ECT, however, may accentuate cognitive problems in a patient who already has mild dementia symptoms (American Psychiatric Association, 2001; Gatz, 1994).

Another major drawback of ECT is that relapse rates are high. Depending on the study, relapses have been reported for between 33 and 80% of patients within 1 year of treatment (Blazer, 2002; Sackeim, 1994; Sackeim et al., 2001). Relapses can be reduced somewhat by following up ECT with medications (Sackeim et al., 2001). The high propensity for relapse may be due in part to the fact that some patients receiving ECT have more severe depressions that have been resistant to medications.

The decision to use ECT is often related to social factors. Historically, people who were given ECT had less education and were believed to have little personal insight into their problems (e.g., Kahn & Fink, 1959). Families of older patients with depression play a major role in the decision to use ECT (Gatz & Warren, 1989). When family burden was higher, and the patient was no longer performing activities of daily living or was behaving in bizarre or deviant ways, ECT was a more likely choice. In many cases, families pressured the patient into giving consent for treatment. There was also little effort to prevent the buildup of stress on these families (Gatz & Warren, 1989).

ECT, then, should be regarded as a tool for use when other treatments are not effective and when an immediate treatment response is critical. Questions remain, however, about the long-term safety of ECT, as well as about its acceptability as a treatment.

Family Issues in the Treatment of Late-Life Depression

Family problems play a role in depression for many older people. A series of groundbreaking studies by Hinrichsen and his associates (Hinrichsen, 1992; Hinrichsen & Hernandez, 1993; Hinrichsen & Zweig, 1994; Zweig & Hinrichsen, 1993) demonstrate the effects that the family has on recovery and relapse rates in late-life depression. These investigations focused on a sample of people 60 years of age or older who suffered from major depression and who had involved spouses or children. Initial treatment with medications or ECT resulted in improvement in 72% of cases. Improvement was related to characteristics of the involved family members, not of the patients. Relatives of patients who had poorer initial responses had more psychiatric symptoms, particular depression and somaticization. Relatives also reported more difficulty helping the depressed patient and assessed their own health as poor.

A small proportion of patients (8.7%) made subsequent suicide attempts over the next 12 months. These attempts were associated with a combination of patient and family characteristics (Zweig & Hinrichsen, 1993). Patients who made suicide attempts had higher socioeconomic status, past histories of suicide attempts, more suicidal behaviors at the time of initial assessment, and poor initial responses to treatment. Their relatives had more psychiatric symptoms and reported more difficulty caring for the patients and more strain in those relationships. These studies establish that the relationship between the patient and family member may be a critical factor in treatment response and perhaps also in risk for a suicide attempt.

Given the importance and meaning of family relationships in the lives of older people, it should not be surprising that key family members can influence the outcome of treatment. Therapists need to keep in mind that the interactions between the patient and key family members can be contributing to depression. One strategy is building up the patient's resources for managing these interactions. As noted, bringing family members into treatment in strategic ways can identify problematic interactions and provide the therapist with a direction for working with the patient. In some instances, a spouse or other family members might want treatment for themselves or might want conjoint therapy. In the former case, the therapist should refer that person to a colleague to avoid a dual relationship. (Dual relationships are discouraged because of the potential ethical problems they can pose; American Psychological Association, 2002). In the latter case, the therapist may also consider referring the couple or family if too strong an alliance exists with the patient for the therapist to be able to function as a neutral party. Moving into couple or family therapy should be done only when it is in the original patient's interest. In some cases, the best outcome for the patient may be to distance him- or herself from a relative, not to try to improve the interaction. Examples of involving family in treatment are presented in the case examples later in the chapter.

Comorbidity of Depression and Medical Illness

Depression is a frequent and important concomitant of medical illnesses throughout the life span. As noted, depression can be a consequence and a cause of illness. Patients can become depressed for a variety of reasons: discomfort or physical distress, disabilities, or the life-threatening consequences of the illness. Illness and disability can cut people off from friends and family and reduce their ability to engage in usual activities. In turn, many diseases and medications have physiological effects that can result in an increase of depressive symptoms. (See Chapter 4 for a list of illnesses that can lead to depression.)

COMORBIDITY OF DEPRESSION AND MEDICAL ILLNESS

I consulted with a colleague on a case of an older woman whom she was treating for depression. I immediately noticed the woman's face, which had the mask-like and expressionless quality typical of PD. Neither her therapist nor her physician had previously noted these symptoms. When these problems were called to the physician's attention, he began an investigation for possible PD and subsequently started her on an anti-Parkinson medication. Her overall functioning improved somewhat in response to the medication, and she was able to make better progress in therapy.

Physiological and psychological processes can set off a downward spiral in some clients. For example, some nutritional deficits can cause depressive symptoms. In turn, the depressed patient may eat less, thereby increasing nutritional problems (Blazer, 2002). Overeating can be a consequence of depression and can complicate other health problems, as well as contributing to a negative body image. Pain and depression are associated in a similar way. The experience of chronic pain can lead to depression, and depressive symptoms can worsen the experience of chronic pain (Blazer, 2002).

Therapists need to know about the possibilities for rehabilitation and retraining. It is also helpful to know how patients with similar medical problems have been able to adapt. With that information, it becomes possible to distinguish between the real and enduring losses clients suffer and their exaggerated reactions. Treatment involves helping clients identify realistic alternatives that allow them to compensate for their losses or make progress in the recovery of function.

To illustrate how to make this distinction between realistic and exaggerated reactions, we draw on our experience in working with older people who have suffered significant vision loss. Many older people have disorders that cause vision problems that cannot be corrected by ordinary eyeglasses. The disorders that affect vision include macular degeneration, which causes a loss of central vision; glaucoma, which is associated with a loss of peripheral vision; and diabetic retinopathy, which can have varying effects on vision. Most older people with vision problems do not become totally blind, but their remaining eyesight may not be sufficient to carry out valued activities, such as driving or reading print with ordinary eyeglasses. It is no wonder that depression commonly accompanies eye disorders in late life (Horowitz et al., 1994).

Although vision loss is extremely disturbing, rehabilitation efforts can help patients regain the ability to perform many different activities. People with vision losses are able to make successful adaptations by learning how to use visual aids that enhance their remaining vision and by making modifications in their environment. A variety of visual aids are available. Examples range from simple and familiar devices such as magnifying glasses to technologically sophisticated equipment such as closed-circuit televisions that enlarge print and reverse the field (showing white on black, rather than the opposite). These devices make it possible for many people with visual impairments to read print and to perform other visual tasks (see Genensky, Zarit, & Amaral, 1992, for a discussion of vision rehabilitation in later life). Environmental modifications can also help people function more effectively. Using lamps that have high illumination and are focused directly on work or reading areas can help someone read print. Increasing the lighting in hallways and stairways can prevent falls. Another modification to prevent falls is placing contrasting color strips on steps. These interventions do not lead to recovery of some abilities, such as driving, but they enable people with visual impairments to perform a wide range of activities that contribute to a meaningful and fulfilling life.

Despite these rehabilitation possibilities, many patients with vision problems reject or minimize the potential for improvement. They often dwell on what they have lost, rather than what may still be possible for them. Compounding the problem, their physicians or other health providers may have told them that nothing can be done to help them. They may complain that their lives are not worth living without their vision and describe themselves in exaggerated terms, for example, calling themselves blind when they can, in fact, see. As in other situations in which depression is involved, clients' beliefs about the events in their lives and their own abilities determine whether they will take the necessary steps to manage their problems more effectively. If they believe that their situation is hopeless, that nothing can be done to help them, or that the only change that would make their lives satisfying again is to be able to see the way they used to, then they do not take the steps necessary to learn how to use visual aids or make environmental modifications that could improve their functioning. Although the severity of vision loss affects how much rehabilitation is possible, it is not the only factor that affects how patients adapt. Sometimes people with relatively good remaining vision make poor adaptations, whereas others with much poorer eyesight make good progress in regaining function. This discrepancy is frequently the result of differences in beliefs—one patient sees the situation as hopeless, another believes it is possible to improve. Treatment of depressive beliefs, then, is a necessary part of vision and other rehabilitation programs.

The therapist works with clients to challenge and reframe beliefs that exaggerate the consequences of their loss. This must be done gently, because the loss is real. Clients will stop treatment if they sense that the therapist is minimizing their disability. Therapists must walk a fine line between acknowledging the loss and challenging beliefs about the consequences of the loss. Other strategies are useful with older adults who have visual impairments. Behavioral interventions that increase pleasant activities can help identify the things that a client can still do, as well as improve mood. Sometimes family interventions are needed, particularly when family members undermine rehabilitation efforts. Clients can also benefit by talking with people who have similar disabilities, either in a group or in a one-to-one situation. The same client who previously rejected a visual aid when it was presented by an optometrist may try it out after seeing another patient use it. Participants in support groups will pass around and try out each other's visual aids. They also share experiences about how they have learned to get the most out of their aids and to solve problems in their daily lives caused by their vision problems. This sharing of information speeds up the rehabilitation process.

How Therapy Can Contribute to Vision Rehabilitation

Phyllis, age 69, had vision problems due to glaucoma and cataracts. Surgery for these conditions was only partly successful, leaving her extremely sensitive to light. Under conditions of bright light, she was functionally blind. As a result, she could not see well enough outdoors during the daytime to cross busy streets safely. Phyllis had been virtually housebound for the previous year, not leaving her apartment except when the senior citizens' van picked her up for trips to the grocery store. On the positive side, her vision was fairly good when glare and illumination were controlled.

Phyllis was referred for treatment at a comprehensive visual rehabilitation program. As a first step, an orientation and mobility specialist went to her house to teach her how to cross streets safely. Phyllis was also fitted with wraparound sunglasses that greatly reduced glare and made it possible for her to get around safely outdoors on sunny days. As a result of these interventions, she could take the bus to the vision center for her appointments, as well as resume other activities.

Despite these initial gains, Phyllis was very depressed and was referred for psychological treatment. Her depression revolved around the belief that there was nothing she could do anymore that was satisfying or important to her. Treatment focused simultaneously on identifying pleasant activities and addressing the ways in which she exaggerated difficulties and minimized the value of things she was able to accomplish. After several sessions of exploring possible activities, Phyllis set a goal to learn how to paint. She had always been interested in painting but never had the opportunity to pursue it. She was able to locate a painting class and to figure out the bus routes for traveling there. Phyllis did quite well in the class, learning how to work around her vision difficulty. She discovered that the light in her kitchen was best for her in the morning, so she set up her easel then and painted. She got a great deal of satisfaction from painting and became quite good at it. She even won a prize in a local art competition. Besides painting, Phyllis gradually became involved in other social activities, including serving as a volunteer at the vision rehabilitation center.

This example is both typical and exceptional. As in many cases, treatment involved challenging and reframing the client's dysfunctional beliefs that exaggerated the consequences of her loss and prevented her from getting the most out of rehabilitation efforts. Treatment also focused on increasing pleasant activities. What was unusual is that the main breakthrough involved a visual activity—painting. This example underscores how important it is not to identify with clients' statements that they cannot do anything anymore or do not see the sense of going on. Although vision loss is frightening, it does not pose an inevitable barrier to many activities.

The opportunities and methods for rehabilitation and retraining vary considerably from one type of disorder to the next, but the basic approach described for vision loss can still be applied. When working with a client who has a particular illness or disability, the therapist needs to become familiar with the disorder and the possibilities for rehabilitation and recovery. An understanding of what is possible helps therapists identify and reframe depressive beliefs, as well as implement other behavioral and family interventions.

Comorbidity of Depression and Personality Disorders

By far, our most challenging clients are those who have depression and a personality disorder (see Chapter 5). Although depression is the initial complaint, it quickly emerges that these clients have long-standing difficulties in many areas of their lives. The particular pattern of problems depends on the type of personality disorder. People with borderline or histrionic disorders, for example, have more dramatic symptoms, usually anxieties and fears, but occasionally paranoia. By contrast, people with a schizoid pattern may feel an emptiness inside that makes it difficult for them to find pleasure in anything or to develop a relationship with the therapist. Of course, the distinctions among the different personality disorder diagnoses can become blurred, and clients can display features of more than one disorder.

Clients with personality disorders are more likely to be alone in old age. Many are estranged from children or other relatives or have ongoing struggles with them. They want their children's attention but drive them away with their behavior. They characteristically place themselves in difficult situations, getting into conflicts and frustrating anyone who might help them. They have difficulty enjoying the positive events in their lives or experiencing positive feelings. Suicide risk can be high in these patients. Most important, their dysfunctional behaviors and cognitions are very difficult to change.

We often find ourselves doing long-term therapy with these clients. Treatment is a balancing act, trying to prevent crises while also building more adaptive behavior. Initially, clients may be mistrustful and even critical of the therapy relationship. If good rapport is developed, they benefit from therapy. A frequent goal is to prevent burnout among their children or other support sources.

Modifications of cognitive-behavioral therapy have been developed for long-term treatment of people with particularly rigid underlying belief systems (Beck, Freeman, & Associates, 1990; Gallagher-Thompson & Thompson, 1996; Linehan, 1993). Cognitive-behavioral therapy for personality disorders emphasizes identifying the underlying themes or beliefs that give rise to and emerge from automatic thoughts. Examples of these underlying themes are "I am no good" and "No one can ever love me."

An assessment instrument called the Historical Test of Schemas (Young, 1994; see also Gallagher-Thompson & Thompson, 1996) can be useful for identifying underlying themes. As a first step, clients create a time line of significant events in their lives. Client and therapist then work together to identify how the client interprets key events. This review can generate evidence that contradicts long-standing schemas. New schemas are developed through a reformulation of the events in the person's life.

Just as therapy is more difficult with clients who have personality disorders, so is the use of medications. The right combination of medications can greatly facilitate therapy, but finding that combination may be tricky. Compared with our other clients with depression, someone with a personality disorder gets only limited relief from medications or does not respond at all. Unlike the unequivocally positive response we see in many depressed patients, those with personality disorders never attain a consistent level of well-being with SSRIs.

These clients also have problems in dealing with their physicians. We often have to interpret their behavior to the physician and the physician's findings to the client. These clients may not get the treatment they need for serious medical problems because they alienate physicians and other medical personnel.

It is possible to make slow progress, but these patients will continue having difficulty and crises. For the therapist, treating this patient is emotionally draining. Therapists need to be realistic about the prospects for improvement and to make sure they keep proper boundaries.

Novel Treatments for Depression: Exercise and Light Therapy

In addition to traditional medical and psychological interventions, a variety of novel treatments have been tried for depressed adults. In many cases the claims are not supported by data, but at least two types of interventions have been promising: exercise and light therapy. Penninx and colleagues (2002) reported that older people with osteoarthritis who participated in aerobic exercise showed significant decreases in depressive symptoms compared with a group engaging in resistance training and a control group. Exercise has also been found to be useful in older patients with major depression (Blumenthal et al., 1999). Light therapy has also been found to reduce depressive symptoms, though the number of rigorous trials is limited (Golden et al., 2005). Both exercise and light therapy may be useful in combination with psychotherapy or medication (e.g., Martiny, Lunde, Unden, Dam, & Bech, 2005).

LONG-TERM OUTCOMES OF LATE-LIFE DEPRESSION

Studies of late-life depression suggest that outcomes are generally positive. Over the long term, between 60 and 80% of patients do fairly well (Baldwin & Jolley; 1986; Frank, 1994; Murphy, 1994). Some people may experience repeated episodes of depression between interludes of good functioning. As discussed earlier, maintenance treatment involving medications, psychotherapy, or a combination of both improves the rate of long-term recovery (Frank, 1994; Reynolds et al., 1999). Factors associated with a poorer prognosis include evidence of cognitive impairment or a chronic physical illness (Murphy, 1994). Age, however, has not been found to be related to poorer long-term prognoses.

LATE-LIFE DEPRESSION IN CLINICAL PRACTICE

The controlled studies that have established the effectiveness of various treatments for depression in late life follow rigorous protocols. In clinical practice, the therapist is often confronted with complex cases that would not necessarily have been included in clinical research trials because of medical or psychiatric comorbidities. Rather than a straightforward depression, the client may have mixed symptoms (e.g., anxiety or paranoid symptoms), features of a personality disorder, and/or a chronic health problem. In these situations it is best to employ all the treatment tools available (for example, using both medications and psychotherapy), rather than to test one approach at a time. The practicing therapist should draw on clinical research in selecting treatments with known effectiveness. But it is also important to respond flexibly, providing an optimal mix of treatment approaches suited to a particular situation.

The cases described here illustrate situations that a therapist is likely to encounter in an outpatient or private practice setting. They illustrate such issues as how therapists must consider and coordinate therapy with medications and/or ECT, how to involve family members to facilitate treatment, and the role of chronic illness.

Recurrent Major Depression

Catherine, age 78, had her first major depression at the age of 64, several years after an uneventful menopause, for which she did not take hormone replacement. She had been prescribed trazodone (Desyrel) at that time, which she said helped her with her mood but slowed her down. Catherine had recently seen a psychiatrist, who had started her on Effexor and a sleeping medication. The current depression was triggered by two strep throat infections, for which she took antibiotics, and a fall that resulted in a fractured leg and arm. Depression is not an uncommon aftereffect of an infection, and antibiotics can trigger a depressive reaction in some individuals.

Catherine described herself as an excellent homemaker, very perfectionistic and extremely hardworking. She had nine children and had cared for eight of them at home by herself much of the time, as her husband had a job that required a lot of traveling. The other child was severely retarded and resided in an institution; she had not seen him in many years. Catherine had grown up on a farm and had a high school education. She married young and helped her husband through college. Most of their children had finished college, and several had professional degrees. Catherine had always felt ashamed of her meager education. When all the children were grown, she took a cleaning job at a large company, because cleaning was something she felt competent to do. Her husband was embarrassed by her job, but she persisted because she received a lot of praise from her employers. When Catherine fractured her arm and leg, she was unable to work and had to quit her job. Her mood plummeted, leading her into a major depressive episode.

The night before her second session, Catherine took an overdose of Effexor and aspirin—only a few pills—with the hope that she would not wake up in the morning. When she did, she was worried that she had damaged her brain with the medication. Catherine came to the session worried and fearful and claiming that she couldn't even commit suicide right. I increased her visits to twice a week, and her husband accompanied her about half the time. She was unhappy with the psychiatrist she was seeing for medication. She said that when she told him about the overdose, he did not seem concerned. I arranged for Catherine to see a different psychiatrist, who started her on Desyrel, because she had responded to it before.

Over the next 2 weeks, Catherine's depression remained severe. She continued to be negative in her thinking, ruminative, and lethargic, and the suicide risk remained high. I discussed hospitalization with her. Her husband had just signed their Medicare benefits over to a managed care plan, which complicated the decision making. Catherine would have preferred to return to the hospital she had been to 12 years earlier. She had received ECT at that time and it had been helpful. However, the hospital she preferred was not covered by her HMO. Catherine was eventually admitted as an inpatient at the HMO hospital. Treatment there consisted of bilateral ECT (which is no longer standard practice because of the high incidence of memory impairment) and medication. She received no individual or group therapy, and the therapeutic milieu was minimal.

After her 10-day hospitalization, I began seeing Catherine again twice a week for structured cognitive-behavioral therapy for depression. She had been started on an SSRI, paroxetine (Paxil), in the hospital, and it helped considerably with her ruminative thinking. Catherine responded well in therapy to written thought records that she could take home with her. I would often include clarifying or affirming statements on them, such as "My full-time job right now is fighting my depression."

As we worked on the thought records and Catherine came to trust me more, she revealed several important historical antecedents to her depression. Her mother had died when Catherine was 12 years old, and she became the only female on the farm. One of the farmhands took advantage of the situation and raped her when she was 16. She did not tell anyone but always felt damaged and inadequate because of it. Catherine's third son was brain damaged at birth. He was so severely retarded that Catherine was unable to care for him, so she and her husband institutionalized him. She felt guilty and responsible for this decision. I reframed this choice as one that allowed all of her son's needs to be well met, which might not have been the case in their home. Catherine described the hospital in which he lives as a good place for him and said that the staff is quite consistent and caring with him. Subsequently, she and one of her daughters went to visit him and found him clean and well cared for, although he did not know them.

Catherine had often felt overwhelmed with the care of all of the children when her husband was gone for extended periods of time, and she compensated for this by developing an overly close relationship with her oldest daughter. This closeness led to significant sibling rivalry among the children that continued to affect family relationships. Her husband was now semiretired, but he was continuing to travel and would be absent for weeks at a time. During the joint sessions, Catherine's husband was able to see that she was lonely with the children gone and that his absences were a problem for her. He began including her in his trips, which Catherine enjoyed because they often went to places near one or another of their children. She did not drive, so she had not been able to visit the children before. Her husband also attempted to become more supportive of the things Catherine did well, and when she was occasionally asked to fill in for her old company, he no longer was critical of her. Ironically, while taking Paxil, Catherine became much less obsessive about cleaning their own home and started to postpone unpleasant tasks, allowing some clutter to accumulate. This is not an unusual reaction to an SSRI. People describe a feeling of "just not caring as much" whether something gets done.

Treatment continued for 8 months: twice a week for 2 months during the acute phase of her depression, then once a week for about 3 months, then every other week. Catherine no longer felt depressed. Then I received a telephone call canceling an appointment because her husband had been in a terrible automobile accident. His car was hit head on. He had multiple fractures of every extremity and spent 3 months in the hospital. He returned home in a wheelchair, within 4 months he was walking with a cane. Catherine now had to deal with the fact that he was at home all the time and with the anger and irritability that accompanied his chronic pain and disability. Catherine managed it quite well, and as of the present time, she has not had a recurrence of her depression. She continues to take Paxil and to have maintenance therapy sessions once or twice a month.

This case illustrates many of the elements involved in late-life depression, such as coordination of therapy with medications and, in this case, ECT; the prominence of family issues; and the occasional involvement of a spouse in therapy sessions. Therapy addressed long-standing issues, such as the rape and the institutionalization of her son, as well as current concerns. The common thread in treatment was the negative beliefs Catherine had about herself. Once the initial crisis was handled, she made excellent progress. Long-term outcome was good, due to the combination of medications and therapy.

Catherine's husband's choice to enroll in an HMO limited her choices for inpatient treatment. We find these kinds of limitations more and more in all of our clients, not just the older ones. The plan Catherine belonged to, however, was generous in its outpatient therapy coverage.

FIRST MAJOR DEPRESSION AT AGE 67

Emily's daughter called initially, telling me that her mother, who had always been a dynamo—getting up at 5:30 A.M. and cleaning the house and starting the laundry before anyone else was up for breakfast—was now not getting out of bed at all. Emily had seen a number of psychiatrists and a psychologist and had not felt that any of them were at all helpful. Her family physician had hospitalized her on a medical ward of the local hospital because she refused to go to the psychiatric unit, but the 3-day hospitalization had done very little for her.

Because Emily was not getting dressed or going outdoors, I decided to do a home visit to assess the situation. This would also give me an idea of the home environment and allow Emily to feel somewhat "special." Emily's home was not only immaculate, but also tastefully and expensively decorated. Her husband, Harry, was very attentive and often finished her sentences for her. Both of them were very worried about the changes in Emily, and both were fairly sophisticated psychologically. They were college educated and very well read. They had both been widowed at early ages and had found one another at about the time their children were grown. Between them they had seven children, ranging in age from 30 to 45.

Emily's symptoms included poor sleep, with early, middle, and late insomnia; poor appetite; loss of libido and loss of interest in activities; anhedonia; lethargy; and an anxious and depressed mood. She described a rapid heartbeat, episodes of sweating, tightness in her chest, and a feeling of impending doom that seemed to come out of nowhere. She was constantly afraid that the feelings would return, adding to her overall sense of dread and hopelessness.

Emily had been receiving medication for her depression, but there had been many confusing twists and turns in her treatment. When her first husband died, Emily had been given diazepam (Valium) to take as needed. For the next 20 years, she took it once or twice a week. As Emily had become more depressed during the past few months, she began taking the medication more often, eventually taking it daily. Then she became worried that she had become addicted to it. She was switched to lorazepam (Ativan), which is a simple substitute for Valium. She took it twice a day; when she ran out, her doctor was on vacation, and the backup physician stopped the medication. When her regular doctor returned, Emily was agitated and upset, and he restarted her on Valium. She did not improve, so she was referred to a psychiatrist, who gave her risperidone (Risperdal), a major tranquilizer, and lithium carbonate, which is used for bipolar disorders. The psychiatrist perhaps interpreted her lack of sleep and agitation as mania. Emily had severe side effects from the lithium carbonate (which, as noted, is no longer recommended for use with older patients). Again a backup psychiatrist switched her to another minor tranquilizer, alprazolam (Xanax), which seemed to help. However, he then switched Emily to clonazepam (Klonopin), supposedly to wean her from benzodiazepines, but she still had significant side effects, especially gastrointestinal distress.

Emily's depression was steadily worsening through all of this, and she felt more and more hopeless. I spent the early sessions with both Emily and Harry, allowing them to describe in detail exactly what was happening and what benefits and side effects the medications were having. It was clear from the history that what was important initially was spending enough time with them both so that they felt heard and understood. I saw them twice a week for about a 3-month period. A considerable amount of time was spent explaining exactly what each medication was, when it would normally be indicated, and what the side effects were. As more and more of their experience was explained to them, both Emily and Harry became involved in problem solving to find the best medication, and Emily was referred to a different psychiatrist, one who was willing to work closely with a psychologist.

The new psychiatrist started Emily on Paxil, with Klonopin in the morning and at bedtime to address her anxiety. Gradually she was weaned from Klonopin to buspirone (BuSpar) in order to reduce her dependence on tranquilizers. She started to experience tremors as the Klonopin was withdrawn, and the psychiatrist prescribed propranolol hydrochloride (Inderal). Inderal is an antihypertensive medication also used in the treatment of tremors. Emily used the Inderal sparingly, but one day she felt shaky and took the prescribed dose. I saw her shortly afterward, and she seemed fine. By this time, she was no longer severely depressed, and she was busy making plans for the holidays. Two hours after my visit, Harry called me, very upset, because Emily had what he called "amnesia." Not only did she not remember seeing me, but she also had no idea who I was. She was not distressed, just completely disoriented. I told them to call the psychiatrist immediately and follow his instructions. He told them she was "overstimulated" from the weekend and that she would be fine in the morning.

Unsatisfied with this answer, I consulted with a geriatrician, who said that this is a known response to Inderal in the elderly and that it should not have been given on an as-needed basis. Rather, if the intention had been to wean her from the Klonopin and treat the tremors, the medications should have been given together and decreased together. Luckily, the delirium cleared by the next day, and Emily had no memory of the episode. Harry decided to throw away the Inderal, and Emily decided she could tolerate the tremors without medication.

At the present time, Emily is doing well, continuing to take Paxil daily, with minimal use of Buspar as needed. Emily continues to have psychotherapy sessions twice a month to deal with these issues and as insurance against a recurrence of depression when it comes time to discontinue the Paxil.

Although the outcome of this case was ultimately successful, it was complicated by what could best be described as an erratic pattern of prescribing psychotropic medications. Without question, some prescriptions involved questionable judgment and had adverse consequences. We would like to say that this type of problem occurs rarely, but that is not the case with older clients. That is the reason that the geriatric mental health specialist needs to be familiar with medications and their effects. The goal is to work collaboratively with prescribing physicians, when possible, and to know when to encourage clients to seek another opinion.

We recommend seeing patients at least once a month as long as they are taking antidepressants, particularly if the medications are being prescribed by a physician who spends only a brief time with them discussing side effects. On a number of occasions, we have been able to head off a recurrence of depression when we have "caught" patients discontinuing medication on their own, usually because they had so few side effects with SSRIs that they underestimated what the medication was doing for them. In these instances, it was a relatively simple matter to get the clients back on course; if they had not been followed, they might have reverted to a major depressive episode.

TREATMENT OF A PERSON WITH DYSTHYMIA

Linda, age 81, is a divorced mother of four who suffers from chronic symptoms of depression. She recently moved to a new city to live near her only daughter. She was referred to me by her geriatrician after several trials of antidepressant medications were unsuccessful due to her complaints about side effects. Linda's symptoms of depression were not severe enough to warrant a diagnosis of major depressive disorder, but they were distressing and disruptive in her life. This pattern of chronic depression meets DSM-IV criteria for dysthymia (American Psychiatric Association, 1994).

Linda is the oldest of five children who grew up in poverty. She was the babysitter, assistant mother, and housekeeper for the family. She married young to escape the home and had her own children right away. Linda's husband was a civilian employee of the military, and when he left her after 30 years of marriage, she was not even eligible to collect Social Security benefits. She lives on the small amount of support her ex-husband sends her, around $400 per month. Her children try to help her financially, but she is very proud and refuses most of their offers.

Linda has a negative cognitive style, anticipating the worst in every situation and using her life experiences to justify her thinking. She has lived with financial insecurity her entire life, although she actually has more security now than she has ever had: She has Medicare for her medical expenses and a subsidized apartment. Still, Linda turns every situation into a negative scenario. Her children surprised her on her birthday by paying her cable television bill for a year. Rather than being pleased or accepting their good intentions, she complained that it wasn't what she wanted, that the cable company would not know what to do with it, and that she would much rather have had something else.

That "something else" is their time. Linda has never asked them directly to spend more time with her; this longing came out after considerable probing in therapy. What she would really like is for each child to call her weekly and have a leisurely conversation with her, letting her be a part of their lives. She has a hard time realizing that her negative style causes them to limit their exposure to her.

Apart from her depression, Linda is healthy and lives independently. Her biggest problem is that she is a chronic complainer, which drives her children away rather than getting them to give her the attention she wants. Linda travels across the country to visit some of her children, and although she enjoys traveling, she does not allow herself to enjoy the visits. Her children's affluence makes her uncomfortable, and she criticizes their lifestyles. In therapy sessions, Linda has recognized that she turns her children off with her complaining, but that was as far as she could get. Her insight did not translate into more positive behaviors.

A main focus of treatment was dealing with the side effects of the medications she was taking for her depression. When Linda took fluoxetine (Prozac), she developed diarrhea, a common side effect, so it was discontinued. Then she tried Paxil, and for about a week she felt as if she had been reborn. She was no longer depressed, ruminative, or negative in her outlook on life. The benefit did not last, however. Ultimately, Linda tried all the SSRIs and Effexor, but with little relief. Finally, I referred her to a new psychiatrist, who spent time listening to her history and started her on Pamelor. When she complained of lethargy, he gave her Ritalin to take in the morning. This combination proved to be effective, helping her feel somewhat better and facilitating some progress in therapy.

Linda has continued in therapy for more than 2 years, though like other older clients, she limits the number of sessions to one a month. The work in therapy, combined with a better drug regimen, has led to a small amount of progress. She now recognizes that her negative beliefs contribute to her dissatisfaction with her children and with life in general. Linda will say during a session, "I know I have to be more positive in my outlook. Help me do it." This awareness is a major step forward for her, as she had shown very little insight into her problems at any point previously in her life. It has not as yet, however, led to a change in her behavior, in part due to the low frequency of her visits.

This case is fairly typical of older people with dysthymia. Though not meeting criteria for a major depressive disorder, the patient's symptoms are fairly constant and related to her cognitive style. Progress in treatment is slow and often involves preventing decline rather than achieving a major break-through.

COMING TO TERMS WITH THE PAST

John, age 73, is a retired economist. The youngest of four children, he was born just before the Great Depression. His father worked episodically during the Depression, and his oldest sister, who never married, also helped support the family. One brother, who was very much a loner and may have been paranoid, died of a heart attack. John was estranged from his remaining brother. John thinks his father may have suffered from episodic depression and that his mother was depressed for the last 15 years of her life.

John's wife, Mary, is an artist who helped found a nonprofit art school. John and Mary have been married for 40 years, and they have three children, a son and two daughters. None of the children lives closer than a 4-hour drive. John feels there is a strain in these relationships, some of which he attributes to himself and some to Mary. He describes both himself and Mary as people who don't like to be told how to do anything, people who think they know the right way to do things. This has led to some conflict in the marriage, and at times Mary has threatened to leave. John also reported conflicts in his relationships with colleagues at work and in his many community activities.

John retired in 1995 and had an episode of depression at that time. In 1996 John saw a psychotherapist for a year, but he felt he did not make progress with him. He had just finished a 4-year project, a book that he had not only written but also typeset and published himself. He had also gotten involved in the stock market, developing theories that he had worked on during his career.

John had irritable bowel syndrome, which had historically worsened in the fall season. He also had high blood pressure, for which he took medication. Just before the initial interview with me, John's internist had started him on Prozac. He reported a long history of morning anxiety, which he felt was a little better with the medication. He had tried a tricyclic antidepressant, Desyrel, with his previous physician, but it had given him a dry mouth and constipation, so he had discontinued it.

John recognized that he was depressed and that he had been uncomfortable with people all his life. With some help, he was able to identify several areas that he worked on gradually over the next 2 years. First, he reviewed his career, in which he felt both an imposter and a failure. Using cognitive therapy techniques, John was able to examine and reframe many of his experiences and reach a measure of peace with what had been an active and primarily successful working life. Having been born during the Depression may have led to a pervasive sense of insecurity about the stability of work, and it certainly caused him to be very conservative financially (a common trait in this cohort). Furthermore, there was a fair amount of psychopathology in his family, which may have colored his interpretation of people and events around him.

The second main focus in therapy was John's relationships with his children. John acknowledged difficulty in getting close to his children, particularly his son. As he examined the relationships, he realized that both he and Mary were very critical of their children and that many of their visits ended in unpleasantness. They had unvoiced expectations of how the children should treat them, then became angry and unpleasant when their expectations were disappointed.

Over the course of treatment, and in collaboration with Mary's therapist, these expectations were identified, and John and Mary were able to be much more direct with their children. By the second year of therapy, John was reporting much less tension during visits and that the children were all talking directly to him, rather than avoiding him as they had in the past.

The third problem area was the marital relationship itself. John felt that he had been very self-absorbed during the course of his working career and not as supportive of Mary as he could have been. Both of them had experienced frustration and burnout in their careers simultaneously, and they had not been able to support one another. During the time this issue was discussed in therapy, John and Mary began to talk about it at home, and they gradually were able to resolve their past disappointments.

Although John initially had a positive response to Prozac, he began having a hard time falling asleep. His physician prescribed BuSpar at bedtime, but it did not help very much. After about 3 months on Prozac, John was switched to sertraline (Zoloft). He was quite willing to stay on medication because he was experiencing not only a lift in mood but also a marked reduction in ruminative thinking. He found himself waking without anxiety, wanting to begin the day, and with a much more optimistic outlook on life. He reported intense dreams that seemed very real, and he used them to help him think about the issues he was working to resolve in therapy. (All the SSRIs can cause intense dream experiences, which people tend to remember.) John has been on Zoloft for almost 2 years now with no adverse reactions. In his words, he had always been overly sensitive to rejection. On Zoloft he has been able to tolerate looking at his own role in creating situations in which he feels rejection and to change his responses.

By the end of therapy John had developed a sense of satisfaction with what he had been able to accomplish in his career, and he was optimistic about continuing to improve his family relationships.

   This case underscores the potential for growth in older clients. As in the other examples, treatment involved addressing current problems, as well as coming to terms with critical events in the client's past. Medication was again important, making possible the progress that took place in therapy. Over the course of treatment, John improved his relationships with his wife and children and developed a sense of satisfaction with himself and his life that he probably had never had before. He was also able to develop new interests and activities.

CONCLUSIONS

Depression has been the most studied of any mental health problem of later life. With classic, uncomplicated cases, a variety of treatments have been found to be effective, including behavioral, cognitive-behavioral, and interpersonal psychotherapies, as well as medications and ECT. With clients who have more complex clinical pictures—for example, a mixture of depression and anxiety, a chronic illness, or a difficult family situation—therapists must find the combination of approaches that best addresses affective symptoms and their correlated cognitive, behavioral, and interpersonal dimensions. Medications are a valuable asset when used judiciously with older adults and a liability when not. Although not everyone responds to treatment, many older people can make significant gains and remain symptom free for long periods of time.

CHAPTER 10

Treatment of Anxiety Symptoms

Anxiety symptoms are quite prevalent among older people. In contrast to depression, however, treatment of anxiety has received much less systematic attention. As noted in Chapter 4, anxiety symptoms can be part of the clinical picture of several disorders. Among older clients, therapists are most likely to encounter generalized anxiety disorders, panic and phobic disorders, and obsessive–compulsive disorder. Although pure cases of these syndromes can be found, the more usual presentation is as part of a mixed pattern of symptoms that includes medical illness and/or depression. Insomnia is a common component as well. In this chapter, we present a general approach to treatment of anxiety symptoms and indicate when special techniques need to be used for a particular diagnostic category. Management of insomnia is also addressed. In later chapters, we look at anxiety symptoms that are part of other disorders, including schizophrenia (Chapter 11) and dementia (Chapter 12).

Late-life anxiety usually does not involve fears about aging. Aging is a gradual process, and people do not wake up suddenly at age 60 or 70 with fears about what is happening to them. Anxiety about growing older is more likely to be found in younger people, who sometimes go to great lengths to maintain a youthful appearance. Older people as a rule are accepting of the changes that have happened. Apart from the overt physiological changes, they feel a psychological continuity in their lives. They may have regrets over things they have done or not done but no anxiety over being old. They also have come to terms with death, though they may have concerns about avoiding a painful or prolonged death (see Chapter 4).

The following example illustrates one presentation of anxiety in later life.

263

PRESENTATION OF ANXIETY SYMPTOMS

Bert, age 74, was referred for a neuropsychological evaluation for possible dementia. The results of the evaluation, in combination with the history, revealed a mix of obsessive–compulsive features and dementia. The referring physician was quite surprised with the diagnosis of OCD, because to him Bert looked like an extremely cautious, slow-moving, slow-thinking person, characteristics that he attributed to age and dementia. However, a careful interview with Bert and his son revealed that this was how he had functioned all of his life. There is a quality in him that people with anxiety often have. In conversation, Bert takes a while to respond, because he is still thinking about his last response when you ask the next question. It is often hard to interact with obsessive–compulsive people because the usual give-and-take in conversation is not there, as they may be overprocessing their answers and thinking about previous responses.

This example illustrates how complex the presentation of anxiety symptoms can be. When anxiety is found in conjunction with medical illness or dementia, it can easily be overlooked. Other clients just look anxious. They appear tense, on the edge of their chairs, and are very ruminative. The prototypical anxious person has often been portrayed in comedy. The appearance, mannerisms, and speech of the anxious character are immediately recognizable, whether in Tony Shalhoub's portrayal of the television detective *Monk*, or any character played by the late Don Knotts through his long career, or myriad other anxious examples. These caricatures are almost painful to watch, and they suggest the interpersonal difficulties that highly anxious people may encounter.

Sometimes, this anxious appearance leads physicians and mental health professionals to overlook new physical problems, ascribing the symptoms to anxiety.

OVERLOOKING NEW HEALTH PROBLEMS IN AN ANXIOUS CLIENT

Mildred, age 75, had a long history of anxiety with obsessive–compulsive features. She was prescribed antianxiety medications in response to an upsurge of symptoms. When the symptoms did not subside, the medications were increased to the point at which she experienced considerable side effects, including excessive sedation and increased memory problems, as well as the original anxiety symptoms. At that point, a more careful evaluation indicated that she had developed parkinsonian symptoms, which had been overlooked due to her anxious presentation. Treatment for PD brought Mildred's anxiety back down to a manageable level.

People with anxiety disorders in old age frequently have had them for most of their lives. They may have adapted to those symptoms and found ways to control their exposure to anxiety-provoking events and their response to them. New symptoms of anxiety are almost always triggered by an adverse event that has disrupted their ability to manage it. The therapist has to help them understand the events that made them lose control and to help them regain a sense of control over these events.

As a result, older clients with anxiety disorders rarely present for treatment as being anxious. Young people will generally seek help for anxiety and related symptoms, but older people do not. Instead, they report whatever event or circumstances disrupted their management of anxiety. Anxiety is secondary to the problem that brings clients in, but it may be essential to treat the anxiety in order to address the life problems that caused them to seek treatment in the first place.

The following example illustrates how a new problem can destabilize the ability to manage long-standing anxiety.

PRECIPITATING TREATMENT FOR AN ANXIOUS PATIENT

Norm, age 73, called a clinic seeking help for his wife. When he indicated that he did not travel outside of his house, I arranged for a home visit. Norm greeted me at the door and showed me into his cluttered and somewhat dirty house. His wife Victoria was in the bedroom, where she spent most of her time. A brief examination indicated that she had little speech and that her cognitive functioning was severely impaired. Norm described a history of gradual decline that had gone on for a few years.

As we talked, Norm went into his own history. When he was 20 years old, he experienced what he believed to be symptoms of a heart attack while standing in a line at a post office. Doctors never found anything wrong with his heart, and, in retrospect, he probably experienced a panic attack. After that event, Norm became fearful of going outside on his own because he feared he might have another "heart" attack and no one would be there to help him.

Norm was able to have a successful career running a small business by arranging for his employees to pick him up and drive him to the office. He had married, and Victoria's presence at home provided him reassurance, because she would be able to help him if his heart symptoms recurred. The precipitant for his call was the realization that his wife could no longer assist him if he needed help.

In Norm's case, his wife's illness undermined his sense of control over his symptoms. Referrals of nursing home residents with anxiety symptoms follow a similar pattern. These individuals functioned adequately elsewhere but did so by arranging whatever they needed to control anxiety. Moving to a nursing home took away their feelings of control and set off their anxiety. Patients with dementia, in particular, may become extremely anxious when institutionalized, as they lack the cognitive and coping skills to make sense of their new environment.

PERSONALITY CHARACTERISTICS AND ANXIETY

Beyond the specific diagnosis, another consideration in treatment of the patient with anxiety is personality. Clinical experience suggests that anxiety disorders can occur in the context of different personality configurations. One pattern might be called the "anxious independent." These individuals are usually perceived by others as highly competent. Their family and friends turn to them to get things done. People who fall into the anxious–independent pattern have usually managed to keep their symptoms in check all their lives by always being organized and prepared for anything that might happen. Treatment of these individuals is usually brief. The focus is on whatever issues or problems caused them to lose control. Once their anxiety is back under control, they will be eager to move on with their lives.

In contrast, people who might be characterized as "anxious dependent" want treatment all the time. Whereas anxiety symptoms of the anxious–independent person may come as a surprise to friends or even family, the anxious–dependent person is more expressive, as they use anxiety symptoms as a way of attracting help or sympathy. Nonetheless, some anxious–dependent persons can be successful in life if they find themselves in situations in which they have sufficient support. As an example, a business executive functioned well while employed because she had three secretaries who performed most everyday chores for her, but she became highly anxious when retirement left her without their support.

Anxiety symptoms have an impact on interpersonal relationships. Similar to depression, anxiety tends to repel other people and erode their support. Some anxious–independent people may attract others to them because of their competence. Even when highly anxious people are successful, however, their efforts to control their anxiety can come at a cost. They may possess an underlying irritability or anger that comes out with family or friends. Though appearing charming and competent to people they want to impress or do not know well, they can become quite nasty with the people close to them, such as spouses or children. The difference seems to involve feelings of control. By working hard to be competent, they can control feelings of insecurity, but when they feel they are losing control, they can get belligerent and angry.

PSYCHOTHERAPY AS A TREATMENT FOR ANXIETY

Psychological interventions have a long history of efficacy for treatment of anxiety. Outcomes are better and more cost effective than medications and have superior long-term effects (e.g., Heuzenroeder et al., 2004; Roy-Byrne et al., 2005). A growing research literature suggests that psychotherapy has similar positive benefits for older people with anxiety disorders, although the amount of improvement is sometimes modest (Fisher & Durham, 1999; Mohlman, 2004; Nordhus & Pallesen, 2003; Wetherell, Gatz, & Craske, 2003; Wetherell, Sorrell, Thorp, & Patterson, 2005). The focus of most of these studies has been on generalized anxiety disorders, although some have included people with mixed diagnostic features. Most studies also have used cognitive-behavioral therapy (CBT), although the components of treatment employed have varied from one study to the next.

Stanley and her colleagues (Stanley et al., 2003) have developed a multicomponent treatment program for older persons with generalized anxiety that has been found to be effective compared with a control group who received supportive telephone contacts. Components of the treatment are:

- Education about anxiety and its treatment.
- Relaxation training, including breathing retraining and progressive deep-muscle relaxation.
- Cognitive therapy techniques such as thought stopping, coping self-statements, and modifying cognitive distortions by developing alternative beliefs and identifying logical errors.
- Problem solving to improve management of everyday situations.
- Progressive exposure to anxiety-producing situations.
- Sleep-management techniques.

Compared with similar protocols for younger adults, Stanley and her colleagues (2003) recommend more treatment sessions for their older patients. One reason is that there is more history to learn about. Another factor is that older people need extra sessions to deal with setbacks, which are more frequent than with younger patients. These setbacks may be the result of a slower rate of learning, or symptoms may be entrenched in medical or situational problems that are more difficult to change.

Mohlman and colleagues (2003) have developed an enhanced version of CBT for older adults. Specific modifications have been incorporated to improve treatment response, including learning and memory aids, such as reminders to do homework; troubleshooting telephone calls; and taking time in treatment sessions to review the concepts and techniques that were discussed in previous sessions. Results indicated that people in the enhanced approach had better outcomes than standard CBT and a control group.

Useful resources for planning treatment include the classic text *Anxiety Disorders and Phobias* (Beck, Emery, & Greenberg, 1985), which gives an overview of CBT and approaches to treatment, and *The Complete Anxiety Treatment and Homework Planner* (Jongsma, 2004), which provides an array of assessment and treatment approaches, including some for older adults. A full treatment manual with detailed descriptions of the multicomponent intervention can be found in Stanley, Diefenbach, and Hopko (2004).

Though we draw on CBT techniques, we have generally taken a less structured approach to treatment of anxiety than is found in the literature. In part, this has to do with individual strengths; that is, we are better at some approaches than others. Experience also plays an important role in developing a more individualized approach. Therapists will repeat those things that work, and in part those are the techniques that the therapist does best. Beginning clinicians should start with a more structured approach and then develop their own style as they gain experience.

Implementing Treatment

The starting point for treatment is gathering a history. Older patients with anxiety disorders have usually had these problems for a long time and have often had treatment in the past. A triggering event disrupts their usual way of managing their anxiety. It is critical to find out what event has tipped the balance and brought the client into treatment—illness, loss of spouse, change in living situation, or some other triggering event. Older clients often seek treatment for whatever set the problem off, but the therapist will have to treat their anxiety to help them respond effectively to whatever problem brought them in. The problems these clients are having are realistic, not imaginary or exaggerated, even though their reactions appear disproportionate.

Another part of the history is to review medical conditions and medications. Even if someone has had past episodes, a new medication or illness might be contributing to the current episode. Medications associated with anxiety symptoms include amphetamines, appetite suppressants, asthma drugs, decongestants, and steroids (Preston et al., 2002). Excessive use of caffeine can also contribute to anxiety.

When the patient has had treatment for anxiety, it is useful to find out what worked and what did not. Treatment can be optimized by building on those strategies that were useful in the past.

Education about Anxiety

A primary component of CBT is educating clients about their anxiety symptoms. Education provides the rationale for treatment and begins to create a framework for reinterpreting symptoms. We recommend beginning by explaining the physiological response to something frightening happening, for example, a near miss while driving. The body's response is a rush of adrenaline, which results in an array of sensations, including dry mouth, sweaty palms, shortness of breath, and rapid heartbeat. This classic fear response subsides gradually once the danger is past. In contrast, anxiety is a fear response that has become stuck on "go." Although an adverse event may have set off the episode, it is the client's thoughts or ideas that fuel the response and prevent it from running its normal course. In other words, once symptoms begin, the client reacts to the anxiety itself and is flooded with adrenaline and the associated sensations. People with a history of anxiety are hypervigilant about physiological arousal and react strongly when they experience these symptoms.

By explaining the basis of anxiety, the therapist provides a framework for clients to learn to normalize and not to overreact to an adrenaline response. The framework also serves as the basis for identifying the specific thoughts that trigger anxiety symptoms—for example, when a client interprets a rapid heartbeat as a possible heart attack. This is a difficult point to make. People with anxiety become quite accomplished at avoiding the situations and thoughts that trigger these feelings. As people age, they become even more skilled at managing these events and avoiding anxiety. As a result, it is often a more difficult process than with younger people to convince them to look at the thoughts that trigger anxiety.

Another facet of education that arises during treatment is helping clients learn to differentiate between real threats that they should be concerned about and reactions only to a thought that they had. In the latter case, it is possible to lower anxiety by changing the thought, as well as the person's reactions to arousal.

Identifying Events and Thoughts That Trigger Anxiety

After laying the groundwork for treatment, the next step involves identifying antecedent situations that trigger anxiety and the thoughts that contribute to these reactions. The therapist should identify which events trigger symptoms and which are the most troublesome or interfere most with everyday functioning. These events may be situations, places, or particular people. A standard approach to pinpointing triggers and identifying situations that are the most troublesome is to ask the client to keep a daily journal of anxiety symptoms for a week. The journal can indicate when symptoms occur, their intensity, the specific antecedents that trigger the episode, and consequences that follow it.

Through discussions with the client, the therapist can then form a hierarchy or ranking of the events. This can be done in a less formal way than in classic desensitization, but the goal is the same. Interventions should start with situations that are the least anxiety provoking so that the client can learn skills and gain confidence before moving on to more difficult problems.

Management of Anxiety Symptoms

Next, the therapist can move on to management of anxiety symptoms. This is done by drawing on relaxation exercises, cognitive skills, and problem solving. Historically, muscle relaxation has been at the heart of psychological treatment of anxiety. The treatment protocols for older adults that have been found to be effective almost all include some form of relaxation. Relaxation, however, can be hard for many older clients. They do not like the feeling of being out of control that can occur during relaxation exercises. People with comorbid medical problems, particularly those who are in pain, also have difficulty with muscle relaxation. Relaxation training can also be time-consuming.

Instead of relaxation, we recommend more emphasis on education with older clients and on teaching them self-hypnosis strategies. The goal of self-hypnosis is to quiet an overruminative mind, helping the client relax. These approaches are also helpful for sleep-onset insomnia, which is very common in patients with anxiety. A simple technique is to count backward from 1,000 by 7s, which requires concentration and focus. Alternatively, patients can be instructed to count backward while sensing things—for example, thinking of five things they can see, hear, and feel, and then four things they can see, hear, and feel, and so on. Another common technique is to imagine oneself in a favorite place, making the scene as vivid as possible by filling in sights, sounds, and smells. These self-hypnosis approaches are effective because the client cannot do them and think anxiety-producing thoughts at same time.

Treatment of anxiety uses similar cognitive approaches to those for depression (Chapter 9), though the therapist needs to be careful not to push clients too hard or too fast. Clients with anxiety will be reluctant to identify their thoughts because they are what makes them anxious. It is sometimes possible to use thought records that identify the specific cognitions that trigger anxiety symptoms, but more often the therapist brings these thoughts out in discussions. Older clients appear less willing to confront these thoughts on their own, but they will do so during a therapy session with the support and encouragement of the therapist. Part of this work involves continuing with education about anxiety. In particular, we try to find examples in the client's experience to demonstrate how the immediate positive consequences of avoiding the sources of anxiety eventually led to negative ones. This is the heart of getting people with anxiety to work with the therapist, helping them see that what they are doing is not successful and that they need to do something else. The therapist, however, must be committed to helping them through this process so that they do not suffer from their anxiety while they examine precipitating events and thoughts.

A wide range of cognitive techniques is discussed in the literature, but we recommend relying most on developing alternative explanations to dysfunctional thoughts. In contrast to work with younger clients, the therapist will need to generate at least some of these alternatives. Older clients appear more entrenched in their thoughts and less willing to confront and change them. Many alternative explanations rely on the information the therapist has given about why people feel anxious, thereby helping clients understand and tolerate their physiological reactions. Normalizing their reactions helps prevent escalation of symptoms into a panic.

Problem solving comprises a variety of strategies for helping clients improve everyday functioning. Clients with anxiety have often become highly avoidant of a wide range of situations. The therapist works to increase their involvement in situations that will be rewarding or pleasurable and for which they have the appropriate social and behavioral skills. When their skills are deficient, the therapist can work with them to shape more adaptive behaviors and accompanying thoughts. Clients may also experience anxiety in their interactions with difficult or aversive people. The therapist can help differentiate between those relationships that are necessary to maintain—for example, with a job supervisor—and situations that can be avoided without any loss or harm. Some situations are simply not worth the time or effort to master, either because they are too peripheral to what is really important to a client or because the other people are too difficult to deal with. In other words, part of the therapy process is learning to differentiate between situations that appropriately produce fear and concern and those that can reasonably be managed. Training clients to be more assertive can be helpful for dealing with those difficult individuals in their lives that they want to or need to relate to. Problem solving can also address lifestyle changes in diet and exercise habits that can increase well-being and decrease anxiety.

Homework is a part of all these techniques. Rather than written homework, however, many older clients do better with an assigned task that helps build these cognitive and behavioral skills. The type of task depends, of course, on the problem that the client is working on. Particularly with anxiety, the principle of taking small, manageable steps is critical for homework. Examples of homework tasks can also be found in Jongsma (2004).

MEDICATIONS FOR ANXIETY

Medications are frequently prescribed for treatment of anxiety. They are used best in more severe cases and in combination with psychotherapy. This section reviews the types of medications commonly used, and the next section describes combined treatment with medication and psychotherapy.

The SSRIs and combination SSNRIs (see Chapter 9) are considered the first choice in treatment for severe anxiety, especially when depressive symptoms also exist (Lenze et al., 2003; Preston et al., 2002; Swartz & Margolis, 2004). The benefits, as well as drawbacks, of SSRIs are linked to the same characteristic of people with anxiety—hypervigilance. People with anxiety are always scanning their environment and their bodies for threats or problems. The SSRIs are effective in anxiety when they reduce patients' hypervigilance. By ruminating less about possible threats, they feel less anxious. Unfortunately, the SSRIs sometimes have the opposite effect. Typical side effects such as rapid heartbeat or sweating can trigger anxiety. The hypervigilant person with anxiety is more likely to notice these effects in the first place and to become upset by them. These symptoms, after all, are similar to the upsetting feelings they have when they become anxious. SSRIs, such as Prozac and escitalopram (Lexapro), are more likely to bring out anxiety symptoms in patients who have tendencies toward anxiety. Zoloft and citalopram (Celexa) are less likely to lead to anxiety (Preston et al., 2002).

Because of the potential for adverse reactions, it is necessary to use the SSRIs cautiously in treating anxiety and only when the anxiety is severe or the tradeoff of benefits and potential side effects is worth it. As with treatment of depression, the therapist can provide information and support as the patient begins medication to improve compliance. Although tolerating the side effects of the SSRIs is also a problem for people who are depressed, people with anxiety have much more difficulty doing so. In some cases, the thought of what the medication might do is sufficient to trigger their anxiety and cause them to refuse medication. As soon as they take the medication, they are monitoring their bodies for side effects.

A class of mild anxiolytics, the benzodiazepines, has been used widely for treatment of anxiety and sleep problems (Table 10.1). In contrast to the SSRIs, which may require a few weeks to become effective, these medications have an immediate impact. When comorbid depression exists, some physicians prescribe a combination of antidepressant and tranquilizing medication to produce a specific therapeutic benefit that would not occur from using

TABLE 10.1. Short-Acting and Long-Acting Benzodiazepines

Short-acting medications	Long-acting medications
oxazepam (Serax)	clordiazepoxide (Librium)
lorazepam (Ativan)	diazepam (Valium)
alprazolam (Xanax)	prazepam (Centrax)
triazolam (Halcion)	clorazepate (Tranxene)
clonazepam (Klonopin)	

Note. Data from Salzman (1992) and Preston, O'Neal, and Talaga (2002).

either medication alone. Besides their effects on anxiety, all of these medications can reduce irritability and agitation (Salzman, 1992).

Concern about significant side effects limits the use of the benzodiazepines (Hogan, Maxwell, Fung, & Ebly, 2003; Salzman, 1992; Swartz & Margolis, 2004). These side effects include:

- *Sedation:* Patients can become overly sedated and, as a consequence, agitated or belligerent.
- *Cerebellar symptoms:* These problems include ataxia, dysarthria, unsteadiness, and decreased motor coordination. Patients who are already unsteady or have other physical problems can become much worse on these medications. Falls that result in hip fractures or other injuries are a particular risk (Cummings & Le Couteur, 2003).
- *Slowing:* Patients show decreased reaction times and perform a variety of tasks more slowly. Slowing, along with poorer coordination, can lead to significant impairment in driving, including a greater risk of accidents (Madhusoodanan & Bogunovic, 2004; McGwin, Sims, Pulley, & Roseman, 2000).
- *Cognition:* Short-term memory can be significantly impaired. Some people taking these drugs appear demented, though full recovery occurs when the medication is withdrawn (Salzman, 1992).
- *Dependence and tolerance:* Some people develop a dependence on the medications. Tolerance can also develop so that a larger dose is required to produce a similar calming effect, increasing the risk of other adverse side effects. Dependence, however, may not be as common as generally thought among patients with anxiety. The risk is greatest among people with a history of alcoholism or other substance abuse or in cases of a family history of substance abuse (Preston et al., 2002).

The bad reputation that these medications have is due in part to overuse among frail older people, for whom the most adverse side effects, cognitive impairment and falls, are more likely. When used for short periods of time and properly monitored, the risks are lower, although as with any drugs there can always be adverse effects (Preston et al., 2002).

Benzodiazepines can be classified into short-acting and long-acting medications (see Table 10.1). Side effects are more likely in long-acting drugs. Short-acting medications build up to therapeutic dosages quicker and are eliminated from the body faster. Long-acting drugs stay in the body longer and can continue producing symptoms for several days or even weeks after they have been discontinued (Salzman, 1992). As most of these drugs are metabolized by the liver, the longer acting benzodiazepines are problematic for patients with liver disease (Preston et al., 2002).

In some situations, however, long-acting drugs may be preferable. They can be given less often, and the effects last longer. A common problem with a short-acting drug that is given at bedtime is that it wears off before the patient would normally wake up, producing restlessness and anxiety on waking. A long-acting medication could be effective in helping someone sleep through the night.

Patients' hypervigilance can also affect the response to benzodiazepines, as the following example illustrates.

HYPERVIGILANCE FOR MEDICATION EFFECTS

Thelma, 62, had a lifelong history of anxiety. She was prescribed a mild benzodiazepine to help increase her control over the anxiety, but she was very reluctant to take the medication because she was so anxious about what the pill would do. Finally, she agreed to take one-quarter of a pill. She came into the next therapy session complaining that the medication caused her to be unable to sleep and to have terrible dreams when she was asleep. The dosage she took, however, could not have caused those effects. As she talked about what happened, it was apparent that she became hypervigilant after taking the medication, keeping herself awake to try to determine what the effects might be. The little sleep she had was disturbed by the intense anxiety she felt before falling asleep about the possible effects of the medication. I talked with her about the effects of the drug and how her thoughts about those effects led to her bad dreams. In effect, the incident provided a dramatic example of how one's thoughts could generate intense anxiety. Thelma agreed to try the medication again and to use self-hypnosis techniques she had previously learned if she had trouble falling asleep. She was then able to use the medication and get some relief from her anxiety.

Another antianxiety drug, buspirone (BuSpar), is chemically different from the benzodiazepines. BuSpar is less sedating and less likely to cause cognitive symptoms. It is mainly effective in generalized anxiety disorders, less so with panic disorders (Jacobson et al., 2002). It is also used to treat anxiety symptoms in people with depressive disorders and may help potentiate the SSRIs. Like the SSRIs, BuSpar does not become effective right away. Latency of response may be between 1 and 6 weeks (Jacobson et al., 2002).

COMBINATION TREATMENT:
MEDICATIONS AND PSYCHOTHERAPY

Combination treatment can be a very effective approach to anxiety disorders. The therapist should consider a referral for medication if the anxiety is crippling and makes it impossible for the person to function. If symptoms are not severe, the goal is to avoid medication if possible or to get patients off it as treatment progresses.

With severe generalized anxiety disorder, it is often necessary to start with an SSRI or other medication before therapy can become effective. Medications can make it possible for clients to begin working on the cognitive and behavioral triggers of anxiety.

The SSRIs are also effective for people with obsessive–compulsive disorder (OCD), but they do not work well except in combination with psychotherapy. Clients have to work in therapy to counter the obsessive–compulsive systems they have built up. The therapist's goal with the older client is not to eradicate the OCD; that is usually not possible. Instead, successful treatment involves shifting their focus from their obsessions to something that will benefit them more. That requires finding a powerful incentive to change what they are doing.

CONTROLLING OCD SYMPTOMS

Hank, age 56, a divorced teacher, had always been concerned about fitness and appearance. In the past few years, he had become focused on his weight and on bodybuilding. He spent every free moment at the gym lifting weights and obsessively planning his diet so that he would ingest a minimum of fat. As a result of his preoccupations, Hank had few friends and enjoyed little in life, and his weight was dangerously low.

I consulted with Hank's physician, who prescribed an SSRI. Hank was willing to try it, because he had reached the point at which he realized his life was not going anywhere. Hank had written a few articles about bodybuilding for a fitness magazine, and so I encouraged him to begin doing research on nutrition and exercise to improve his articles. As he learned more about nutrition, he became less preoccupied with fat. I also encouraged Hank to go to writing workshops and conferences on nutrition and fitness. He began meeting people with similar interests and developing friendships. Overall, he felt his life was now much better than it had been. When Hank terminated treatment, he told me, "You know, I am still as obsessive–compulsive as ever. Now I am using it for something to my benefit." Treatment did not eliminate his cognitive style but helped direct it in a more adaptive way.

For panic attacks, the SSRIs are also useful, but a short-acting anxiolytic combined with education and problem solving represents an optimal combination treatment (Preston et al., 2002). Patients are instructed to take the medication at the start of a panic attack. The therapist assures them that they will not be able to continue to have the panic attack once they take the medication. This reassurance can prevent uncontrolled release of adrenaline, which is what patients are afraid of. Once patients understand this process and no longer need to fear uncontrolled anxiety, the therapist can engage them in identifying triggers so that they can prevent panic attacks in the future. The medication provides clients with a safety net, something they can fall back on if they need it. We have many patients who carry the medications for years but do not use them. This approach can also be effective for simple phobias and agoraphobia without panic attacks, but it is less so for social phobias.

TREATMENT OF INSOMNIA

Insomnia is a common complaint among older people. Aging can affect the sleep cycle, leading to increased time in falling asleep, less deep sleep, and more frequent awakenings, as can a variety of diseases and medications (Kryger, Monjan, Bliwise, & Ancoli-Israel, 2004). Other factors can induce insomnia or make it worse, including use of caffeine, nicotine, or alcohol (Regestein, 1992). Daytime naps and lack of exercise also can contribute to insomnia.

People with anxiety and/or depressive disorders are especially likely to report insomnia. In a study of people with generalized anxiety disorder, Belanger and colleagues (Belanger, Morin, Langlois, & Ladouceur, 2004) reported that 48% had difficulty falling asleep, 64% woke during the night and had trouble getting back to sleep, and 57% woke too early in the morning. These sleep difficulties were almost always associated with ruminations.

Older people who complain about sleep problems to their physicians are often prescribed one of the benzodiazepines. These medications can have short-term benefits for sleep, but they lose their effectiveness after 20 to 30 days (Regestein, 1992). With prolonged use, they can actually make sleep problems worse. As with other problems, insomnia should be carefully evaluated before medications are prescribed.

Behavioral and cognitive-behavioral approaches have been found to be effective in treatment of insomnia, performing at least as well as medications in the short run and having better long-term outcomes (Morin, Colecchi, Stone, Sood, & Brink, 1999; Smith et al., 2002). These approaches are also helpful in treatment of insomnia in people with comorbid medical and psychiatric conditions, including cognitive impairment (Rybarczyk, Lopez, Benson, Alsten, & Stepanski, 2002). Combination treatment does not improve outcomes over CBT alone, but as with treatment of anxiety disorders, short-term use of medication might be helpful in individual cases.

Several behavioral and cognitive strategies are used for treatment of insomnia. Sleep restriction involves limiting the time a person is in bed to sleep. A patient who reports sleeping only 6 hours, for example, would be initially allowed to spend only 6 hours in bed, though that time could subsequently be expanded. Stimulus control is used to build an association between the bedroom and sleep. Use of the bedroom is limited to sleep and sex. Clients are instructed not to read or watch television in bed or to carry out other activities in the bedroom. They are also advised to go to bed only when sleepy, to get up if they cannot fall asleep after more than 15 or 20 minutes, and to get up at the same time every morning. Other behavioral techniques include avoiding daytime naps, increasing daytime exercise and exposure to natural light, taking a hot bath before bedtime, and using relaxation or self-hypnosis techniques before bedtime (Engle-Friedman, Bootzin, Hazlewood, & Tsao, 1992; Morin et al., 1999; Regestein, 1992). Cognitive strategies explore dysfunctional beliefs associated with difficulties falling asleep, particularly an individual's worries that not getting enough sleep will have dire consequences for his or her health and functioning (Morin et al., 1999).

ANXIETY IN NURSING HOMES
AND OTHER INSTITUTIONAL SETTINGS

In contrast to clients seen in private practice, who usually do not initially complain about anxiety, referrals in nursing homes frequently concern anxiety. In that instance, however, it is the staff, not the patient, who has identified the problem as anxiety. The usual referral concerns a resident who is making excessive demands on the staff. In a typical scenario, the patient may have shown some anxiety symptoms and have been prescribed a short-acting benzodiazepine. The effects of the medication wear off quickly, leaving the resident feeling anxious or anticipating the reoccurrence of symptoms. The resident then begins asking for medications all the time and making other demands. These constant requests become a burden to the staff, who want an intervention that will make these residents less demanding.

The first treatment should optimally combine behavioral intervention and staff education (see Chapter 14). Staff members need to learn how to avoid reinforcing the very behaviors they are objecting to. Often, the only way a resident can get attention from staff members is to have a problem (Baltes, Kindermann, Reisenzein, & Schmid, 1987). Staff members rarely approach residents who are not having problems. This creates a vicious cycle in which only problem behaviors are reinforced. Staff education should also include training in differentiating between emotional responses, such as agitation, irritability, loneliness, and boredom, all of which may be interpreted by busy staff members as anxiety.

The etiology of anxiety in these cases is partly due to the setting. Anxiety is about perceiving threat. Being ill and having to go to a nursing home is a very anxiety-producing event. In particular, placement is associated with a loss of control. Residents in a nursing home do not control even the most basic elements of their daily life, such as the choice of a roommate (or whether to have a roommate at all), when and how often to bathe, when and what to eat, and so on. People with ordinary anxiety may become increasingly anxious after placement due to this loss of control.

One approach to the immediate problem of a demanding, truly anxious patient is to work with the physician to change to a longer acting medication and to create a schedule for administering it. Telling patients about the medication schedule will lead them to stop continually asking the staff members. Of course, interventions that help residents experience more control over other aspects of their environment can also be helpful (see Chapter 14).

We conclude with some examples of treatment of older clients with anxiety disorders.

___

DESENSITIZATION OF A LONG-STANDING PHOBIA

Norm, a client who had been a lifelong agoraphobic, was introduced earlier in the chapter. Treatment began by addressing caregiving issues, including obtaining a medical evaluation of his wife and helping to facilitate a reconciliation between Norm and one of his daughters. Norm's growing understanding of his wife's limitations led him to request treatment for his agoraphobia.

Treatment combined classic desensitization and cognitive-behavioral strategies to help Norm understand his reactions to bodily sensations. A hierarchy of anxiety-provoking situations was constructed. Norm learned to do progressive muscle relaxation and used a tape of the exercise to practice between sessions. He gradually was able to go outside by himself, first just to his front gate, then to the end of the block; eventually he mastered the kind of situation in which he had first experienced his symptoms, standing in line at a post office or a supermarket. He learned and practiced alternative thoughts for interpreting the anxiety he experienced in these situations. He eventually became sufficiently at ease in these situations that he was able to begin conversations with the other people standing in line with him. At the end of treatment, Norm still restricted the distance that he would travel by himself, but he had reached all of his treatment goals.

MANAGING THERAPY OF AN ANXIOUS PATIENT

Laura, age 68, was a retired teacher who was referred for memory testing because she was sure she had AD. When I started testing her, she got so anxious and upset that she refused to continue and decided she didn't want to know whether she had AD after all. Laura told me, "I'm a teacher. I give tests, and I don't take them."

A year later Laura came back for treatment after her physician had prescribed an SSRI. He had prescribed this because she had been going to him with a lot of medical complaints that were not founded. In the first session, Laura acknowledged how anxious the testing had made her. She described how she been an anxious person her whole life. She handled her anxiety by being overprepared, overcareful, and a perfectionist. In that way, Laura could control the events in her life and avoid feeling anxious. That strategy worked well for her in some ways. She was successful in her work, and her family and others relied on her to get things done. The cost was that she was always tense, had sleeping problems, and tended to be negative. Her children perceived her as a critical parent.

As Laura had grown older, she had started focusing on her memory problems all the time. She could remember every memory problem she ever had. She believed that her memory problems helped explain any mistakes she made. Laura reasoned that if she had AD, it did not matter whether she made mistakes.

Laura's husband did have a serious medical problem—PD. She was very fearful of what would happen to both of them in the future. She focused all her fear, however, on whether she had AD. Laura continued to be ambivalent—she both wanted and did not want to know whether she had AD.

Laura had a similar approach–avoidance conflict about therapy. As a result, I took a very cautious approach to treatment, seeing her infrequently, about five or six times a year, and giving her control over the schedule. This has gone on now for about 4 years. She comes to these appointments with a long list of problems in her family. These are real-life problems. Laura's goal had been to keep everything perfect in her life and her family. If she did that, she would not have to feel anxious, and people would not realize she was not the competent person she appeared to be—a perfect teacher, wife, mother, and member of the community. Unfortunately, there have been many problems in her life and her family that she could not control. As Laura grew older, she probably had less energy to try to fix all these problems, but it was more acceptable to her to think of herself as having AD. That way she did not feel responsible for the problems she could not fix.

The SSRI that Laura took, Zoloft, appeared to calm her down, but she felt it made her more forgetful. The effect of the medication may have been to slow down her ruminations, which she had used to help her keep striving to be perfect in the past.

Laura probably could not have tolerated a structured or intensive treatment. Her overriding psychological issue is feeling in control. Although she comes to therapy intermittently, she does not share her problems with anyone else. There is no one else she would let know about her imperfections. Laura uses the treatment sessions to unburden her imperfections, takes very few directives, and then leaves. Laura is probably atypical, but other anxious clients seem to do better when they control how often they come to therapy. They have to decide when to let go of things. It is very anxiety producing for them to think about coming to therapy to talk about the things that make them anxious. Some do more therapeutic work than Laura does. In the end, though, she is able to use therapy to shore up the control she feels in her life and to be effective in addressing the real problems she faces.

CONCLUSIONS

This brief overview of treatment of anxiety disorders touches on the most common ways that anxiety can present in later life and provides a framework for treatment. Often, clients initially focus on the events that have happened in their lives to upset their control of their anxiety, rather than on the anxiety itself. Psychological interventions are an essential component of treatment of anxiety with older adults. Either by themselves or in combination with medication for more severe cases, these treatments have shown promising results. The goal that many patients have is to restore the control they have had in their lives for managing their anxiety. Through education and the use of a variety of cognitive and behavioral techniques, they can learn to understand and manage their symptoms more effectively.

CHAPTER 11

Treatment of Paranoid Symptoms

Paranoid symptoms are a prominent feature of several disorders found in later life. These disorders include early-, late-, and very-late-onset schizophrenia, paranoid personality disorder, delusional disorder, obsessive–compulsive disorder, delirium, and dementia (see Chapter 5). Regardless of etiology, paranoid symptoms are very disruptive, both to older patients and to the people around them.

An older man complains that he is awakened during the night by a light shining on him through his bedroom window, but his wife maintains that the room is dark all night. A woman claims that she hears music playing wherever she goes. She moves from one apartment to another to get away from the music, but it has started to bother her in her new home, making her nervous and upset. Another woman believes that an intruder has been breaking into her home, messing it up and stealing things, but there is no evidence that anyone has broken in.

These examples illustrate some of the patterns of paranoid symptoms in later life. People with paranoid symptoms and other types of hallucinations and delusions are often upset and frightened but usually have little insight about how they are distorting reality. This combination of delusional beliefs and lack of insight is very disturbing to other people, can weaken family support, and may cause some service providers to refuse to help them. A person who has psychotic symptoms is more likely to be stigmatized as crazy than someone who is depressed.

Despite the disruptiveness of paranoid and other psychotic symptoms, treatment can reduce or eliminate symptoms and make the problem more manageable. Treatment depends in part on the etiology of symptoms, but there are elements that are similar regardless of type of disorder. Psychological treatment takes place on the levels of, first, building a relationship with the client and second, when appropriate, working with family, community, and/or institution staff so that they can respond in ways that help contain the symptoms. A basic step is to establish a trusting and accepting relationship, which is a challenge because clients are suspicious and their symptoms are often blatant and disturbing distortions of reality. It is possible, however, to enter into the world of the person with paranoid symptoms, to identify the pain or other emotions that lie behind their distortions, and thereby to establish the trust needed to make treatment successful. Another feature of treatment is coordination of medical and psychological approaches, especially when medications and health problems are involved in onset of symptoms or when medications are part of the treatment plan.

Treatment of older people with paranoid symptoms should be guided by the principle of minimum intervention (Kahn, 1975). The goal of treatment is to identify and treat any reversible components and, if that is not possible, to reduce the negative ramifications of paranoid beliefs, allowing a person to function as well as possible despite some paranoid thinking. When possible, clients with paranoid symptoms should be helped to stay in their homes, because an unwanted move usually only heightens their symptoms. This type of approach can prevent the breakdown of a fragile support system.

The number of clients with paranoid symptoms that a clinician is likely to see varies by the treatment setting. Few clients with paranoid symptoms are willing to fill out all the forms and go through the thorough evaluations that are often required by a teaching facility. These clients are more likely to be encountered in community mental health programs and occasionally in private practice. Paranoid symptoms can also be a problem in nursing homes and similar settings. A useful source for planning treatment is Cognitive Therapy of Schizophrenia (Kingdon & Turkington, 2005), which contains many approaches likely to be helpful for management of paranoid and other psychotic symptoms in later life.

EARLY-ONSET PARANOID SCHIZOPHRENIA

People who have paranoid schizophrenia early in life grow old, and their problems sometimes persist or are exacerbated by losses and other stresses in later life. With long-standing paranoid schizophrenia, the main concerns for clinicians are to continue treatments that were effective in the past, to help the person's support network cope with symptoms, and to identify and address any new problems or stressors that may be upsetting the client and exacerbating symptoms. Treatment that focuses on these new problems and stressors can lead to an overall improvement in functioning, as in this next example. (See Chapter 5 for details on symptoms and assessment of schizophrenia.)

OLD AND NEW PROBLEMS IN A CLIENT WITH PARANOID SCHIZOPHRENIA

Margaret was a woman in her late 70s, who had a long history of delusions and hallucinations that she reported as being continuous but that also worsened periodically. She first sought help because she believed she was being harassed by people who lived in the apartment next to her. Margaret claimed that her neighbors had computers that were constantly making noise and were reading her thoughts. She asked for help in finding another apartment so that she could escape the computer people. I discussed with Margaret's therapist whether a move would reduce her symptoms or whether they would recur in the new setting. Although neither the therapist nor I thought the move would be helpful, we decided it would be best to provide her with information about available housing. Margaret arranged a move for herself and her daughter, who lived with her. Her therapist was accepting and empathic, so when the computer people "tracked down" Margaret at her new residence, she returned to treatment.

Treatment focused on giving Margaret support and empathy and helping her build adaptive skills to resist the intrusions by the computers. Her therapist never confronted her about her symptoms. Reality testing dealt with alternatives to help her cope better, never with whether the computer people were really tormenting her. The goal of treatment was to minimize the disruption the symptoms caused in Margaret's life and to prevent decompensation that might lead to hospitalization or even nursing home placement.

During the course of treatment, Margaret frequently talked about her daughter, who was in her late 30s. Margaret described her as mildly retarded and needing her care and supervision. At one point, Margaret became ill and needed to be hospitalized. Although the hospitalization went smoothly, she became increasingly symptomatic following discharge. Her therapist recognized that she was worried about what might happen to her daughter if she should die and that Margaret expressed this concern by worrying more about the computer people. Other clients with paranoid symptoms have experienced exacerbation of delusional ideation that masks a real concern.

The therapist suggested working with Margaret and her daughter to identify programs that might take care of her daughter, including special housing and employment. Both mother and daughter welcomed this intervention. The therapist arranged for a colleague to conduct a psychological assessment of Margaret's daughter to determine her level of functioning. Based on the test results, it was concluded that the daughter was not retarded but had low-normal functioning (full scale WAIS-III in the mid-90s). She had never worked and had always been dependent on her mother, but that appeared to be due more to their enmeshed relationship than to limited cognitive abilities. With that in mind, a therapist was assigned to work with the daughter to identify appropriate job and skills training for her and to help her make contact with these programs. Both mother and daughter were pleased with this outcome, and Margaret's paranoid symptoms subsided. Resolution of a reality-based and age-related concern—what would happen to her daughter when she died—led to a stabilization of the situation. Although never symptom free, Margaret was able to continue functioning at home at probably the best level possible for her.

Antipsychotic medications have typically been part of the treatment of people with long-standing paranoid symptoms. Long-term use of these medications becomes increasingly problematic in later life, because the risk of tardive dyskinesia increases with age. The older class of antipsychotic medications, which includes haloperidol (Haldol) and thioridazine (Mellaril), have significant anticholinergic effects that can lead to memory problems, excessive sedation, and other complications among older adults. A new class of atypical antipsychotics, which includes risperidone (Risperdal), olanzapine (Zyprexa), quetiapine (Seroquel), and aripiprazole (Abilify), has largely supplanted the older medications, but tendencies still exist toward oversedation, extrapyramidal side effects, and other adverse events. Also, few controlled studies of use of these medications with older people with paranoid or other psychotic symptoms exist except in the case of dementia (see Chapter 12). The potential gains in symptom relief from use of these medications must always be weighed against side effects (for reviews, see Jacobson et al., 2002; Jeste et al., 2004; Lohr, Jeste, Harris, & Salzman, 1992).

PARANOID SYMPTOMS AND PERSONALITY DISORDERS

Paranoid symptoms can be part of a long-standing personality disorder. Individuals with these disorders often have histories of paranoid beliefs. Based on these histories, some of them meet the criteria for paranoid personality disorder. For other individuals, paranoid symptoms have been intermittent in the past or have occurred only during stressful situations. For them, the onset of symptoms in late life marks a change rather than continuation of old patterns. The most common feature in these cases is a history of poor social adjustment. Patients are usually estranged from their families and do not have close friends. As they grew older, their social isolation increased. Employment often provided structure and social contact in their lives that is lost with retirement. Most of these patients are women. When they were younger, they had been able to get attention from men because of their physical attractiveness. Now, however, like other older women, they are largely invisible and feel ignored. Clients have even described being bumped into by someone as though they were not there and not being waited on in restaurants. Depression is often mixed with their suspiciousness and delusions.

Treatment follows a similar protocol to that for early-onset schizophrenia—develop a supportive relationship, address age-related concerns, and coordinate use of medications.

A CLIENT WITH A PARANOID PERSONALITY DISORDER

Marie was in her late 60s when I saw her. She suffered from a paranoid personality disorder and her suspiciousness and distrust of other people often threatened to undermine the precarious balance in her life. When she was younger, she had been very attractive, and as a result she received a lot of attention from men. As she got older, men no longer noticed her, and she became increasingly isolated. Marie had married a man who, based on her description of his behavior, probably had paranoid schizophrenia. The marriage was short-lived and explosive, but they had a daughter, whom Marie raised. Once the daughter reached adulthood, she tried to have as little to do with her mother as possible. Now, however, Marie's health was failing, and she had moved to the city where her daughter lived to be closer to her and to get help from her. Her daughter was upset about having her mother so close to her, and Marie, in turn, was upset by her daughter's ambivalence toward her.

Treatment had three goals. The first was to provide Marie with support and acceptance to lessen her isolation and fears. A second goal was to help her set boundaries with her daughter. I discussed the importance of not putting too much stress on her daughter so that she would be able to provide Marie with assistance when she really needed it. As is the case with people who suffer from other personality disorders, Marie required many repetitions of this idea before she was able to use it to control her behavior. A third goal was to prevent Marie from becoming overly upset or suspicious about everyday occurrences in her life. When she became too upset, her functioning deteriorated and she needed hospitalization, which she did not tolerate well. Marie frequently struck up conversations with strangers and made new acquaintances easily. But then she would dwell on something that a new friend had said during a conversation, taking an innocuous statement and interpreting it as threatening or hostile. I spent a considerable amount of time in therapy sessions helping Marie reinterpret these interactions.

The therapist sometimes becomes the target of the suspicions of clients with paranoia, and that would happen periodically with Marie. It was important to check periodically to see how she was reacting to what I said. She would frequently dwell on an innocuous statement made during the therapy session and give it a hostile interpretation. Complicating the situation was the fact that Marie's attacks on me sometimes did make me feel hostile or angry, and Marie readily detected these feelings because of her hypervigilance.

Overall, treatment was used to sustain Marie at her current level of functioning. There was little progress in reducing her paranoid symptoms, and antipsychotic medications that had been frequently used in the past had little effect. Though Marie did not improve with treatment, exacerbations of symptoms were short-lived, and it was possible to prevent psychiatric hospitalization on several occasions. Some improvement also occurred in her relationship with her daughter.

The best approach with older clients with paranoid symptoms is to be very accepting of how they view the world, not to challenge it. To help develop empathy for them, the therapist can view their complaints as a problem in living rather than as strange or psychotic. It is not possible to convince them that their beliefs are distorted; for example, that people are not out to harm them. Instead, the therapist can help them feel a bit more secure and reduce the worries associated with their paranoid beliefs. Trying to see the world through their eyes will often reveal that a lot of depression and pain is associated with their fears and preoccupations. When a depressive component exists, antidepressant medications can sometimes be useful as part of the overall treatment.

ENCAPSULATED PARANOID DELUSIONS

Some older people have encapsulated paranoid delusions, such as the belief in a plot or conspiracy directed against them. This delusion involves one domain in their lives, and they have no other symptoms that would warrant a schizophrenia diagnosis. This pattern can be seen in someone who has functioned well in life, with steady employment and possibly a long-term marriage, who experiences a traumatic event that triggers the delusion. Some people with borderline personality disorders also have encapsulated delusions.

ENCAPSULATED PARANOID DELUSION

Lilly, age 64, was referred for treatment of migraine headaches. The treatment involved relaxation training, and she had been doing very well with this approach. At that point, I asked her to be part of a training videotape to demonstrate the use of this treatment. Lilly got very frightened and mistrustful and explained, "I can't do that, because the CIA is after me. You know they send messages at the bottom of the TV screen. And you can always tell which cars they have because there is a little mark on the bottom of the license plate." This was astonishing to me, because I had seen no indication of paranoid tendencies until that point. This was, in fact, the first time Lilly had mentioned her belief to anyone. It came out only because of the request to videotape a session. I discussed her belief with her in a few subsequent therapy sessions, after which she did not want to talk about it anymore.

Lilly had had a successful career as a teacher. She had been married briefly, had a son, and raised him. Her son had been involved in drugs as a teenager and died of a drug overdose in his early 20s. He had been the focus of Lilly's life, and his drug-related death was unacceptable to her. Much of her delusion had to do with her son's death. She maintained that the CIA had murdered him because he knew something he should not know.

The therapy relationship for the original problems continued for some time, and Lilly experienced continued improvement for her headaches and related health problems. The therapy relationship was supportive, and she had a great deal of trust in me. She stopped treatment when she moved out of the area to be closer to relatives. I continued to receive Christmas cards from Lilly every year until her death, with no indication that the delusion had ever come out again or that her functioning had become impaired because of it.

Lilly's delusion was very important because it helped her accept her son's death. Most of the time, the clinician does not encounter this type of delusion. Clients complain about problems such as depression or, in this case, migraine headaches. When a delusion is brought up, the therapist needs to be accepting. As in this example, an encapsulated delusion does not necessarily interfere with functioning as long as the client does not dwell on it or talk openly about it to family and friends. If the delusion becomes public and upsets the client's family, the therapist can encourage them to accept rather than challenge the disputed belief. There usually is little harm in these beliefs, and they can be allowed to recede into the background.

PARANOID BELIEFS
AND OBSESSIVE–COMPULSIVE DISORDERS

Paranoid symptoms may be part of an obsessive–compulsive disorder (OCD). People with OCD can be so hypervigilant that their obsessions take on a paranoid quality.

The pattern in which obsessive and paranoid thinking are intertwined is found among hoarders. Hoarders are people who fill their homes with possessions or objects, never throwing anything away. They usually do not seek help for this problem, so clinicians encounter them in the process of community outreach or home visits or when neighbors or health authorities complain about the condition of their homes. The most extreme instance of hoarding we have seen involved a couple who had collected newspapers and magazines for many years and had so filled their house that there were only small passageways left between one room and the next. Everywhere else were piles of newspapers stacked high. The clutter had piled up to such an extent that the house had become unlivable, and the couple lived in a trailer parked in the driveway. Because the couple were not asking for help with their hoarding and because there was no immediate threat to health or safety, no treatment was initiated.

The outcome in this example is typical. Most hoarders see their behavior as appropriate and do not want help for it. Hoarding is one of those characteristics that fall under the rubric of an eccentricity. It is annoying to family members, who often want mental health professionals to intervene, but unless there is an imminent danger, little can be done. We have treated hoarders for other, sometimes related problems but without much impact on their hoarding behavior. As mental health professionals, we have to differentiate between problems that are a threat and lifestyle decisions. Although we would not choose to live the way hoarders do, they have the right to make that choice as long as it does not harm anyone else.

There is an obsessive component to this kind of collecting, but it often also indicates suspiciousness toward other people, as in the following example.

SUSPICIOUSNESS AS PART OF AN OBSESSIVE–COMPULSIVE DISORDER

Marvin was a 78-year-old man who saved virtually every piece of paper that came into the house, including junk mail. He was convinced that he could not throw anything away because he might need it in the future. Marvin's house had not been cleaned for many years. He did not want anyone to come in because he was ashamed of what they would find and because he was mistrustful of having someone in the house. At one point, a neighbor came in to clean. Afterward, whenever Marvin could not find something, he accused the neighbor of having stolen it. Although suspiciousness was part of the overall problem, his obsessive–compulsive disorder remained the bigger treatment issue. Marvin was also depressed, and when he was treated with an SSRI, both his depression and hoarding improved somewhat, although he still accumulated excessive amounts of paper in his small and dirty home. Marvin did not view his hoarding as a problem, and so treatment focused on other, more pressing issues.

SENSORY LOSS AS A CONTRIBUTING FACTOR

Paranoid thinking often appears to be triggered by sensory loss. Hearing impairment is more likely to be involved, though vision loss can also play a role (Rabins, 1992). The mechanism by which sensory loss leads to paranoid thinking is misinterpretation and distortion of input. A person with hearing loss who is having trouble understanding conversations may come to believe that other people are talking about him. Someone with poor vision may believe that she cannot find things around the house because someone has come in and stolen them.

Treatment of paranoid thinking associated with vision and hearing loss proceeds in the same way as for other paranoid symptoms—development of a trusting relationship and judicious use of medication. Every possible way of correcting or compensating for sensory losses should be explored. A person with hearing loss may benefit from a hearing aid or from training to overcome difficulties in using an aid that had previously been prescribed.

Environmental changes can also be helpful. Background noise is particularly problematic for people with typical late-life hearing loss. Cutting down on background noise in the home (e.g., turning off televisions or radios when no one is listening to them) can help. Avoiding situations such as noisy restaurants may reduce misunderstandings. The person's comprehension may improve if other people speak slowly and distinctly and use complete sentences. Talking at a low pitch is more important than speaking loudly. Encouraging family and friends to talk one at a time and to talk individually with the person with hearing loss can also help. For vision loss, a variety of aids, ranging from magnifiers to closed-circuit television systems for reading, can improve functioning (Genensky et al., 1992). Improving lighting and contrast can also be helpful.

PARANOID BELIEFS AND SEVERE HEARING LOSS

John, age 80, was brought to a clinic by his family because of their concern over his increasingly bizarre and troubling behavior. He believed that he had heard on television that the bank was going to repossess his house. John became increasingly preoccupied and disturbed by this thought. He insisted that his wife turn off all the lights during the evening, and he prowled the house with a knife to prevent the bank officials from breaking in and seizing his house. John had also become suspicious of two of his sons, whom he thought were plotting against him. John's family was worried that he would mistake his wife in the dark for a bank official and injure her. They were also concerned about the poor quality of her life as a consequence of his eccentric behavior.

John had a profound hearing loss, but, as in many of these cases, no prior history of paranoid thinking. The family physician had prescribed a neuroleptic, which was appropriate for John's symptoms, but the family was reluctant to try it. I talked with John about the medication that his doctor had prescribed. To overcome his reluctance to take it, I followed the suggestion of one of the pioneers in the study of late-life paranoia, Felix Post (1973). I told John that it was important to take the medication because it would make him stronger. John was willing to take the medication and experienced an immediate decrease in symptoms.

I also talked with the family about making environmental modifications to maximize John's ability to hear. This was a big family, and family gatherings tended to be large and noisy. Some of John's paranoid beliefs about his sons developed during these gatherings, when the amount of background noise caused him to misinterpret what they were telling him. His sons had also tried to argue with him over his fears about the bank repossessing his house. I recommended that everyone be reassuring about the house, but in a general way, without disputing John's belief that the bank was a threat. I also recommended that family members talk to John one-on-one and in situations in which there was a minimum of background noise. A hearing aid was not possible because of the type of hearing loss. His family made the recommended changes. Follow-up a few months later indicated that the situation was stable and that John had had no recurrence of paranoid thinking.

MULTIPLE ETIOLOGIES FOR PARANOID SYMPTOMS

There can be other antecedents of paranoid symptoms in older adults. A major loss, such as death of a spouse or retirement, can trigger paranoid thinking. Especially when a married couple had an enmeshed relationship, the death of one of them can lead to paranoid thinking in the other. The surviving partner may not be skilled at interpreting what other people do in relationships. Add to that a little vision or hearing loss and considerable potential exists to misinterpret social communications. For example, a widow goes to a senior center. If no one makes a place for her to sit, she might interpret that as hostile. She might also misperceive gestures and expressions. She might say, "I saw the look on that woman's face. She doesn't really want me here. I'm not wanted."

ONSET OF PARANOID SYMPTOMS FOLLOWING THE DEATH OF A SPOUSE

Donna, age 56, had married young and had always been very dependent on her husband. She had never been employed and did not have many friends or interests outside the home. When Donna's husband became severely ill with cancer, she visited him in the hospital every day. As she did not know how to drive, it took her an hour and a half each way by public transportation to see him. After a long illness, he died, leaving no insurance and few assets. Donna was referred for therapy by the chaplain at the hospital, who was concerned about how she would put her life back together.

Treatment initially focused on depression and on building skills that would help Donna become more independent. After a few months, she felt ready to get involved in social activities and identified dancing as something she enjoyed. She started going to a social club that held weekly dances, and she obviously enjoyed the activity and the attention she received from the men there. One of the men she danced with developed an interest in her. When he made a comment to Donna that seemed, in her retelling, to be a very indirect sexual innuendo, it upset her and caused her to reject him. The prospect of getting involved sexually was very frightening to her. Donna then became preoccupied with the belief that he and the other men were all talking about her and saying bad things about her because she would not sleep with him. She became increasingly distressed and was reluctant to go back to the group.

Because the therapist had a good relationship with Donna at this point, she was able to introduce cognitive approaches to look at these critical events in other ways. Though Donna's belief that the men in the club were talking about her did not change, she identified another dance group and began going there with no recurrence of the problem. She continued to work in therapy on developing better social skills and reality testing so that she was less likely to overreact to advances from men at the dances or misinterpret other communications.

Gradually, Donna became more skilled at taking care of other issues in her life (e.g., managing her finances, getting part-time work). She continued to attend dances and to enjoy them as a social outlet. She liked the attention from the men she danced with but continued to maintain a distance from them.

In this example, the key factors were the client's long dependence on her husband and her lack of social sophistication. When her dancing partner became sexually interested in her, she overreacted and felt that all the men there had turned against her. The therapy relationship was used to help lower her fears and to build more adaptive social skills.

PARANOID SYMPTOMS IN DELIRIUM

Paranoid symptoms are often observed in delirium. Delirium should be suspected when delusions or other paranoid symptoms develop suddenly. The clinician must first ask what has changed recently—medications, the client's health, or anything else. Although delirium can have many different causes (see Chapter 3), the most common triggers are medications and illnesses. Heart and antihypertensive medications, antibiotics, and steroids frequently are involved in development of paranoid delusions and other delirium symptoms, though many other medications can be involved as well.

DELIRIUM WITH PARANOID SYMPTOMS PRECIPITATED
BY A CHANGE IN HEART MEDICATIONS

Jean had been prescribed Inderal, a medication used for heart disease and for hypertension after a heart attack 20 years earlier. At that time, she developed the belief that her neighbors were transmitting radio waves into her apartment, causing her to become increasingly agitated. With discontinuation of the medication, the psychotic symptoms ceased, and Jean was discharged. She had no similar problems during the following 20 years. Her current physician did not have this history, and although Jean remembered the episode clearly, she did not recall the name of the medication. When her physician made a change in her medications, prescribing Inderal, Jean developed the paranoid delusion that her daughter was going to kill her. She believed that she had to kill her daughter in order to defend herself.

My evaluation revealed the psychotic episode 20 years before and the fact that the current onset of symptoms coincided with Jean having started the heart medication 3 months earlier. With this information, Jean's physician discontinued the medication, and the symptoms went away.

A couple of points should be emphasized about this example. First is the importance of history. The events of 20 years earlier provided a clue to the present episode, as did the sequence of events (i.e., change in medication) that led up to the onset of symptoms. It is continually surprising how often history is overlooked. Careful reconstruction of the sequence of events that has led up to the sudden onset of paranoid delusions or other delirium symptoms provides valuable information about the cause. Second, this case illustrates the role of medications in delirium and associated psychotic symptoms. Unless trained in geriatrics, physicians are not necessarily familiar with the mental changes associated with medication reactions and can easily ascribe these symptoms to other causes. Older patients with medication-induced deliriums have been labeled as schizophrenic, demented, or just "old." By developing good working relationships with physicians, a therapist can encourage them to review the medications as possible contributing factors to a sudden onset of paranoid symptoms.

Onset of a Delirium with Paranoid Symptoms Following Treatment with Steroids

Pat was a client I had seen for awhile for psychological concerns. She had been a smoker and had developed bronchial problems. She was hospitalized for these problems and placed on prednisone. She subsequently became increasingly suspicious and fearful while on the medication. Pat was discharged on a decreasing dosage of the medication. Once she was discharged from the hospital, I dealt with her fears by talking with her daily on the telephone. I gave her reassurance that the bad things that she feared would not happen. I explained that her fears were the result of the medication, not of how people felt about her. By hearing this frequent reassurance, Pat was able to tolerate the suspiciousness until the medication was eliminated and the symptoms went away.

In this example, the patient had some degree of insight and could use verbal reassurances that her fears were due to the side effects of the medication. Her insight contrasts with cases of paranoid beliefs due to other causes. In both lifelong and late-onset paranoia, patients show little or only fleeting awareness of the distortions that are involved in their beliefs. Even with a reversible delirium, insight may be limited.

PARANOID SYMPTOMS IN DEMENTIA

Paranoid symptoms are very common in dementia. One type of paranoid symptom appears to be the result of a process by which patients fill in gaps caused by their memory loss. They may accuse someone of stealing a wallet or purse they have misplaced. These beliefs can be adaptive in that, by accusing someone else of causing their problem, patients can avoid recognizing the problems they are having finding and remembering things.

Another type of symptom reported by patients with dementia is imaginary visitors who come into the house. Occasionally, these visitors are benevolent; for example, a child who comes to visit. More often, the visitors are threatening and frightening, and they steal things from the patient. These types of problems should be differentiated from illusions that are experienced later in the dementia process. A later stage patient may report seeing small animals running across a dimly lighted room. These illusions are not experienced as frightening and do not have a malevolent or threatening component. They are primarily upsetting to the family.

When a patient with dementia develops paranoid symptoms, the first concern is to rule out a comorbid delirium. Given the increased susceptibility that patients with dementia have to delirium (see Chapter 3), this possibility should be considered, especially when sudden change in functioning occurs. Once a delirium is ruled out, treatment takes place at several levels: patient, family or other involved people, and environment. When the patient's dementia is not too severe, the clinician can develop a supportive relationship and, as in other cases of paranoid symptoms, use the relationship to provide reassurance and reduce fears. As with paranoid symptoms due to other etiologies, it is best not to confront patients with dementia or try to get them to change their beliefs. Rather, the therapist can respond to the affective components of their delusions—the fear, anxiety, or depression that accompanies the belief that someone is stealing from or threatening them. Medications may be considered, but the response is unpredictable with dementia (see Chapter 12).

The main focus of treatment is typically the family or other caregivers. Often the problem is the family's reactions to paranoid complaints, not the complaints themselves. It is especially problematic when the patient makes accusations against someone in the family. Families typically respond to paranoid symptoms by trying to change the patient's beliefs. Reasoning with patients or even demonstrating that an object was not stolen does not usually reduce these complaints. Arguments over the facts are not successful, because the patients' beliefs are embedded in their diminished ability to process information. These beliefs help patients understand their increasingly confusing world, and they hold onto them in the face of obvious and repeated contradictions. The therapist can work with the family or other caregivers to avoid confrontations and arguments over the facts. As an alternative, they can learn to respond to the emotions the patient conveys in these communications (see Chapter 13 for a more detailed discussion).

Finally, a structured routine can keep patients occupied while minimizing opportunities to misplace or lose valued objects. Keeping patients busy also tires them out, reducing their anxiety and agitation. Simplifying the environment can also be beneficial. Caregivers might be encouraged to straighten up a messy home. In a neater setting, patients may still lose objects, but families have an easier time finding them. Good illumination in the home is also helpful, especially in late afternoon or early evening, when these problems can be greatest.

PARANOID OR REAL?

In many instances, paranoid-sounding complaints can seem plausible. It is important to consider whether there is a basis in fact to these complaints. When clients complain that someone is stealing from them, there is always a possibility that it has happened. Older people are taken advantage of by strangers or even family members. The situation can be more complicated when a client's complaint has both a basis in reality *and* an exaggerated, paranoid component.

PARANOID COMPLAINT OR FACT?

In a first visit, Ellen complained about intruders who had vandalized her house and property. I had recently seen two other clients who had reported similar stories that turned out to be imaginary. One of those clients suffered from long-term paranoid schizophrenia, and the other had dementia. Ellen was upset when talking about the intruders, and so her story was disjointed and many of the details were not clear. Rather than assuming that she was delusional, however, I conducted a home visit, which revealed gang activities in the lot next to her house. Some gang members had, indeed, vandalized her property, just as she described. Needless to say, treatment was quite different from an intervention for a paranoid disorder.

SHIFTING ETIOLOGIES OF PARANOID SYMPTOMS

The concluding case is one of the most complicated we have ever followed. This case illustrates the importance of assessment and the potential for multiple etiologies in cases of paranoid beliefs. It also illustrates how a multifaceted treatment approach can enhance a client's strengths and support independent functioning.

The Changing Nature of Paranoid Ideation

Eleanor, age 72, was seen at a clinic specializing in problems of older people. She initially said that she needed help in finding a job. When I questioned her about it, she told a fragmented story about a recent hospitalization. According to Eleanor, she had gone to the county hospital for treatment of a medical problem and had been held against her will on the psychiatric ward. She described a nightmarish sequence of being wheeled into the deep recesses of the hospital and put through an apparatus that examined her brain (probably a CT scan). She was afraid the doctors had put something into her brain during that procedure. Despite this odd story, Eleanor had no current overt psychotic symptoms and no gross cognitive impairment, as determined by brief mental status testing. She lived alone and claimed to have no living family.

A treatment plan was developed to explore her concern about working and her financial worries (she was afraid she would be evicted from her apartment for failing to pay the rent). The sessions would also be used to assess her further to understand better what had happened during the hospitalization and to respond to her fears that it might happen to her again. Although medical records might have clarified what happened during the hospitalization, Eleanor did not want me to contact the hospital and would not sign a release so that her records could be obtained.

Some progress was made in a few treatment sessions toward developing a therapeutic relationship and exploring Eleanor's concerns about money. Her counselor learned that Eleanor received a small Social Security check as her only income and that her landlord wanted to evict her because she was sometimes late with the rent. The counselor inferred that her behavior made the threat of eviction more likely, but her stories were disjointed and difficult to follow.

Eleanor then failed to keep an appointment and did not answer telephone calls. After failing to contact her, her counselor visited Eleanor's apartment building. When there was no answer at her apartment, the counselor talked to a neighbor, who described how Eleanor had been taken away in an apparently psychotic state by an ambulance. For a few nights before this incident, she had been waking her neighbors by standing in the hallway and yelling loudly and in an incoherent way. The neighbor did not know where she had been taken.

After about a month, Eleanor phoned the clinic to speak to her counselor. She was now residing in a nursing home, where she had been brought by the ambulance. She wanted the counselor to help her get back to her apartment. After talking with the nursing home staff, the counselor agreed to make visits there.

From discussions the counselor had with Eleanor in the nursing home, the sequence of events leading to this episode—and possibly to the previous one—

became apparent. Eleanor's financial concerns had been quite serious; she ran out of money toward the end of each month. As a consequence, she had no money for food and stopped eating, which preceded her bizarre behavior. Our provisional diagnosis was that the episode was a delirium, given her psychotic and disorganized symptoms, their episodic pattern, the association with poor nutrition, and her apparent full recovery. She did, however, remain somewhat suspicious of other people, including the nursing home staff, whom she felt were trying to keep her against her will.

For their part, the staff at the nursing home felt that Eleanor could not live independently and were annoyed when they found out about her efforts to move. The physician at this facility had diagnosed her as having AD and was opposed to her moving, though once again our cognitive testing revealed no obvious deficits. She had by now lost her apartment but had persuaded her brother (she had previously denied having any relatives) to move her possessions into storage. We talked with her brother, who indicated that he was involved reluctantly and that he preferred to leave her in the nursing home, where she would not be a bother to him. He described his sister as having led a marginal life, able to support herself in the past by working at low-paying jobs but otherwise isolating herself and being suspicious of others.

Despite the opposition of the nursing home staff, Eleanor insisted she wanted to move. Our assessment was that she was capable of living independently, and so her therapist provided her with names and phone numbers of low-cost retirement homes. Eleanor preferred that type of housing because meals would be provided. In a few weeks, she was able to locate a retirement home she liked and arranged to move.

After the move, she functioned well for a while. The retirement home provided congregate meals and a small amount of supervision, allaying our concerns about a possible recurrence of a delirium. Nonetheless, Eleanor soon became suspicious of the management at the home. She was also having difficulty tolerating the close contact with other residents. The therapist and I were worried about the risks involved if she went out on her own, but she was insistent. Again taking the initiative, she found an apartment and arranged the move. To address our concerns about her nutrition, her therapist looked into the possibility of having meals delivered to her and, with Eleanor's consent, arranged for home-delivered meals. This worked out well, though at one point we needed to intervene with the agency, which was threatening to discontinue the meals because Eleanor was refusing to make a "voluntary" donation.

The therapist followed Eleanor for several more months. Although remaining suspicious of many people, Eleanor had a good relationship with her therapist and would call when she needed help. Retesting indicated that her cognitive functioning was stable.

This case illustrates many important features of late-life paranoid disorders. From both Eleanor and her brother, we learned that she had a long history of poor social adjustment and suspiciousness toward other people. This suspiciousness became obvious in her relationships with the staff in the nursing home and with staff and residents in the retirement home. Complicating the situation, however, were the two apparent delirium episodes. In retrospect, these episodes were triggered when Eleanor ran out of food and stopped eating. The bizarre behavior during those two episodes was never observed in any other situation. Thus this case involved both lifelong paranoid beliefs *and* recent episodes that were part of a delirium. The contribution of several different factors to paranoid symptoms underscores the importance of a careful assessment. Knowing only Eleanor's history, it might be concluded that her problems were long-standing, possibly due to paranoid schizophrenia. The physician at the nursing home also ignored history and mislabeled her problem as AD. The implications of diagnosis should be evident. If Eleanor had AD and declining cognitive functioning, then keeping her in a protected setting might be justified. But repeated testing and Eleanor's own competency in arranging moves showed no evidence of dementia.

Given Eleanor's suspiciousness and history of fragile interpersonal relationships, our first emphasis in treatment was development of a supportive, trusting relationship. A therapist could not become too close or intrusive yet had to be perceived by Eleanor as a strong enough ally to be her advocate. What Eleanor wanted most was to remain independent. She had, in fact, initially sought help in finding a job. In the end, we responded to this initial request in an indirect way, helping her find a stable living situation in which she could afford food and rent and remain on her own.

Like many people with odd or abrasive behavior, Eleanor often alienated potential helpers. We sometimes had to run interference for her, as we did with the home-delivered-meals program. Agencies that serve the elderly are often not used to dealing with people with serious psychopathology. In these cases, developing cooperation between mental health and aging services is especially valuable.

Eleanor's case illustrates the often delicate balance between independence and dependence in older clients. A clinician's primary goal should be to design interventions that are consistent with clients' values. There are many circumstances in which taking protective actions are necessary, of course. But when the older person is competent to make a decision, the clinician should value and support independence to the extent possible. The decision to place someone in a protected setting is frequently couched as a medical decision, much like a prescription for medication. Often, however, this decision concerns values about lifestyle and quality of life, including the risks that someone is willing to take by continuing to live in a less protected setting. Clients may prefer to live in ways that clinicians or family disapprove of, accepting the accompanying risks as the best way to live out their lives. The pressure on the client and the clinician in these situations can be tremendous. But there are risks associated with protected settings as well, and the best decision involves balancing risks in the broader context of the client's values.

CONCLUSIONS

Paranoid symptoms in later life are a complex and challenging problem in geriatric practice. The starting point is conducting a careful evaluation that differentiates among the various possible etiologies. Symptoms can be the manifestation of a lifelong disorder (paranoid schizophrenia, paranoid personality disorder) or a worsening of a long-standing personality disorder with little or no prior history of paranoid symptoms. Symptoms can also be a response to sensory loss, dementia, and delirium. Identification of the probable etiology is always the first step in treatment; interventions depend in part on the etiology. Successful treatment requires a full range of treatment skills, including developing a supportive therapeutic relationship with the client, the client's family, and other professionals; bringing in aging services when needed; and examining values and choices in complex situations.

CHAPTER 12

Treatment of Dementia

Trapped by their memory loss in an increasingly bewildering present, patients with dementia become unable to recognize their surroundings and the people around them. Though they need help, they sometimes lash out at anyone who tries to assist. Their families can become overwhelmed by the need to provide around-the-clock care and supervision of an increasingly unreasonable person. Not surprisingly, dementia is the major reason older people are placed in nursing homes or other institutional settings. Just as care of these patients can be overwhelming for families, it also places considerable burden on the staff in institutions, who all too often have insufficient resources and training to do the job asked of them.

Although the effectiveness of treatments for the underlying disease is still limited, timely and well-planned interventions can help patients, their families, or institution staff to function as well as possible. This chapter begins with a framework for treatment of dementia. Next, treatment approaches developed specifically for early mild dementia are described. We then examine the use of medications, cognitive training, and behavioral interventions. The focus on dementia continues in Chapter 13, which addresses family caregiving, and in Chapter 14, which describes consultation in nursing homes and other institutional settings for people with dementia and other residents.

FRAMEWORK FOR TREATMENT OF DEMENTIA

How a problem is conceptualized determines expectations for treatment. If dementia is viewed as a medical illness for which no treatments are available to stop or reverse the course of the disease, then it follows that mental health professionals can do very little. Alternatively, dementia can be conceptualized as an interaction of biomedical, psychological, social, and environmental processes (Figure 12.1). Even though the biomedical components of dementia cannot currently be altered to a significant degree, it is possible to intervene at the psychological, social, and environment levels. These interventions will not restore a person to health, but they can make a substantial difference in how patients function, as well as in their quality of life and in how well their caregivers are able to manage.

We illustrate this approach through the most troubling problem associated with dementia—behavior problems. Neurodegenerative illnesses such as AD can increase the likelihood of disturbed or agitated behavior in several ways. Neurons are lost in key regions of the brain, leading to corresponding deficits in neurotransmitters involved in the regulation of mood and behavior (Kirby & Lawlor, 1995). Cognitive deficits associated with dementia also make problem behavior more likely. Patients may misunderstand what other people say to them, be unable to communicate effectively, or become frightened by their inability to recognize people, places, or things. They also have more difficulty initiating activities and keeping occupied. These changes create an increased probability of behavior problems. Whether and how often these problems occur, however, is partly dependent on social and environmental cues and reinforcers. In other words, despite their dementia, patients remain embedded in a context, and their behavior often is a response to specific events.

The following example of the interaction of patient and environment should be familiar to anyone experienced in dementia care. A patient is walking down the hall of a nursing home. A staff member comes up from behind and starts talking to the patient before making eye contact. The patient star-

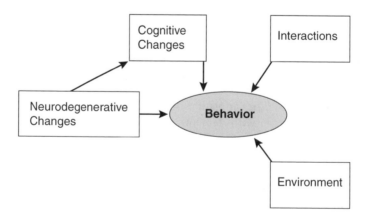

FIGURE 12.1. Model of behavior problems in dementia.

tles, swings out, and hits the staff member. Viewing the incident as due to the disease, the staff concludes that patients with dementia get violent. If seen as an interaction, however, the incident takes on a different meaning. The patient's outburst was due to an encounter between a person with a cognitive disorder who startles easily and a staff person who was not skilled in dealing with dementia. Viewing the problem in this way reveals a straightforward solution: If the staff member had walked around and made eye contact before speaking, the patient would not have struck out. As this example illustrates, dementia does not cause violent behavior, but it does lower patients' inhibitions against striking out when startled.

Sleep problems, which are very common in dementia, provide another example of the complex interactions between disease and environment. Changes in sleep are in part due to damage in regions of the brain that regulate sleep and waking (Bliwise, 1994). Sleep problems, however, are more common among patients who nap during the daytime. A combination of structured activities and decreased opportunities for unscheduled naps during the day may improve sleep during the night for patients with dementia, as they do for the rest of us (Zarit, Stephens, Townsend, & Greene, 1998).

Dementia, then, increases the likelihood of a variety of problems, but when and how often they occur is related to interactions within a particular setting. Even in advanced dementia, events trigger problem behaviors, and how people respond can reinforce these behaviors. Viewing the behavior of patients with dementia as the outcome of an interaction creates the possibility for many types of intervention. Sometimes it is possible to intervene directly with patients, for example, by using medications or even psychological interventions. More often, it is possible to change how other people respond to the patient or to make alterations in the environment that lead to better functioning. The main goal is to identify treatable or modifiable aspects of the situation.

Good dementia care also means focusing not just on the disease but on the person. In his influential book, *Dementia Reconsidered*, Thomas Kitwood (1997) argued that people with cognitive impairment are stigmatized and viewed as not being fully alive. This perception creates pathological interactions that account at least in part for the behavioral and emotional problems of people with dementia and also lead to tolerance of poor and degrading care. To alter these negative interactions, Kitwood proposed a person-centered approach for people with dementia. Person-centered care emphasizes the basic humanity of someone with dementia (Woods, 1999). It gives people a voice in their own care when caregivers learn about their past preferences, as well as their personal and cultural identities. Person-centered care also emphasizes that people with dementia communicate through their emotions. Misunderstandings result when people with dementia are expected to be able to communicate in a primarily cognitive way. Rather than responding to a person's cognitions or behavior, which are faulty attempts to communicate, we need to identify underlying emotions and to respond at that level to the person's intent.

INTERVENTIONS FOR EARLY, MILD DEMENTIA

An increasing emphasis is now placed on early diagnosis of dementia. This trend reflects the availability of medications that may slow the progression for a while in some patients. Early diagnosis is important because more effective treatments, when they are developed, will in all likelihood need to be administered as soon as possible in the disease to stop the degenerative process.

Early intervention represents a window of opportunity to incorporate the patient's perspective into treatment (Kuhn, 1998). Treatment can address the patients' immediate concerns and emotions raised by diagnosis and can include their input about the care they would like to receive as the disease worsens. It is also an opportunity to help the person with early-stage dementia and his or her caregivers find better ways to work together, thereby heading off some of the predictable problems in communication that arise later in the disease.

It is critical to these interventions that patients retain an awareness of their diagnosis and the problems they are experiencing. Awareness makes it possible to engage them in an active way (Zarit et al., 2004). Although we use the term "early stage," the stages of disease remain imprecise, and there can be considerable heterogeneity at every stage. Not everyone in the early stages of dementia has this awareness, but some patients may retain awareness for a long time. Awareness can also fluctuate, which poses another challenge for treatment. Other interventions for early-stage patients (e.g., certain medications, adult day care) may not depend on awareness.

Early-stage interventions can also address some of the risks associated with diagnosis. These risks include the possibility of false positive diagnoses, depression and withdrawal, inappropriate manipulation of assets by family members seeking to protect an inheritance, and adverse side effects of medication (Iliffe & Manthorpe, 2004). A risk of suicide is also greatest early in a dementia, when patients still retain the capacity to plan and carry out an attempt.

Should people diagnosed with mild cognitive impairment (MCI) be included in early-stage programs? As noted in Chapter 3, many people diagnosed with MCI progress to dementia, but some do not, and the guidelines for diagnosis remain vague. For those reasons, we recommend working with patients with MCI, and possibly also their families in individual counseling sessions that can address their concerns and monitor changes in functioning. We would not place these individuals in a group with people who have confirmed dementia diagnoses. The focus in a group would be on dealing with the consequences of inevitable decline, not on the uncertainty that an MCI diagnosis entails.

One-to-One and Dyadic Counseling with Early-Stage Patients

Patients in early and sometimes even middle stages of dementia who have an awareness of their deficits can participate actively in counseling. Early in the dementia process, patients are often depressed or anxious in response to the changes in their intellectual functioning. It is appropriate to see them for individual therapy as long as they have adequate short-term memory to recall ideas and events from week to week. There will inevitably come a time when the dementia progresses beyond that point and the primary caregiver must become involved.

Treatment of early-stage patients usually arises following an assessment that confirms the findings of dementia. It is usually true that the patient and family have been aware of problems for quite some time before an assessment is sought. Performing the assessment and giving feedback is the beginning of a long process. Based on the assessment, we make recommendations in three major areas: (1) for the referring physician, for example, if medication is involved or additional tests are indicated; (2) for the patient regarding compensatory strategies and addressing depressive or anxiety reactions to the diagnosis and its implications; (3) for the family about how to optimize the patient's independence and manage current problems and to alert them to potentially dangerous situations that might arise in the future.

The implications of a diagnosis of AD are catastrophic, so a frank discussion with patients about their illness can have adverse consequences. Some families, in fact, do not want to tell patients about the diagnosis, and many physicians advise families not to tell patients what is wrong. It is better, however, to answer patients' questions truthfully. Ethically, they have a right to know. Furthermore, catastrophic reactions to the diagnosis are quite rare. Patients are either able to handle the information or conveniently forget it. That is not to say that patients cannot react badly to finding out they have dementia. Suicidal thoughts may arise, and clinicians should respond as they would in any other situation, including hospitalization if the risk is great.

Whenever possible, we recommend working with patients and caregivers together, because that will allow better continuity of care as the dementia worsens. The goals for these sessions include providing information to them about the disease and potential treatments, improving communication, learning strategies for coping with memory loss, learning how to deal with family and friends concerning memory loss and other changes in those relationships, identifying how the person with dementia might maintain a sense of usefulness, and discussing feelings of grief and loss (Clare, 2002; Kuhn, 1998;

Moniz-Cook, Agar, Gibson, Win, & Wang, 1998). Clare (2002) observes that treatment needs to help the patients and caregivers strike a balance between fighting the disease and accepting it and the limitations it imposes.

The following case illustrates how working with a couple from the outset can be useful as the disease progresses.

THE SHIFTING FOCUS OF TREATMENT

Patrick, age 57, had taken early retirement when his memory began to fail. A thorough evaluation led to a diagnosis of AD. His wife had kidney disease and was just beginning dialysis. They came to therapy together, but she made it clear that they were in therapy so that Patrick could talk about his feelings. He was depressed and withdrawn, but as he became more comfortable in the setting, he opened up more. Although they came every 6 or 8 weeks for financial reasons, therapy became an important stabilizing factor for both of them.

Over several years Patrick declined to the point that he could no longer participate actively in the sessions. When his wife became eligible for a kidney transplant, she placed him in an assisted living facility. By this time, he was unable to remember where his wife was or when she would be back. For a period of several weeks, I was able to see Patrick at the facility and also to consult with staff there to help him through this crisis. Much of the focus was on providing concrete ways to remind him about where his wife was and when she would see him again. Examples included putting a note on his door and marking a calendar. The reminders helped keep Patrick calm and reduced the burden on staff.

In this case, the relationship I developed with Patrick's wife led her to turn to me at the time of her kidney transplant. Although Patrick's memory was too poor at this point for him to participate in therapy, he still remembered me, and I could give him support and reassurance in the assisted living facility. Because I knew him well, it helped me formulate effective strategies that the staff could use for reassuring him.

When working with a dementia patient and caregiver, we recommend alternating between conjoint and individual sessions with each person. This pattern allows shorter sessions with the patient when his or her attention span would preclude an hour-long session. It also makes it possible to build a strong relationship with the caregiver, which is important for the long haul. When the patient is not present, caregivers can express the full weight of their frustrations and despair over the diagnosis. Similarly, people with dementia may use their sessions to voice annoyance with their spouses or other caregivers or to reveal something about themselves that they want to discuss privately.

The conjoint sessions are useful in other ways. The therapist has the opportunity to observe directly how the pair is interacting. It is possible to determine whether the patient's memory deficits are exacerbating existing communication problems. The interactions may also reveal how the illness has changed the balance of power in the relationship. Clinicians need to be aware of this shift and avoid allying solely with the caregiver, which will only increase the growing imbalance in the relationship. Instead, interventions should bolster and validate the patient's position in the relationship while allowing his or her caregiver to take over responsibilities as needed.

One frequent source of tension involves the caregiver's taking over activities that the patient used to do. Patients often feel threatened or upset when this happens, or they resist and argue with their caregivers over whether they can continue performing a task. Conjoint sessions can clarify which activities the caregiver really needs to take over. Patients can sometimes identify what they would like their caregiver to say or do when they need help.

In time, the patient's ability to participate in individual and conjoint sessions decreases, and the focus of treatment shifts to the primary caregiver and other family members. The therapist cannot ethically continue to see a person with dementia once the disease precludes his or her ability to participate in treatment. The person can, however, continue to be part of conjoint or family meetings. Taking the time to focus on that person in these sessions can still have a supportive effect, even though he or she can no longer work on current problems.

A recent study looked at the benefits of engaging people with early-stage dementia and their caregivers in a process of planning for the future (Whitlatch, Judge, Zarit, & Femia, in press). Participants included both married couples and parent–child dyads. The dyad met jointly, as well as individually, with a counselor. As is typical in many early-stage interventions, the counselor reviewed information about dementia and about services available with the patient and caregiver. The innovative feature of the treatment was to engage the dyad in a discussion of their preferences for care when the patient needed more assistance. The two individuals first explored their values and preferences for care. The focus then moved to developing a specific care plan that listed who would provide help for different kinds of tasks, such as managing the finances or assisting with activities of daily living. For this step, the counselor used a visual aid consisting of three large circles, one marked with the caregiver's name, one marked as other family members and friends, and one marked as "paid helpers." The counselor would write in the appropriate circle who the pair decided should do a particular task. Through the use of the circles, it would become apparent to the caregiver, and almost always to the person with dementia as well, that the caregiver would quickly become overloaded with all the care demands he or she was expected to handle. That would lead to a revision of the plan so that more family members and paid helpers would be included. The counselor would then write down the final plan for the patient and caregiver and put it in notebooks they used during the treatment. The long-term goals were to incorporate the patient's perspective into a plan for care and to give caregivers permission to get additional help if needed.

A patient without family supports is extremely vulnerable. In these cases, the therapist often must navigate a difficult course between what the patient wants and the types of support and help that may be needed.

In these situations, the therapist must be careful to keep the client's best interests in mind and not just push for a convenient solution. Some people with dementia may insist on remaining at home, despite increasing problems in caring for themselves. In those cases, I take a careful look at the amount of help that might be available and how much risk there would be if the client remains at home. It is important to keep in mind that while something bad might happen to a person with dementia who remains at home, a different set of hazards are encountered in institutional settings. When the risk associated with living at home becomes too great—for example, that a client might harm him- or herself or someone else, or fail to provide for his or her own basic needs—then placement would need to be considered. In that case, the therapist's role is to find a solution that best suits the client, given his or her background and preferences, and then to help the client through the transition. If a client steadfastly refuses to choose a facility, I would need to involve the appropriate public agencies in his or her care. This process, however, is less likely to incorporate the client's own preferences in selecting a place to live.

Sometimes, of course, conflict or even abuse may occur in the family. In the following case, the person with dementia was vulnerable to financial abuse because of his memory loss and suggestibility. He could be involved actively in resolving the situation because he still had the ability to understand the choices facing him and to indicate his preferences.

Addressing Financial Exploitation

Irving, age 79, was a widower with two children, both of whom lived 3 or 4 hours away. Irving had been a successful medical professional. He had VaD and was aware of his short-term memory problems, although he tended to minimize them. After the initial evaluation and feedback, he felt no need for further treatment.

About 2 years later, Irving's older daughter called to begin family therapy with him. She had just discovered that her younger sister had been systematically obtaining "loans" from her father for her usually ill-fated business ventures. By the time the older daughter discovered the loans, her sister had gotten nearly $1 million from Irving. Her concern was both that he might endanger his own financial security and that he was being influenced to distribute his estate in a way that was inconsistent with his true intent.

Irving, the older daughter, and I met several times to discuss the loans. Irving was genuinely surprised that the total was as high as it was. It had not been his intention to give her so much money. Finally, he agreed to turn his finances over to a financial planner and to have his older daughter approve any additional transfers to his younger daughter. This arrangement was worked out with his lawyer and with the lawyer his younger daughter had retained.

In this case, Irving had the capability of understanding what his resources were and how he wanted to manage them. The effects of the dementia, however, had made him highly suggestible, and he also had troubling remembering how much he had given to his younger daughter. The result of these sessions with his older daughter was to determine his preferences about how the money should be managed and to help him make a decision.

The therapeutic possibilities are as varied as individuals, their diseases, their caregivers, and their circumstances. The keys to providing a high quality of psychological care are flexibility and adaptability. Although these are challenging cases that require creativity and ingenuity, there is also the potential for great personal satisfaction in building a therapeutic connection to the person with dementia and helping ensure the best possible care.

Group Treatment in Early Dementia

Support groups for early-stage patients and their family caregivers can be found in many communities and have been reported to be very helpful (e.g., Goldsilver & Gruneir, 2001; Mason, Clare, & Pistrang, 2005; Yale, 1991, 1999; Zarit et al., 2004). As noted, these groups should be used for people with a confirmed diagnosis of a dementia, not for someone with mild cognitive impairment or who is worried about memory loss. As with other group treatments, the opportunity to interact with other people going through the same process is a major benefit. Patients can overcome the sense of being isolated and gain support from one another. They may also learn better ways of coping with their problems. Yale (1991) recommends using here-and-now experiences in the group to build coping strategies. For example, if one member loses track of the topic being discussed, she asks other participants if that happens to them. Other topics covered in these groups include discussions about possible treatments, looking at how the disease has affected their lives and family relationships, concerns about the future, attitudes toward death, and how to maximize one's remaining abilities and to engage in satisfying activities (Yale, 1991; Zarit et al., 2004). Summaries by the leader at the start and end of the session can help participants orient themselves to the group and help them recall previous discussions.

A major focus in groups can be reminiscence, which draws on memories not yet affected by the disease. Reviewing prior accomplishments and activities can build esteem in the face of this catastrophic process. Mason and colleagues (2005) report that social contact in the group and sharing personal stories is a major source of support to participants.

Group leaders need to be prepared to address communication and behavior problems. Denial is a common response in patients with dementia. Even when participants have been selected based on their awareness of their diagnosis and memory loss, denial can be a problem (Zarit et al., 2004). Denial can be adaptive. Group leaders should not conduct a frontal attack to try to break through it. They should consider carefully whether anything valuable will be gained by overcoming a patient's denial. Often the answer is no. Instead, patients should be helped to deal with information they cannot handle in a gentle and sometimes indirect way. The group can have a general discussion of these difficult areas, taking the focus off the individual.

To date, only limited evaluations have been done of the effectiveness of group treatments for people with dementia or their caregivers. One treatment approach, Memory Club, consisted of a 10-session structured program that allowed for both separate and joint discussions for patients and caregivers. Patients and caregivers both evaluated the intervention positively, but caregivers found the group format and interactions more helpful to them than patients did (Zarit et al., 2004). Similar to reports by Mason and colleagues (2005), less sharing and mutual support took place when patients met separately from their caregivers, and leaders had to take an active role in keeping discussions going. The biggest value of Memory Club may have been the opportunity for caregiver and patient to discuss common concerns together. Patients could tolerate frank discussions about dementia and its long-term consequences and were able to share some of their concerns with their caregivers.

MEDICATIONS FOR DEMENTIA

Medications for dementia can be divided into two broad categories: those used as primary treatments for the disease and those that address associated symptoms, such as behavior problems and depression.

Medications as Primary Treatment

The main class of medications for treatment of AD is the cholinesterase inhibitors (Table 12.1). These medications also have been reported to have benefits in other types of dementia, including VaD (Malouf & Birks, 2004) and DLB (McKeith, 1997). Improvement is found when the medication is administered in earlier stages of the disease. The current prescribing practice is to place patients on one of these medications as soon as the diagnosis has been made or, in some cases, at the point at which MCI is determined and to keep patients on them for the duration of their illness. Maintenance of patients on these medications is based on the assumption that they will experience a drop in functioning once the drugs are removed.

TABLE 12.1. Cholinesterase Inhibitors Used in Treating Alzheimer's Disease

Generic name	Brand name
tacrine[a]	Cognex
donepezil	Aricept
rivastigmine	Exelon
galantamine	Reminyl

[a]No longer widely used because of side effects.

These prescribing practices and the optimistic claims of spokespersons for the drug companies are surprising in light of the data, as well as of clinical experience with these drugs. Most studies show that patients have modest, short-term improvements with these medications compared with controls. These benefits include mild improvement in memory, slowing of functional decline, and global ratings of improvement made by clinicians and families (AD2000 Collaborative Group, 2004; Birks, Grimley Evans, Iakovidou, & Tsolaki, 2000; Birks & Harvey, 2003; Loy & Schneider, 2004). The amount of cognitive gain is small, about 2 to 4 points on the 70-point Alzheimer's Disease Assessment Scale—Cognitive (ADAS Cog), a composite measure of several cognitive functions. Improvement in the behavioral symptoms of dementia has been reported, although the results are modest (Sink, Holden, & Yaffe, 2005). Improvement lasts between 12 weeks and 1 year, although some reports suggest that benefits may remain for up to 2 years. A preventive study found a small delay in progression from MCI to AD with use of donepezil (Aricept) after 1 year, but no differences were found after 3 years (Petersen et al., 2005).

One of the most comprehensive long-term studies of donepezil found only a small initial difference in cognitive functioning between people who received the medication and a control group (less than 1 point on the MMSE; AD2000 Collaborative Group, 2004). Less than 10% of patients showed a moderate or good cognitive response to medication (an improvement of 2 or more points on the MMSE), and these patients subsequently tended to decline more rapidly than individuals who had had no initial medication response. Over the long term, there were no differences between treatment and control groups on cognitive, behavioral, or functional measures or in rates of nursing home placement. The authors conclude, "The findings of disappointingly little overall benefit from donepezil cannot be taken lightly" (p. 2114).

Side effects of the cholinesterase inhibitors are generally mild and mainly involve gastrointestinal symptoms. Some patients may retain some awareness while on the medications and become depressed as a result.

The other current medication for AD is memantine (Ebixa; see Chapter 3). Studies with both early- and later-stage patients have found mild improvements in cognition, behavior, and functioning over a 6-month period (Areosa, Sastre, et al., 2005). Mild positive benefits were also found for people with VaD. As with the cholinesterase inhibitors, the magnitude of change is small.

Given these findings, what position should clinicians take with patients and their families? We certainly do not discourage families who want to try the medication, because some patients do benefit and serious side effects are rare. On the other hand, we would support the decision to discontinue a medication if the patient has not responded or has continued to deteriorate. The evidence does not support the belief that patients will deteriorate at a faster rate if the medications are withdrawn or that long-term use conveys any other benefits. It is also worth noting that the medications are expensive, and the cost can add to the burden on families without any benefit.

The limited effects of these medications are not unexpected. They treat only a symptom of AD, changes in neurotransmitters, not the cause of cells sickening and dying (see Chapter 3).

Medications for Secondary Symptoms

The other main use of medications with patients with dementia is to treat behavior problems, including agitation, aggression, and depressive symptoms (sometimes called behavioral and psychiatric symptoms in dementia—BPSD). The standard for treatment of BPSD has long been low doses of antipsychotic medications. There has, in recent years, been a movement from the older neuroleptics, such as Haldol, to a group of medications called atypical antipsychotic medications (e.g., Risperdal, Seroquel, and Zyprexa) that have a lower profile of side effects. Although these medications are widely used, questions about their safety and efficacy are increasing. In a comprehensive review, Sink and colleagues (2005) found evidence for efficacy of only two antipsychotic medications, Zyprexa and Risperdal but noted that improvements were modest and that there was an increased risk of stroke associated with the use of these medications (see also Ballard & Cream, 2005). The U.S. Food and Drug Administration (FDA) issued a black-box warning in 2005 based on findings of increased mortality among people with dementia in a 10-week trial of atypical antipsychotics. Deaths were mainly due to cardiovascular problems (e.g., heart failure) and infections (e.g., pneumonia). The FDA further indicated that these drugs were not approved for treatment of BPSD (www.fda.gov/cder/drug/InfoSheets/HCP/risperidoneHCP.htm). The reader should check this and other appropriate websites for the latest information on research and safety warnings.

Though the findings of increased risk of mortality are recent, concern about the efficacy of the antipsychotic medications for BPSD is long-standing (e.g., Lohr et al., 1992; Schneider, 1996; Schneider, Pollock, & Lyness, 1990; Sink et al., 2005). Why, then, do they remain the treatment of choice? Ballard and Cream (2005) suggest a number of reasons that physicians continue prescribing these medications for BPSD. Physicians believe they should do something for BPSD, and prescribing is the easiest option. In choosing that route, they may not be aware of the risks involved and are influenced by marketing efforts that downplay adverse effects. A placebo effect can also reinforce use. Some patients' behavior does improve on the medications, but controlled studies have shown that people who do not receive the medication are as likely or nearly as likely to improve. BPSD generally fluctuates, and some incidents may resolve themselves quickly without intervention. In some cases, oversedation may be taken for improvement. Finally, physicians are neither knowledgeable nor skilled in behavioral and environmental interventions that are the main alternative to the antipsychotic medications. Given the limitations of these medications, treatment of BPSD is an area in which behavioral specialists have an important role to play.

Because many patients with dementia are likely to be taking antipsychotic mediations, it is important to be familiar with the side effects. The main side effects are:

- Excessive sedation
- Hypotension
- Anticholinergic effects (dry mouth, constipation, urine retention, increased memory impairment)
- Extrapyramidal symptoms (motor restlessness and muscular tension)
- Parkinsonian symptoms (bradykinesia, rigidity, tremor, and loss of postural reflexes)
- Acute dystonic reactions (spasms of the face, neck, back, or extraocular muscles)
- Tardive dyskinesia (random jerking of facial muscles, which impairs talking and eating; Lohr et al., 1992)

Paradoxical effects, such as increased agitation and medication-induced delirium, can occur. Anticholinergic and other side effects are less pronounced but not eliminated in the atypical antipsychotics (Sink et al., 2005). Ballard and Cream (2005) note an increased risk of falls and that drug mechanisms may actually worsen memory.

Patients with DLB are particularly vulnerable to adverse effects of all the neuroleptic medications. The effects include sedation, increased confusion, rigidity, immobility, and increased mortality (Ballard & Cream, 2005).

Although data are limited, the benzodiazepines (see Chapter 10) are an alternative to antipsychotic medication for certain behavior and sleep problems. These medications should be used with caution in dementia because they can produce excessive sedation, may increase the risk of falls, and can make cognitive functioning worse (Mulsant & Pollock, 2004; Salzman, 1992). Ativan can lower anxiety and agitation in some patients with dementia. Another antianxiety drug, BuSpar, can also have positive benefits (Sakauye,

Camp, & Ford, 1993). BuSpar is less sedating than the benzodiazepines and is less likely to cause cognitive symptoms (Salzman, 1992).

Finally, use of antidepressant medications for depression in people with dementia has been increasing. Evidence of their efficacy is limited, and the results are mixed (e.g., Reifler et al., 1989; Teri et al., 2000). Patients with dementia can do well on an SSRI during the daytime and a low dose of a tranquilizer at night to help with sleep. These patients are less depressed and less agitated. Some patients who are not depressed have shown improved behavior on these medications. Like any other medication, however, antidepressants can have adverse effects, and more evidence of their efficacy is needed.

Medications, then, are widely used in treatment of people with dementia, but their efficacy as either a primary treatment or for managing of symptoms is limited. The modest benefits have to be weighed against the risks, particularly in the case of neuroleptics. It is likely that new medications, particularly for primary treatment of AD or other dementias, will become available in the next few years that will alter this equation and provide additional tools for treatment. In the meantime, behavioral, cognitive, and environmental interventions remain promising strategies, with potential for improvement and little risk of adverse effects.

COGNITIVE STIMULATION

Cognitive symptoms are such a prominent part of dementia that it is logical to try to train patients to compensate for these deficits. Cognitive training strategies have had some success with head trauma patients. Cognitive stimulation and training have been used with dementia since the 1960s. Reality orientation came into wide use in nursing homes. Orienting information, such as the date and the weather outside, would be posted in prominent places on wards, and some residents participated in classes in which they reviewed such things as the date and the name of the president. There is some evidence that experimental trials of reality orientation have an effect on cognition and behavior (Spector, Orrell, Davies, & Woods, 2000), although it is hard to generalize from these trials to the rather lackluster way in which orienting information is handled in most nursing homes. A variety of other cognitive stimulation and memory strategies have been tried, including training in repetition, use of imagery, organizing and categorizing information, and practical strategies that provide reminders to patients about things they need to do. Although early trials were disappointing, more recent efforts have resulted in improvements in cognitive functioning that are of about the same magnitude as those shown with the cholinesterase inhibitors (e.g., Quayhagen & Quayhagen, 1989; Spector et al., 2003).

Camp and his colleagues (Camp, Foss, O'Hanlon, & Stevens, 1996; Camp & Schaller, 1989; Camp & Stevens, 1990; Camp et al., 1993; Hayden

& Camp, 1995) developed a program of cognitive intervention using spaced retrieval to improve memory in dementia. This method involves training patients in a behavior (e.g., checking the calendar) and then gradually increasing the interval between trials until patients can perform the action independently. This method relies on external aids rather than internal cues that are often difficult to establish for someone with dementia. This approach also emphasizes the use of implicit over effortful memory—for example, learning through repetition or application of words rather than by trying to memorize a list. Implicit memory processes appear spared to some extent in dementia (Lustig & Buckner, 2004), and their use in training results in gains in memory functioning (Clare, Wilson, Carter, & Hodges, 2003).

Spector and her colleagues (2003) developed a group approach to cognitive training. Their program uses orienting information to remind participants about factual information such as the purpose of the group. Cognitive stimulation is provided through discussions of topics that draw on past knowledge and current experiences. The discussions included visual, as well as verbal, stimuli. The overall focus of training was not on learning specific facts but on encouraging participants to process information in an active way. A randomized trial of this 14-session program was conducted for people with dementia who used adult day care or resided in institutional settings. Participants who received the cognitive intervention showed significant improvements compared with controls on the MMSE and the ADAS-Cog and on a quality-of-life measure. A follow-up study found that adding a series of maintenance sessions after the end of the 14 original classes resulted in further gains in cognition (Orrell, Spector, Thorgrimsen, & Woods, 2005).

These results are encouraging and suggest a role for cognitive stimulation and rehabilitation in dementia care. The major questions for cognitive training, as well as for cognitive-acting medications, are whether improvements in cognition make a difference for everyday functioning now and down the road and whether the cognitive gains are maintained over time. The goal, of course, would be to build a buffer against the devastation of dementia that allows people to function at a higher level for a longer period of time. The work by Camp and colleagues and Spector and colleagues both demonstrated immediate generalization to everyday functioning. More work of this kind is needed. Combining memory training with use of cholinesterase inhibitors to enhance performance is another promising direction (Lowenstein, Acevedo, Czaja, & Duara, 2004).

The effects on caregivers also need to be evaluated. In a memory-training study that involved both dementia patients and their caregivers, patients improved significantly in memory performance, but caregivers were more depressed at the end of the intervention (Zarit, Zarit, & Reever, 1982). The reason for this paradoxical finding is that the training program emphasized to caregivers how much patients could *not* do. Rather than giving caregivers hope or helping them manage everyday situations better, the training program confirmed the seriousness of their relatives' illness. What caregivers found valuable about the classes was the opportunity to get together with other people in their situation, a point we come back to when we discuss support groups in Chapter 13.

In everyday practice, we focus mainly on developing practical memory strategies rather than cognitive stimulation. We engage in problem solving together with patient or caregiver or with just the caregiver to identify strategies that make it easier for the person with dementia to remember. This may include the use of reminders, such as calendars, or encouraging caregivers to keep the house straightened up. Cognitive stimulation could be done in a group format, though, as noted, without raising expectations inappropriately for patients or caregivers.

Behavioral Interventions

Behavioral strategies are a promising and powerful approach for managing problem behaviors in dementia, with none of the side effects of medications. Medicare regulations in the United States mandate consideration of behavioral intervention as the first step in treatment of BPSD. Surprisingly, the amount of research on behavioral approaches with patients with dementia has been extremely limited. There have been some encouraging demonstrations of the use of behavior management with a variety of problems, including agitation, depressive symptoms, insomnia, verbal disruptions, and urinary incontinence (Burgio, 1996; Hinchliffe, Hyman, Blizard, & Livingston, 1995; McCurry, Gibbons, Logsdon, Vitiello, & Teri, 2005; Stokes, 1996; Teri & Logsdon, 1991; Teri et al., 1997, 2003).

Over the years we have used a basic framework for behavioral interventions in dementia called problem solving. The main elements of this approach are described here. Chapters 13 and 14 focus on how to apply these techniques with family caregivers and in institutional settings.

Problem solving is carried out in a series of steps, as shown in Table 12.2. Information is obtained from family members or from staff members, if the person lives in an institution. The starting point is to identify a problem and determine when it occurs. Some staff or family members may not describe

---

TABLE 12.2. Problem-Solving Process

1. Pinpoint a behavior and assess when it occurs and how often.
2. Identify antecedents and consequences.
3. Identify possible strategies for intervention (brainstorm).
4. Select a strategy (use pros and cons).
5. Plan and rehearse implementing the strategy.
6. Try out the strategy and evaluate it.

behavior problems in a clear or precise way. Asking questions can bring out a more detailed description. It is also helpful to ask caregivers to collect a behavior record of their observations over the course of a few days. Using a form to record problems (Figure 12.2), caregivers write down when the targeted behavior or other problem occurs. The goal is to identify when and how often a problem occurs. Caregivers also record what happened right before the problem (antecedents) and what occurred afterward (consequences). Antecedent events may trigger or set off the problem behavior, and consequences may reinforce the problem. Teri and her colleagues (1997) have a helpful mnemonic to help families remember this process: ABC—Antecedent, Behavior, Consequence.

Examples of common antecedents and consequences of problem behavior in dementia are shown in Table 12.3. Problem behaviors may be triggered by many different events. Agitation and restlessness frequently follow periods of inactivity or daytime naps. Other common antecedents of behavior problems are discomfort, pain, or hunger. Patients may not be able to say that they are hungry or thirsty or that they are in pain, but these feelings are expressed in increased behavior problems. A study of physical assaults by patients in a nursing home during bathing found that confrontational and disrespectful ways of talking to the patient, failure to prepare the patient for the task, unexpectedly spraying the patient with water, touching the patient, and hurrying the patient through the shower were predictors of violent behavior (Somboontanont et al., 2004).

Caregivers' responses to the patients can have consequences. Caregivers may inadvertently reinforce problem behaviors. They may ignore patients when they are not causing any problems but give them attention when they act out.

Once caregivers have clarified when and how often a problem occurs and have provided information about possible antecedents and consequences, it is possible to consider solutions. Solutions may emerge out of the pattern that has been observed. For example, if a patient becomes upset following a period of inactivity, the problem may be headed off by introducing activities. The caregiver and clinician talk about ways of doing that. Similarly, if the consequence of a behavior is that the patient gets attention, caregivers can identify ways of giving attention for positive behaviors instead. Some common interventions are shown in Table 12.3. Buettner and Fitzsimmons (2002) have written a useful book with a wealth of ideas about interventions for behavior problems.

Rather than suggesting specific solutions, however, the therapist helps caregivers review the information they have gathered and to identify their own interventions. This approach builds on caregivers' own problem-solving abilities. Sometimes caregivers feel too frustrated or hopeless to come up with solutions. They may have some ideas but reject them as not likely to succeed. The therapist can encourage them to brainstorm. They should say anything

Time of Day	Problem	What Went Before	What Happened After

FIGURE 12.2. Daily record of behavior problems.

TABLE 12.3. Common Antecedents, Consequences, and Solutions for Behavior Problems

Common antecedents of behavior problems (triggering events)
- Interactions with caregiver or other people
- Boredom/understimulation
- Napping
- Frustration/stress
- Overstimulation
- Anxiety
- Pain
- Hunger/thirst
- Illness
- Medication

Common consequences of behavior problems (reinforcers)
- Attention
- Stimulation
- Contact
- Food
- Comfort

Useful strategies for intervening with behavior problems
- Modify how people interact with the patient
- Increase the patient's activities
- Reduce daytime naps
- Give comfort, reassurance
- Reinforce positive behaviors
- Treat pain
- Make sure the patient is not hungry or thirsty
- Treat illnesses
- Evaluate medications

that comes to mind and not censor any thoughts. In that way, they can generate ideas that they might otherwise prematurely reject.

Once the caregiver has generated possible solutions, he or she makes a decision about which one to try. At this point, some caregivers express reservations about the solution and indicate a reluctance to try anything. They may be angry and frustrated at having to make so much effort and getting so little in return. Other caregivers feel hopeless and believe that nothing can make a difference. It is important to empathize with these feelings—they are quite understandable given the circumstances in which caregivers find themselves. But the therapist should not dwell on these emotions. Instead, he or she must direct the caregiver back to the problem.

When caregivers are unable to make a choice or to make any change, we use the method of "pros and cons" (Beck et al., 1979). We give the caregiver a piece of paper with two columns, one marked "pros" and the other "cons." We discuss the advantages and disadvantages of each solution, and the caregiver writes them down. Writing down these responses cuts down on endless ruminations and clarifies solutions that may actually be worth trying. For caregivers who believe that anything they do will make the situation worse, the pros-and-cons comparison may be between doing one specific new thing and doing nothing. The goal is to get the client to engage in some new action as a way of disrupting old patterns of behavior.

Once a solution has been identified, caregivers can be encouraged to mentally rehearse the steps involved in carrying it out (Beck et al., 1979). This type of cognitive rehearsal ensures that the caregiver can actually carry out the plan. A caregiver may, for example, decide to respond calmly when the patient asks the same question over and over and then distract the patient with an activity. In rehearsing this approach, it may become evident that the caregiver is too angry to answer the question in a patient manner. The caregiver and therapist can then work to resolve these feelings or develop a different approach for the problem.

When caregivers have a plan they are comfortable with, the next step is to try it out. As with other behavioral interventions, they should schedule a specific time and place in which to try the new response. The caregiver should continue monitoring the targeted problem to find out whether the new response results in a change in the frequency of the behavior. If the intervention is successful, the targeted behavior will decrease. If not, caregiver and clinician can look at other possible solutions.

Another possible solution for problem behaviors is medications. As discussed, the options for medications are currently limited. By using medications within a problem-solving framework, it is possible to evaluate their effectiveness. Caregivers can obtain a baseline of how often targeted behavior occurs prior to the introduction of a medication and then how the frequency changes after the patient has begun taking the medication. These records indicate clearly whether the medication is having its intended effect. Medications that are not effective or that are producing adverse effects then can be discontinued.

Behavioral solutions need to be practical and workable. As an example, the assessment may suggest that increasing the patient's activities is likely to reduce agitation, but the family caregiver may be too exhausted or angry to do so. In that case, other resources can be identified for increasing activities, such as enrolling the patient in a structured adult day care program or finding someone who can take the patient out for walks. Interventions should also be specific and detailed—that is, caregivers should know exactly what do and when they should do it. They should, of course, actively participate in development of the plan, understand it, and be willing to carry it out.

Sometimes problem solving results in a decrease in frequency of a problem but not its elimination. Some caregivers may become discouraged and dwell on the remaining incidents. For example, increasing a patient's activity during the day might reduce the number of nights that he wakes up the caregiver from 6 to 2 days a week. The caregiver, however, might complain that she has gotten no relief because she is still being awakened, thus ignoring the fact that the problem happens less often. In that situation, the therapist can use the caregiver's written records to demonstrate that there has actually been improvement and can discuss the significance of bringing the problem partly under control.

One of the most promising applications of behavioral methods has been for treatment of depressive symptoms among patients with dementia. In a series of studies, Teri and her colleagues (1997, 2003) have demonstrated that several approaches are useful in reducing depression. In the first study (Teri et al., 1997), caregivers of people with dementia and comorbid depression were randomly assigned to one of four treatment conditions: (1) increasing pleasant events, (2) behavioral problem solving, (3) advice and support (control condition), and (4) a wait list. The first treatment, pleasant events, drew on behavioral approaches for treatment of depression in people without dementia (see Chapter 9). Family caregivers completed a special inventory, the Pleasant Events—AD, to identify potentially reinforcing behaviors for their relatives. With a therapist, they then planned out how to increase the number of pleasant events that dementia patients engaged in. This intervention addressed the patient's difficulties in initiating and sustaining satisfying activities. The second treatment, problem solving, taught caregivers to use the behavioral approach described previously. Both the pleasant-events and problem-solving treatments reduced depressive symptoms in the person with dementia compared with the control groups. The amount of improvement among patients was similar to that found with antidepressant medication (Teri et al., 1997). Of particular note, the caregivers' own reports of burden and distress also decreased in those conditions. By learning how to interact more effectively with patients, caregivers themselves may experience more pleasant interactions and perhaps a greater sense of competency in their role.

In a second study, Teri and colleagues (2003) examined the benefits of an exercise program for people with dementia. In the treatment group, caregivers learned how to initiate an exercise program for their relatives, while a control group received standard medical care. An important finding was that caregivers in the treatment group were able to implement the exercise program. Participants in the combined exercise-and-behavior-management condition improved their performance of everyday activities and showed less depression posttreatment compared with controls. These differences were still significant 2 years after treatment.

One of the problems in dementia is that patients cannot plan, initiate, and sustain behaviors. Strategies such as increasing pleasant events and instituting regular exercise can engage patients in meaningful ways. As an alternative to using the family caregiver as the change agent, the person with dementia could attend a day program that provides structured activities. Adult day services can provide needed relief for caregivers (Zarit, Stephens, et al., 1998). By engaging patients in activities, these programs may also affect behavior and mood. In a trial of the effects of day care on behavior of people with dementia, it was found that depressive behaviors decreased over time in a treatment group compared with controls (Femia, Braungart, Zarit, & Stephens, 2004). The effects were greatest on days that participants attended day care, but they also generalized to non-day-care days.

Finally, Teri's group (McCurry et al., 2005) has applied behavioral techniques to management of another significant dementia-related problem, nighttime awakenings. In this trial, caregivers in an active treatment group received training in sleep hygiene techniques. These techniques included setting a consistent bedtime and waking time, implementing a relaxing and quiet bedtime routine, spending time outdoors during the day in natural light, restricting caffeine and other stimulants, and reducing naps. Compared with a control group who received written information about sleep and dementia and sleep hygiene, patients in the treatment group had fewer nighttime awakenings, spent less time awake during the night, and showed less depression. These gains were still evident at a 6-month follow-up.

CONCLUSIONS

The behavior of people with dementia needs to be viewed as an interaction. Although the underlying disease alters the probability of disturbed behavior, the occurrence and frequency of problems depends in part on how other people respond to the patient and on environmental characteristics. Using this framework, we described emerging treatments for early-stage patients, the use of medications, cognitive stimulation, and behavioral interventions. Although there is as yet not much that can be done to alter the degenerative course of dementia, the available studies show encouraging results that interventions can minimize behavioral disturbances and maximize patients' remaining abilities.

CHAPTER 13

Family Caregiving

When people develop disabilities in later life, families are the first line of defense. Family caregivers provide extensive care, often at considerable personal sacrifice to their own health and well-being (e.g., Aneshensel et al., 1995; Anthony-Bergstone, Zarit, & Gatz, 1988).

The first part of this chapter reviews research on family caregiving. As a first step in planning interventions, it is important to understand the stresses of caregiving, particularly what the most difficult problems caregivers encounter are and what helps make the situation more manageable. The second part of the chapter describes comprehensive approaches to treatment of family caregivers. Much of the emphasis is on families of patients with dementia, which is the most challenging and stressful of care situations. These strategies, however, can be applied with minor changes to other caregiving situations.

FAMILY STRESS AND ADAPTATION

Over the past two decades, extensive research has been conducted on family caregivers. At the risk of oversimplifying the complex research findings on family caregiving, we have identified eight points that capture the major themes and results of this work:

1. Caregiving is stressful.
2. The amount of demands on the family are unprecedented.
3. Many different people become caregivers.
4. Caregiving stress is a multidimensional process.

5. Social support and coping buffer caregivers against stressors.
6. Caregiving affects other family relationship dynamics.
7. Caregiving involves continuity and change.
8. Placement is not always the answer for caregiving stress.

Caregiving Is Stressful

Care of a disabled older person is very stressful, especially when the person suffers from AD or another dementing disorder. Study after study has documented the negative effects that caregiving has on the health and well-being of families. Caregivers are more likely to be depressed and angry and possibly also to have poorer health than age-matched controls who are not involved in caregiving (Anthony-Bergstone et al., 1988; Gallagher, Rose, Rivera, Lovett, & Thompson, 1989; Kiecolt-Glaser, Dura, Speicher, Trask, & Glaser, 1991; Schulz & Beach, 1999; Schulz, O'Brien, Bookwala, & Fleissner, 1995; Vitaliano, Persson, Kiyak, Saini, & Echeverria, 2005; Vitaliano, Zhang, & Scanlan, 2003). Perhaps the most dramatic evidence of the toll that caregiving takes is the fact that caregivers who experience strain in their roles have higher rates of mortality than age-matched controls who are not caregivers (Schulz & Beach, 1999).

The Amount of Demands on the Family Are Unprecedented

Although families have always provided care for their disabled elders, the convergence of several trends has resulted in dramatic changes in the conditions and context of caregiving that have made it potentially very stressful. First and foremost, caring for an elder used to be a rare event in a family's life, because most people did not survive to old age. Now, as more people live into their 70s and 80s, ages when rates of disability and the need for assistance steadily rise, caring for an elderly relative has become a frequent occurrence. Second, the period of time that people live with disabilities at the end of their lives has increased (Cassel et al., 1992). As a result, families care for older relatives for a longer period of time, and the disabilities that their relatives have are more severe now than they were in the past. Patients with dementia, for example, once had a relatively short period of decline. Now it is not uncommon for people to live 10–15 years or even longer after the onset of this illness (Aneshensel et al., 1995). While demands placed on families have been increasing, their resources for providing care have shrunk. Family size is smaller, so the burden of care falls on fewer people. Furthermore, women's participation in the workplace means that they cannot readily incorporate caregiving responsibilities into their daily schedules as in the past. Instead, care of an older parent represents one more demand on top of an already overfull schedule of work and family responsibilities. Increased rates of divorce may also reduce the commitment of potential caregivers to a spouse or a parent. The sum of these trends, then, is that more people require more extensive assistance for longer periods of time than ever before, whereas the family's resources for providing this help are often limited.

Many Different People Become Caregivers

The media image of a caregiver is a daughter who is balancing care of a parent, work, and her own family responsibilities. That pattern happens, but the most likely person to take on caregiving responsibilities is a husband or wife (Stone, Cafferata & Sangl, 1987). Husbands, in fact, become caregivers almost as frequently as wives do. Children get involved in a secondary way when both parents are alive or as primary caregivers when a parent is single or widowed. Usually, it is a daughter or daughter-in-law who handles most of the care, but occasionally sons assume the primary care responsibilities. When an older person has no children, sometimes other relatives get involved, including siblings and grandchildren, or even a close friend. Friends and neighbors can also provide regular assistance.

How the caregiving experience plays out depends a lot on the relationship of caregiver and care receiver, as well as the caregiver's gender. The commitment of a spouse is different from those of children or other relatives. Spouses are often more willing to make personal sacrifices to keep a husband or wife at home but paradoxically are also less likely to hire paid help to relieve some of the strain on them. Caregiving daughters who use support services such as adult day care may actually keep their parents at home for a longer period of time than a spousal caregiver who becomes overwhelmed by the demands of the situation (Zarit, Stephens, Townsend, Greene, & Leitsch, 1999). Understanding the meaning of the caregiver's commitment is sometimes the key to helping that person make changes in the situation.

Gender also makes a difference in how caregiving is approached. Husbands often take on their responsibilities as if they were a job (Miller, 1990; Zarit, Todd, & Zarit, 1986). They see their role as performing instrumental tasks and take satisfaction from doing so. The biggest challenges they face are mastering household routines and getting support from children and other family members. In particular, when a father has played a domineering role in the family, daughters often harbor lingering anger toward him and withhold help and other support.

Wives, by comparison, are more likely to be affected emotionally by their husband's illness (Miller, 1990; Zarit & Whitlatch, 1992). They will feel depressed but also sometimes resentful and angry that this burden has been placed on them. Compared with husbands, they are more likely to feel helpless and trapped in their role, scared to make changes that might improve their circumstances. Because so few sons have been studied, we know less about how their involvement may differ from that of daughters.

Caregiving Stress Is a Multidimensional Process

The stresses of caregiving can be best understood as a multidimensional process. No single measure of stress or burden can capture the impact on caregivers. Rather, the changes in an older person's health and functioning set off a chain reaction that affects families in many different areas—financially and emotionally, as well as in how they carry out other roles and responsibilities. How this stress process plays out, however, depends on characteristics of the older person's condition, as well as the family's own resources in responding. As a result, the impact of caregiving can vary widely from one family to another.

We have found the stress process model of caregiving, developed by Pearlin and his associates (Aneshensel et al., 1995; Pearlin, Mullan, Semple, & Skaff, 1990), to be particularly useful in understanding caregiving stress and identifying helpful interventions. The starting point is the changes caused by the older person's illness and disabilities, called "primary stressors." Primary stressors include the amount of care needed for daily activities and any behavioral, cognitive, and emotional disturbances that caregivers must cope with. Another primary stressor is the caregiver's growing sense of loss of the relationship with the person (Aneshensel et al., 1995). The impact of those problems on caregivers varies considerably. Some caregivers, for example, find dealing with their relative's incontinence to be overwhelming, whereas others view it as just one more task to manage.

Research confirms this varying impact of behavior problems on caregivers (e.g., Aneshensel et al., 1995; Zarit et al., 1986). Objective measures of primary stressors, such as the extent of disability or number of behavior problems, account for a surprisingly small portion of variance of subjective strain and well-being. Subjective measures, however, which incorporate the caregiver's perception of the impact these events are having, are more informative markers of the threat to the caregiver's health and well-being.

The demands placed on caregivers in dealing with primary stressors can spill over into other areas of the caregiver's life, leading to what Pearlin and colleagues (1990) call secondary stressors. The time and energy involved in providing care puts strain on other roles and responsibilities. Caregivers may find themselves pressured in dealing with spouses or children. They may experience conflict with other family members over how they are providing care. The time demands may interfere with their work roles and with leisure activities. This spillover can also have psychological consequences, leading to what Skaff and Pearlin (1992) have called "the loss of self," in which the caregiver's identity becomes absorbed in the caregiving role. However, rather than assuming that caregiving places a strain on a particular role, such as work, the clinician should determine whether, in fact, those responsibilities have become stressful. Some caregivers who are employed outside the home actually report that work gives them a break from their responsibilities at home (Aneshensel et al., 1995).

Social Support and Coping Buffer Caregivers against Stressors

As we have seen, caregivers respond differently to similar events or stressors. The reasons for this variability provide the keys to identifying interventions that can help. Two main factors have emerged in the literature that appear to protect caregivers from the stressors in their role: social support and coping.

People who receive more help from their families generally do better in the caregiving role than those without help. Types of support can include assistance with caregiving tasks, as well as emotional support (Aneshensel et al., 1995). Sometimes family help comes with a price, however, or family members may argue over providing care or the costs of care (MaloneBeach & Zarit, 1995; Semple, 1992). The most common type of help that caregivers receive is advice, which, however well-intentioned, often misses the mark and leaves them feeling more, not less, distressed (MaloneBeach & Zarit, 1995).

Formal, paid services can provide another source of help. These services can reduce the stress on caregivers (Zarit, Stephens, et al., 1998), but sometimes they can make care more difficult. The help provided by community agencies can be unpredictable or intrusive and unresponsive to the caregiver's needs (MaloneBeach, Zarit, & Spore, 1992). The service system, particularly in the United States, is complicated, and caregivers often do not understand how agencies decide what type or how much help they will receive, and they do not understand the complex reimbursement system. Caregivers also complain that they have no say over when help is provided or who provides it. In other words, formal agencies provide help to people who are faced with uncontrollable stress in a manner that makes them feel an even greater lack of control over their situation. Caregivers who are reluctant to use paid services sometimes are making a realistic appraisal of the help that is available.

Coping is the other main factor that appears to protect caregivers from stress—that is, the beliefs and skills that they bring to the management of stressors. Some caregivers do a very good job, for example, in managing disruptive behaviors, calming the patient down, or distracting him or her. By contrast, other caregivers respond to the same behaviors in confrontational or controlling ways that actually increase the patient's agitation or disruptiveness.

As an example, one caregiver reported being awakened at 2:00 A.M. by her mother, who needed help to go to the bathroom. This occurred after a long, tiring day during which the caregiver spent almost all of her time assisting her mother or other family members. Now that she was awake, her mother, who was suffering from dementia, thought it was morning and time to get up. Rather than confronting her or angrily telling her to go back to bed, her daughter instead reminisced with her about pleasant times they had spent together when the daughter was young. In a short while, her mother went back to sleep. Many caregivers do not have the patience or skill to take that calming approach, but getting upset or arguing with the patient would have made the situation worse and kept both patient and caregiver awake longer.

We expand on these approaches for coping with stressful behaviors later in the chapter. Our point here is that some resources, particularly support and coping, are protective against the stresses in caregiving. These resources are also potentially modifiable; that is, we can do things that increase the support available to caregivers and to help them use more adaptive strategies for managing stressors. Even though the older person's illness cannot be treated, addressing these modifiable aspects of the stress process can lead to better outcomes for caregivers.

Caregiving Affects Other Family Relationship Dynamics

Beyond issues of family support and conflict, caregiving can awaken or intensify relationship issues within the family. The altruistic motivation to help can become enmeshed with unresolved feelings about the caregiver or other family members. A caregiving daughter, for example, might feel frustrated because the assistance she gives to her parents brings criticism rather than the approval she has always sought. One child taking on the caregiving role can also reawaken sibling rivalries. When one spouse helps another, the commitment may be tinged with anger from old issues in the relationship. Some wives, for example, feel a resentment at having to care for their husbands when they believe that the husbands were never concerned about their needs.

These kinds of relationship issues create an emotional context for the exchanges that take place in a particular family. As we show, it is not necessary, nor may it be possible, to fix these long-standing conflicts, but gaining an understanding of how these issues affect the current situation can be very useful in providing support to the primary caregiver.

Caregiving Involves Continuity and Change

Both continuity and change characterize the caregiving role. For many families, caregiving stretches over a period of several years. It is not uncommon, for example, for families to care for someone with dementia at home for a period of 10 years or more (Aneshensel et al., 1995). During this sustained effort, stressors emerge and recede in importance. Some caregivers do well despite fluctuations in stressors, and others may wear down. Still others may make adaptations that improve their situation.

Part of our commitment when working with caregivers is to be there for them when their situations change. We have seen caregivers on and off throughout the whole course of their relatives' illness and even beyond, as they cope with bereavement.

Placement Is Not Always the Answer for Caregiving Stress

Because caregiving is so stressful for so many families, shouldn't the role of professionals be to encourage placement in a care facility outside the home? Many clinicians have, in fact, viewed their role that way. However, emotional, practical, and financial considerations may make institutional placement a complicated decision.

From an emotional perspective, placement is often the most difficult decision families have to make. Caregivers often have made a commitment to keep their spouses or parents at home as long as possible. They may even have made a promise to that person or to themselves never to use a nursing home. Once placement is made, caregivers are likely to feel guilty, which is reinforced if other family members criticize their decision. A caregiver may also feel lonely after placing his or her spouse in a care facility. Their commitment to their spouses may prevent them from seeking out friends and social activities. In turn, their friends may not know what to say or whether to include them in social gatherings. The lack of social conventions surrounding the role of spouses who have placed a relative in an institution contributes to their isolation (Rosenthal & Dawson, 1991).

Placement has some practical limitations. Although it relieves caregivers of the stress of everyday care routines, it introduces some new problems (Aneshensel et al., 1995; Zarit & Whitlatch, 1992). Caregivers now have to travel to visit their relatives, which can be difficult for older spouses. Their roles in the facility also become ambiguous. They may provide assistance to their relatives, only to get in the way of staff members. Or they may feel that they know the patient's needs best, only to find that staff members have their own way of doing things and do not listen to their advice. They have to learn how to interact with their relatives and with staff members at the facility, an issue we return to in Chapter 14.

Finally, finances may cause problems. In the United States in particular, people must pay for their own institutional care. Medicare pays only for short-term institutional care following a hospitalization. Some people have long-term care insurance, which offsets the cost of nursing homes, as well as community-based care. To qualify for government assistance under the Medicaid program, people must spend down their assets first. A spouse can retain only a portion of joint assets, and so placement can have a distressing financial impact. It is also illegal to hide assets or transfer them to another family member as a way of qualifying for Medicaid. Even with these restrictions, Medicaid has been overburdened with costs of nursing home care, and many states are looking into how they might impose further restrictions.

Given these considerations, it is not surprising that research on the transition to placement has found that placement does not lower emotional distress among family caregivers (Aneshensel et al., 1995; Zarit & Whitlatch, 1992). Stress does not end at the institution's door. The problems caregivers must manage are often as complex and stressful after placement as before.

For that reason, I do not push people into placement. Many caregivers are willing to make sacrifices to keep their relatives at home. I view my role not as convincing them that they need to place their relatives but as giving them permission to make that decision when they feel the time is right. In the meantime, I work with them to bring in resources that can make the situation more manageable.

Implications for Treatment

Family care is a complex, ongoing process characterized both by considerable individual differences and by key transitions such as nursing home placement that require families to make new adaptations. There are no simple formulas for understanding caregiving nor simple stages that reduce it to an uncomplicated pattern. Research on caregiving provides a framework for viewing the broad phenomenon, for conducting assessments to identify the particular strengths and problems within a given family, and for pinpointing potentially modifiable features of the stress process.

DEMENTIA AND FAMILY CAREGIVING: TREATMENT APPROACHES

I have provided treatment to caregivers in each of the four major phases that characterize their experience: (1) transition to the caregiving role; (2) carrying out the caregiving role when the families' efforts are directed at maintaining the person in the community; (3) transition from community care to institutional placement; and (4) bereavement. As might be expected, treatment issues differ considerably across these four phases. I address my approach to each phase, with most of the emphasis on the period of active community care.

Transitions into Caregiving

Researchers probably know the least about the transition to the caregiving role. Research and clinical interventions typically take place after families have been providing care for a while. Meeting families first in the earliest stages of care creates opportunities for interventions that can prevent problems later on. These interventions can involve the patient him- or herself, as described in Chapter 12 for the person with dementia, or can focus mainly on how caregivers structure the situation so that they do not become over-whelmed at a later point.

At some period an older person may begin to need assistance but insist on remaining independent. Adult children, however, may grow increasingly concerned about their parents' health and safety. The key issues are likely to concern getting appropriate medical care, managing money, safety issues at home and when driving, getting help in the home, and making a change in one's living situation. Their children give them advice about what they need to do, which the parents ignore, sometimes politely and sometimes with an argument that brings in lots of old baggage.

When parents are at imminent risk, I work with adult children to address that immediately. If no immediate danger exists, I often find myself coaching children on how best to communicate with their parents. I stress four points. First, I help clients understand the issue of role reversal. Their parents raised them and were in charge, and now, however unrealistic it may seem, they are reluctant to become dependent on their children. My goal is for clients to appreciate the difficulty their parents are having in accepting their limitations and dependence. Second, I emphasize communications skills. Rather than reasoning or arguing with parents, I teach adult children how to listen reflectively. In that way, they come to better appreciate their parents' opinions and feelings and may be better able to come up with a solution that pleases everyone. Just getting out of the cycle of advice giving and argument will improve the situation. Third, I stress patience. I remind clients that getting their parents to make changes will take time. I encourage them not to attempt too much all at once but to take one step at a time. I make sure that they feel good when they can accomplish these small steps. Fourth, their involvement may re-awaken sibling rivalries. They may become increasingly resentful of siblings who do not help or who get more of their parents approval or money; conversely, their siblings may resent them.

One of the most difficult questions is whether to move one's parent or parents. The decision has considerable emotional significance for everyone involved. As a result, even the best of intentions can lead to an intense family struggle.

In some circumstances, parents and children reach a mutual decision to move. When an older person actively participates in the decision, fewer postrelocation problems are likely to arise. In situations in which clear risk exists if the parent continues living alone—for example, the parent suffers from dementia and does not eat regularly or wanders away from the house and gets lost—then the children have to make a decision that goes against the parent's wishes. Many cases fall in between those extremes. One parent may have dementia and the other may insist that he or she can manage, despite evidence to the contrary. Or a parent may be competent but frail, so that there are risks with remaining at home that the parent is willing to take but that worry the children.

The issue of a move is especially complicated when adult children and their parents live at some distance from one another. Children will often bring up the issue because they have grown increasingly concerned that their parents can no longer care for themselves. The parents may live alone, with diminishing ability to manage by themselves, and with their local support network shrinking as friends and neighbors die or move away. Sometimes they live in homes and neighborhoods that have deteriorated.

A major reason that children living at a distance will push for a move is difficulties in coordinating medical care or social services. Parents may not follow through with medical care or other help. We often have talked with children who arranged for home care for their parents, only to find out that their parents fired the help after one or two visits. Sometimes the paid helpers are not reliable, failing to show up at scheduled times or not following through on treatment plans. The stress on children can be intense if the parent has frequent health crises or other emergencies.

Often, when discussing a move, adult children focus just on the rational arguments, such as safety issues, and not on the emotional and tangible losses that the parent might experience in a move. One cost of moving for the older person is losing contact with neighbors and friends. Families may underestimate the extent to which their parent depends on these interactions. Sons and daughters may assume that a frail older person will be able to replace friends of a lifetime in a short period of time, but that is often unrealistic. Instead, they find that their parents have become totally dependent on them for social interactions. An older person who is demoralized or depressed over the move or who has limited mobility is especially likely to have a very difficult time making new friends outside the family. Another drawback to relocation is that the familiarity of one's home and neighborhood may enhance some competencies. An older person who is able to drive safely on familiar streets may not be able to learn his or her way around a new locale. Other daily routines, such as cooking and shopping, can become disrupted by a move, especially if the older person is now sharing a house with his or her children. Moving someone with cognitive impairment is always difficult because of the problems that person will have in learning new routines and surroundings. An argument can be made for moving patients with dementia early in the course of the disease, rather than later, because they may still have adequate cognitive resources to make the adjustment.

There are no perfect solutions to these dilemmas. The most important thing for the clinician to avoid in this situation is becoming an advocate for one party—either the adult child or the parent. Instead, we want older people and their families to explore their alternatives and to consider all the ramifications of a move. In that way, they can make plans that incorporate the older person's needs and preferences if they decide to go ahead with a move—for example, choosing senior housing that offers an active social life for a parent who likes a lot of social interaction.

As an alternative to relocation, caregivers can hire a private care manager, who will make all the necessary arrangements to support an older person at home. Care managers are becoming increasingly available in the United States. (This service is often provided through public services in European countries, and it can be found on a limited basis in publicly supported services in the United States.) The care manager may arrange for help in the home, home maintenance, transportation to the doctor or other appointments, and so on. Many care managers are very committed and involved with their clients and make sure their needs are taken care of.

Caregiving in the Community: A Comprehensive Treatment to Reduce Stress

Over the years, we have developed a model for treating caregivers who are assisting an older person at home that is designed to address the modifiable aspects of the stress process. This model (Figure 13.1) emphasizes both the specific clinical techniques used to help caregivers build resources for managing stress and the different forms that treatment can take (Zarit, 1996; Zarit, Orr, & Zarit, 1985; Zarit & Zarit, 1982). Many of the approaches can also be applied when working with families and staff in institutional settings (Chapter 14).

The starting point in the model is assessment of the patient and caregiver. The model includes three treatment techniques—providing information, problem solving, and providing support—and three treatment modalities—counseling the caregiver, family meetings, and support groups. Though designed specifically for caregivers of patients with dementia, many features

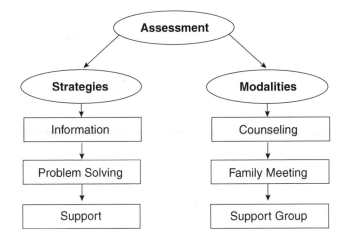

FIGURE 13.1. A model of interventions with family caregivers.

of this approach have wider applications. Empirical tests of this model have found it to be effective in reducing strain on the family caregiver and reducing inappropriate placement into nursing homes (Mittelman et al., 1995; Mittelman, Ferris, Shulman, Steinberg, & Levin, 1996; Whitlatch, Zarit, Goodwin, & von Eye, 1995; Whitlatch et al., 1991). From that perspective, it is a cost-effective intervention; the expense of the clinical intervention is offset by delaying more costly care in a nursing home. Psychological benefits from treatment have also been found to be sustained for a period of 3 years after initial contact (Mittleman, Roth, Coon, & Haley, 2004).

Assessing Caregivers

The initial assessment is used to identify the primary caregiver, to determine the main problems the elder is experiencing and their impact on the caregiver, and to set some preliminary goals. Caregivers sometimes seek treatment for themselves, but the most typical situation is their bringing their relatives for an assessment. In that situation, I begin my assessment with the designated patient, getting as much information as possible from him or her and then supplementing it with information from the caregiver.

How to proceed depends on the older person's competency. Many older clients are fully competent to provide information and make decisions themselves. In those cases, it can be determined whether or not the older person perceives a problem and wants treatment. Depending on the presenting problem, the focus may be just on the older client or on the dyad of client and caregiver. In other situations, it can be quickly determined that the client has a limited ability to provide information or participate in treatment. In those cases, the focus shifts to the caregiver. Even when older persons cannot report information accurately, however, we always treat them with respect and give them time to tell their stories.

Part of this process involves determining who the primary caregiver is. Most of the time, that will be the person who comes to the appointment. Sometimes, however, a son or daughter may take their parent to the appointment, but it is their other parent or stepparent who provides most of the help. That person should be involved as soon as possible.

An important part of the assessment is to find out about the older person's medical condition. Among the useful facts are (1) onset and course of symptoms, (2) physicians' diagnoses, (3) past and current treatments and their effects, and (4) other medical problems and medications (see Chapter 6 for details of assessment).

Besides evaluating what has been done medically, I assess the family's understanding of the patient's illness, symptoms, treatment, and prognosis. As discussed later, obtaining information about these issues is often an important part of treatment.

Another focus of the assessment is identifying what features of the situation are stressful to the caregiver. The caregiver may find it difficult or taxing to provide assistance to the patient. The demands on his or her time may be excessive or the patient may interrupt frequently with requests for help or attention. In cases of dementia, the caregiver may find it difficult to manage cognitive and behavioral symptoms.

A similar approach should be taken in assessing secondary stressors—that is, the extent to which caregiving may affect other roles and activities. I do not assume secondary strains in employment or in other family relationships but instead determine which problems are actually present.

In some instances, the initial interview may raise questions in my mind about the caregiver's cognitive functioning. I do not routinely recommend assessing the caregiver's cognitive functioning, because that is a distraction and may upset the caregiver. I do conduct an evaluation, however, if the caregiver requests one (which usually can then be used to give reassurance that nothing is wrong) or if I observe evidence of forgetfulness that goes beyond everyday memory lapses.

Another focus of the assessment is the wider family network. The clinician should determine who the important family members are and what their current involvement and view of the situation is. Friends and neighbors may also provide support. Among the points to consider are how much help family members and other helpers provide, how much contact they have with the caregiver and the care recipient, what their understanding of the patient's condition and the caregiver's needs seems to be, and whether conflict exists between the caregiver and other family members. Semple (1992) has identified three areas of family conflict: (1) the patient's diagnosis and treatment, (2) the amount and type of care the caregiver is providing, and (3) the amount of help provided by other family members. As in any family situation, the clinician must recognize that he or she is hearing one side of the story and that the perspective of the other family members may be quite different.

I also determine what formal services the caregiver or care recipient have used, what has been helpful, and what has not worked out. Before clinicians suggest that caregivers use formal services, they should know what a caregiver has previously tried and whether or not a particular service worked out.

Finally, I evaluate caregivers' emotional distress. This assessment can be done clinically or by having the caregiver complete a rating scale or form, such as a depression inventory or caregiver strain measure. The advantage of obtaining this type of measure is that it provides a baseline against which subsequent treatment can be evaluated. The possibility of suicidal and homicidal thoughts should be evaluated as well. Clinicians can conduct a standard assessment of these issues and also follow up on any statements or behaviors by the caregiver indicating a possible risk of suicide or homicide.

Following the initial evaluation, I set goals for treatment with the caregiver. Goals include clarifying issues of diagnosis and treatment, exploring ways of lowering stress on the caregiver, exploring the use of formal services, and treating behavior problems of the patient.

Sometimes the goal is broader, such as in cases in which a family member is trying to decide about taking on the caregiving role. Usually, this situation involves sons or daughters, as spouses routinely assume this role for one another. Adult children may be asking whether they should provide care themselves or find a setting in which their parent can be helped, or they may be trying to decide which of the children will take on the role. There are no right or pat answers to these questions. Families must make these decisions consistent with their own values and in light of the resources available to help them with caregiving. Clinicians should be nonjudgmental and make sure that their own values do not color the decision. They can also provide families with information about care alternatives for their parents. Families often view the situation as a dichotomy between providing all the care themselves or putting a parent in a nursing home. Telling families about community resources such as adult day care programs gives them options that might better suit their parents and themselves for the time being.

Treatment Techniques

PROVIDING INFORMATION

The starting point of clinical intervention is making sure that caregivers have a basic understanding of their relatives' illness and the treatment and care options available so that they can make informed decisions. I usually begin by finding out what they know about their relatives' illness and answering their questions. Families typically report that they did not get much information from physicians at the time the diagnosis was made and that they would have liked more (Aneshensel et al., 1995). I help families get the information they want. I provide information myself and also give caregivers books, pamphlets, and information about websites that explain the illness they are dealing with. If there are technical questions I cannot answer, I refer them to their physicians or to an appropriate specialist.

When dealing with progressive disorders such as dementia, the clinician needs to be honest but tactful in providing an accurate picture of treatment options and the long-term course of the disease. I answer questions that families ask, but I also do not press on them information about the progression of the disease that they are not ready to hear.

Families of patients with chronic and incurable diseases may seek out experimental or alternative treatments. These treatments provide hope in the face of a bleak prognosis. I always encourage families who are interested in participating in a clinical trial of a new treatment to do so. But I also discourage them from trying unproven treatments outside research settings that may be of questionable value. Some of these treatments are outright scams, and others have no effect or may even have adverse effects.

The most important type of information addresses caregivers' understanding of their relatives' behavior. Families often misunderstand or make incorrect attributions about the patients' behavior. These misunderstandings increase stress on the caregivers and may also inadvertently contribute to the patients' problems. As an example, a patient with dementia may ask the same question over and over again. Caregivers may conclude that patients are trying to annoy them or that they are too lazy to listen to the answer or that they could correct the problem by trying harder.

The first impulse for most families is to try to correct these cognitive errors. In attempting to reason with patients with dementia, however, families are falling into a logical trap. They are trying to get patients to recognize the facts of a situation, but the patient's ability to understand facts has been diminished by the disease. No matter how much families reason or argue with patients, they cannot win the argument. What is particularly frustrating for families is that their relatives often can argue in a logical way while totally ignoring the evidence, as shown in this rather remarkable example.

THE FAILURE OF REASONING IN DEMENTIA

Lillian, who was caring for her husband, Joe, recounted an argument she had had with him. Joe had always loved horses and had taken care of several horses after his retirement. Because of his progressive dementia, he could no longer continue doing so. One day Joe began to insist that there were two horses in the garage and that he had to give them food and water. He began carrying water out to the horses and insisted that Lillian buy feed for them. No amount of arguing dissuaded him. Finally, exasperated with these continual arguments, Lillian told Joe that she would go out to the garage with him so he could show her the horses. If she could see the horses, she would buy feed for them. They went out to the garage, and she said she could not see the horses. Joe insisted they were there. When she asked if she could touch them, he put her hands on their two automobiles. Totally exasperated at this point, Lillian asked, "If there are two horses here, wouldn't the garage be filled with manure by now?" He replied, "No, not with how little we're feeding them."

As this example illustrates, the cognitive distortions of the patient with dementia are relatively resistant to reasoning and even to demonstrations that they are incorrect. Yet this patient responded to the caregiver's points in a logical way. This apparent logic engages caregivers, and they persist in trying to reason with patients who can no longer respond to a factual argument.

In these situations, it is important to help families see that their relatives' ability to respond to the facts of a situation is limited and that they need to do something else. I work with caregivers on a two-step approach. First, I want them to think about why someone with a memory-impairing disease behaves this way. Second, I encourage them to think about what someone with memory loss might be feeling in this situation. I illustrate this approach with three common problems: paranoid accusations, desire to see one's mother, and desire to go home.

Paranoid accusations are common in dementia and usually have their basis in the patient's increasing memory loss (see Chapter 11). Typical accusations involve someone coming in and stealing money or other valuable objects. Instead of arguing, caregivers are encouraged to view the problem as due to memory loss, to realize that patients cannot remember misplacing the object, much less where the object is. Caregivers can ask themselves what the patient must be feeling and then respond to those feelings. The patient's emotional reaction is valid and real, and he or she may be upset, frustrated, or fearful. Caregivers can address the patient's feelings by empathizing (e.g., "You're upset that you can't find your money") or by responding in ways that are calming (e.g., reassuring patients that they have plenty of money).

The next example demonstrates paid caregivers struggling with a similar reality-based issue.

A Dementia Patient Wants to See Her Mother

I once consulted in a special care unit for dementia patients on a case in which one resident, Sonia, wanted to see her mother. The staff believed their role was to reorient patients to reality, but no amount of telling Sonia that her mother was dead had an effect. Staff members then decided that they would try to trick her. When Sonia asked to see her mother, they had her dial a number on the phone, which rang in another part of the unit. A staff member answered and told Sonia that her mother was in the bath and could not come to the phone. Although her memory deficits were pronounced, Sonia remembered this conversation, and 5 minutes later she told the staff, "My mother is surely out of the bath by now. Can I call her again?" Finally frustrated with their inability to reason with Sonia or to trick her, the head nurse consulted with me, and we came up with an alternative. The next time Sonia asked to see her mother, the head nurse asked her to sit down, have a cup of tea with her, and talk about her mother. That approach had a calming effect and reduced the frequency of her requests to see her mother. Other strategies for this problem would be to look at old photographs or reminisce with the patient about her mother.

The desire to go home is a similar problem. Even patients who have lived in the same house for a long period of time may insist that they are not at home and that they want to go home. We have known families who take the patients back to the homes they grew up in, only to find out that they do not recognize the houses. Sometimes a family can distract a patient by taking him or her out for a walk or a ride; on returning to the house, the patient recognizes it. A more general solution is to respond to the patients' feelings. In wanting to go home, patients may be expressing insecurity or bewilderment that the present is not making sense. A calm, reassuring response can lower the patient's anxiety. Reminiscing, looking at old photographs, or diverting patients to other activities can all be helpful.

One other issue that I address in the early stages of treatment is the family's legal and financial situation. Families facing extensive costs for long-term care should get informed advice about these matters. In particular, spouses need to be aware of how they can protect a portion of their assets and income if their husbands or wives go into nursing homes. Families also need to have power of attorney for their relatives (see Chapter 15). If families do not have a lawyer to turn to, we refer them to someone who specializes in elder law.

PROBLEM SOLVING

The heart of intervention with family caregivers is problem solving (see Chapter 12). Caregivers are taught to use problem solving to manage problem behaviors, as well as other stressors in their lives. The following example shows the use of problem solving in management of agitated behavior.

THE USE OF PROBLEM SOLVING

Helen was caring for her husband, Jim, who was suffering from AD. Her biggest problem was that Jim became agitated between 4:00 and 6:00 P.M. every day. During this time, he would rearrange the furniture in the living room, throw things on the floor, and generally make a mess. While he was doing this, Helen was busy preparing dinner. On the suggestion of her therapist, Helen began keeping a record of her husband's agitated behavior for a week. Reviewing the records together, Helen and her therapist noted that the problem had not occurred on one day during the previous week. They then explored what was different about that day. During the afternoon, the couple had gone out for a ride. They had done this other afternoons as well, but on this particular day Jim had said he was hungry. They stopped for a sandwich. Later that day, Jim was not agitated. Based on this information, Helen and her therapist came up with the hypothesis that Jim's late-afternoon agitation might be triggered by hunger. Helen then came up with a solution that suited her. She decided to serve dinner at 5:00 P.M. rather than at 6:00 to see if that made a difference. She continued to keep records the following week, and they indicated that Jim's agitation in late afternoon was greatly reduced.

This example illustrates a number of important points about problem solving. Based on the initial information about agitation during late afternoon, several hypotheses could have been generated—for example, that this problem was part of the later afternoon delirium called "sundowner's syndrome" and that better illumination might help. The hypothesis that emerged came from focusing on what was different on the day the problem behavior did not occur. It was also built on an understanding of the effects of dementia on behavior. Patients sometimes do not report hunger, thirst, or even pain, and their discomfort can be a trigger for disturbed behavior. The solution in this case emerged from the observations the patient's wife made and drew on an understanding of how dementia affects behavior.

Because caregivers are asked to carry out these interventions, it is important to gain their cooperation. Problem solving can never be a mechanistic technique but must be integrated into the relationship the therapist has with the caregiver. Sometimes a caregiver's reluctance may be due to a lack of understanding of dementia, particularly the fact that people with dementia have a limited ability to make changes in their own behaviors. Although patients can sometimes seem annoyingly willful, they cannot take control of their own behavior as they might have done in the past. Caregivers who do not understand this often respond with anger or resentment when asked to make changes. It is critical for them to realize that *they* are the only ones who can make a change in the situation. Another obstacle to implementing problem solving is feeling helpless or hopeless or too angry with the patient to put the energy into changes. These problems are discussed later.

Solutions can lose their effectiveness over time. At that point, it is important to reassess the situation to find out what has changed and to try a new approach. Caregivers, however, may react to changes catastrophically, feeling that they have lost the little control they had or believing that the situation is now unmanageable. It is important to help them interpret a change as a normal setback. Before they give up, caregivers can try to find out whether there is something different they can do to improve the situation.

Therapists can use problem solving to pinpoint times when a caregiver feels especially stressed or emotionally drained and to identify the specific event or sequence of events that gives the caregiver trouble. Solutions can include finding better ways to manage the triggering events or getting relief for the caregiver before the amount of stress builds up too high.

We have emphasized problem solving as a series of steps, with progress monitored through the use of written records. This framework can be used without formally going through each step. Clinicians who are not experienced with behavioral approaches or with dementia, however, should go through the whole sequence to make sure that the solutions that emerge are specific to the targeted problem and its context. Another advantage of the formal sequence is teaching caregivers how to use the approach themselves. Problem solving can complement the way caregivers deal with difficult situations. Caregivers learn new skills that replace approaches that are not effective in managing a patient with dementia.

PROVIDING SUPPORT

The third treatment technique is providing support. Support emerges naturally from a therapeutic relationship that is empathic and nonjudgmental. A therapist's support can help a caregiver explore difficult issues and gain confidence to make changes.

In order to prepare for the challenges they will face, caregivers must also be able to get support from family, friends, and formal service providers. Support includes assistance with caregiving tasks and emotional support. Through discussions with the therapist, the caregiver can usually identify types of support that would be helpful or that the caregiver would be willing to use. The clinician helps caregivers explore ways of obtaining this kind of help. Caregivers often hold back from getting the help that they need, however, because of perceived practical and emotional barriers. Some of their reasons for not using a particular type of assistance may be realistic, and some might be exaggerations of the possible negative consequences.

Accepting help from family and friends is difficult for many caregivers. Some are reluctant to ask for help because they believe that they should be able to manage on their own. Caregivers may feel embarrassed or ashamed of the care recipient's behavior or their own need for help. A caregiver may not want to burden his or her own children by asking for help and may even try to protect them from knowing how bad the situation has become. In other instances, caregivers believe that they should not have to ask for help, that their family should know what they need.

Caregivers erect similar barriers to accepting help from formal agencies. Caregivers may be concerned that the helpers are not reliable or do not have adequate training. They may also say that the care recipient will not accept help or will become angry at the caregiver for getting help.

When caregivers need help but are reluctant to get it, clinicians should work with them in a collaborative way to identify the reasons for their reluctance. Using a cognitive-behavioral style of gentle questioning (Beck et al., 1979; see Chapter 9), the therapist can help caregivers identify the thoughts that make them feel reluctant or anxious about getting a particular type of help. They can then generate alternative ways of looking at the situation. For example, a caregiver may feel that if her children wanted to help, they would have offered to do so. Through examination of this assumption and alternative ways of looking at the situation, the clinician may determine that the caregiver's children do not actually know what help she needs. It can also be suggested that by not helping, the children are missing an opportunity to do something for and with their father while they still have the chance. Of course, the particular way of reframing the caregiver's thoughts about accepting help depends on the situation.

Caregivers often fear that making any changes in their situation will upset the patient in some way. The clinician needs to recognize that the caregiver's reluctance to use help is often based on unspoken fears that it will make things worse. Through questioning, the clinician can help caregivers identify their fears and instead help them see the potential for positive outcomes. The clinician can talk about the experiences of other caregivers who had similar worries, but where the use of help worked out well.

When caregivers are reluctant to get help despite a high level of stress, the clinician can explore what their goals are and the consequences of not getting help. Most involved family caregivers want to provide help for as long as they can. By helping them to look at the consequences of trying to do everything themselves, the clinician can help them see that they will burn out quicker.

Another objection that caregivers may raise is that they are the only ones who can provide help, that no one else can do it right. The clinician can suggest that it is important for the patient to see other people or to have a change of scenery. Identifying the potential benefits for the patient is helpful when caregivers believe that they are being selfish for seeking help.

Again, these ways of reframing the acceptance of help are suggestions, not formulas. The clinician needs to hold a collaborative and supportive discussion with the caregiver. This discussion should never become badgering or bullying, and clinicians need to be prepared to accept the idea that caregivers may choose to handle a situation in a less than optimal way. By building a supportive and accepting relationship, the clinician leaves the door open for the possibility that the caregiver will become more willing to get help over time.

Caregivers are sometimes reluctant to use services because of practical and realistic barriers. Some service programs are not adequately prepared to handle difficult clients, and a few are incompetent at everything they do. Clinicians can be more helpful to their clients if they have an idea of how various community agencies function. That way, they can assist caregivers to differentiate real barriers from the caregiver's own worries and fears.

Sometimes one can find solutions to real barriers. A typical problem with home health agencies is that they may send a different person for each visit, which can be disruptive for both the family caregiver and the care recipient, especially when the latter has a memory disorder. The caregiver may be able to approach the agency about having the same person come each time or to find another agency that is more cooperative.

Treatment Modalities

COUNSELING

Much of the work we have described takes place in one-to-one counseling sessions with the caregiver. An important part of these sessions is developing a therapeutic relationship that gives caregivers the security to examine the problems they are facing and to try out new approaches for managing them. A delicate balance needs to be established regarding expression of emotions. Caregivers often feel angry, depressed, worried, hopeless, helpless, guilty, or frustrated and may have no one else to talk to about these emotions besides the therapist. These feelings are keys for identifying what problems are the most pressing and where clinicians should intervene. Some caregivers, however, find it hard to move beyond ventilating their frustrations. The clinician needs to create an environment in which the caregiver feels safe in expressing strong emotions but is not encouraged to dwell on them.

The goal of treatment is to find ways to address modifiable features of the situation that contribute to caregivers' distress. Of course, some things cannot be changed, such as their relatives' illness and the sense of loss they may be feeling. It may seem to a caregiver that the only way of dealing with these feelings is to leave the situation, which can be a frightening thought. The clinician must be able to show him or her how taking small, concrete steps can make the situation better, even though the patient's illness has not been cured.

Treatment can address a variety of other issues, including ambivalence over assuming the caregiving role, long-standing problems in the relationship between the caregiver and care recipient, and feelings of guilt. Many caregivers need the opportunity to clarify what their role should be and to set limits to their involvement. If caregivers can articulate what they believe is the right thing for them to do, then it is possible to work with them to develop a plan to do that and to let go when it is the right time. Clinicians need to convey that there is no right way to be a caregiver, that caregivers must decide what is best for them.

The duration of counseling can be brief and problem focused or long term. Some caregivers need just to be pointed in the right direction, and then they can begin managing better on their own. Those caregivers make considerable progress in 5 to 10 sessions. No matter how competent the caregiver may seem, however, the door should be left open for her or him to come back if the situation changes. Other cases are more complicated. Caregivers may be feeling high levels of distress or have inadequate coping strategies for managing the situation. Family relationships may be difficult or complicated. We have found that in these instances weekly sessions for a sustained period of time are useful. When the situation is stabilized, the time between sessions can be lengthened, though regular sessions can be resumed during a crisis.

FAMILY MEETINGS

Families are the most important source of support and assistance to care-givers. Unlike formal agencies, which operate within a bureaucratic frame-work, family members can help in flexible ways and outside business hours. But families may not provide help when the caregiver thinks it is needed or may disagree with the primary caregiver about the care their relative should get. These nonsupportive interactions can be especially debilitating to care-givers already under a great deal of pressure.

We have found that working directly with all relevant family members is the best way to build support. We do this through a family meeting. A care-fully orchestrated family meeting can reduce misunderstandings and conflict over care and allow the family to develop a plan to provide ongoing support for the primary caregiver. A single family meeting with telephone follow-up usually suffices (Zarit, Orr, & Zarit, 1985), though some treatment protocols use several family sessions (Mittelman et al., 1995; Mittelman, Epstein, & Pierzchalla, 2002).

Planning for the family meeting begins with the primary caregiver. The clinician needs to learn about the family structure and relationships before the family meeting even while recognizing that the caregiver's perspective is lim-ited. From a family systems perspective, it is useful to get a sense of how a family functions—for example, who is influential and who is not, who is close to and distant from whom, and what roles the caregiver and care recipient have had in the family. It is also important to identify conflict over caregiving issues, as well as disagreements over other issues that might interfere with the family's pulling together to support the caregiver. The clinician and the care-giver should explore what kind of help the caregiver would like to get and what is realistic to expect the family to provide. Issues concerning the patient's diagnosis should be clarified before the family meeting, because that will often be a topic of discussion.

The caregiver decides whom to invite to the family meeting and when and where to hold it. Family meetings can be held in a clinician's office, though we have had more success when they are held in a family member's home. Fami-lies are less likely to respond defensively at home than when called to a mental health professional's office. By going to their home, the clinician demonstrates a commitment to the family that engenders trust.

In the family meeting, the clinician recapitulates the process the caregiver has been going through, moving from providing information to problem solv-ing and support. As a first step, it is important that everyone has the same information about the diagnosis and the possibilities for treatment. Family members may have partial, distorted, or incorrect information. In cases of dementia, the primary caregiver usually accepts that the illness is irreversible before other family members do; they may continue to question the diagnosis or bombard the caregiver with suggestions about possible treatments they have heard or read about. Although meant to be helpful, these suggestions are frequently experienced by the caregiver as an added stressor (MaloneBeach & Zarit, 1995). Clinicians can address these issues in a gently authoritative and nondogmatic manner. Especially in cases of irreversible disorders such as AD, it is important to assure everyone that everything possible is being done. Because the media frequently report the results of new research on possible treatments for AD and similar diseases, families may want to continue their search for a cure. As was done earlier with the caregiver, the clinician needs to provide honest answers about the prospects of treatment without dashing all hope. The goal is to reframe people's wish to do something from searching for a medical cure to providing support and assistance.

When the family understands the care recipient's condition, the meeting can turn to the caregiver. The clinician can ask the caregiver what is stressful and what kinds of things can help. In some cases, it is the first time the family has thought about the caregiver's situation. When the caregiver's needs are expressed, the family's own problem-solving ability comes into play. Usually, there is someone in the family who is an organizer and problem solver and who takes over at that point to develop a plan. The plan can include having family members provide emotional or instrumental support or helping arrange for or pay for formal help. The tasks that the family agrees to do should be specific and scheduled. It should be clear what each person will do and when. The clinician makes sure that no one has overcommitted and that all the tasks are achievable within the proposed time frame.

The best kind of plan involves giving everyone in the family some responsibility. It is important that people do not argue over whether someone is doing too much or too little. The clinician should emphasize that each person can contribute in a different way and that every kind of help is important.

GIVING EVERYONE A TASK THAT IS IMPORTANT

Lynn was caring for her mother-in-law, who was suffering from dementia. She had been providing most of the care for her mother-in-law but could no longer do so because she was going back to work. Her husband, Martin, was too angry with his mother because of long-standing problems in their relationship to spend more time with her. The patient's daughter, Rose, wanted to do more for her mother, but she was ill herself and lived some distance away. Rose felt guilty that she could not spend more time with her mother.

A family meeting was held, with Lynn, Martin, and Rose attending. I worked with them to construct tasks they each could do. Lynn said she could continue to visit her mother-in-law (who lived in a retirement home) but would go less frequently. Martin was willing to talk to the manager of the retirement home about his mother's condition in order to see what additional support the home might provide. He would also talk with his uncle, who lived in the same retirement home, encouraging him to spend more time with the patient. This was something he thought his uncle would be willing to do. Although Rose could not visit, she could talk with her mother on the phone. When she expressed guilt over not doing more, I stressed to her that this was an important and valuable activity. Follow-up indicated that the plan worked: The family was satisfied with the arrangements they made for their mother and with each other.

The clinician's role in a family meeting is to be neutral and supportive. Already having a relationship with the primary caregiver, the clinician should be sure to note other people's perspectives and observe how the family functions and makes decisions. Caregivers who are strong may be perceived as not needing help and may even have alienated potential helpers. On the other hand, when caregivers are perceived as weak, other family members may deprecate what they have done or blame them for some of the current problems. In these situations, the therapist must keep the focus on how to stabilize the care situation without getting into discussions of the caregiver's or anyone else's personality.

The therapist should use but not try to change family process. Family meetings are not family therapy and should not be used to treat long-standing problems or to redress the balance of power within a family. That is not what the family asked for help with, and it is not necessary to addressing the problems at hand. Rather, the clinician should focus on caregiving issues, identifying common family goals (e.g., providing more support) and developing a plan to reach the goals.

It is possible to work with families who have long-standing conflicts yet can reach an agreement on care-related issues. For example, one family we worked with was so divided into two warring factions that it seemed that a meeting could not be held, because no one could be identified to host the meeting who would be considered acceptable by everyone else. Finally, a distant relative who got along with both sides agreed to hold the meeting. Despite all the conflict, the meeting had a positive outcome. For the first time, all the children of the patient learned how severe their mother's disabilities were. As a result, they were able to rally around their stepfather to provide help. After their stepfather mentioned his need for occasional respite, one daughter pulled out her calendar and began assigning each of the five children to spend one weekend a month caring for their mother. Another reminded the group about the positive role their stepfather had played in their lives when they were teenagers. They agreed on a schedule and also planned to hire help with cooking and cleaning for their stepfather. Follow-up indicated that everyone fulfilled his or her obligations.

This example also shows how families can be creative in generating their own solutions. However, family meetings are not always helpful. It is probably not advisable to conduct a family meeting with severely disturbed families who have poor boundaries, disordered communications, and little history of success in dealing with common tasks and problems. In some families the conflict over care may be too intense for a family meeting.

When Differences Are Too Great for a Family Meeting

George was the primary caregiver for his mother, who was living in a nursing home. He had made the decision to maintain her old home, at considerable expense, because he felt it was good for her to be able to visit it. George's brothers were furious with him and believed that he was squandering the inheritance that was due to them. They had not provided any help with caregiving and, according to George and his wife, were concerned only about their inheritance.

George tried to arrange a family meeting, but his brothers declined to attend. Their refusal to come actually had a positive effect, confirming for George and his wife that his brothers were not interested in their mother's well-being. George and his wife now felt more comfortable with their decisions and felt that they were doing the right thing for their mother.

Family meetings may be small or large, depending on the number of relevant people who should be invited. We have had meetings with just one other person and meetings with as many as 25 people. We have even held family meetings in which some of the participants came from overseas. In one such case, the key person providing emotional support to the caregiver was her sister, who lived in Europe but was visiting home when the family meeting took place. During the meeting this sister expressed how bad she felt that she could not help more. The caregiver was able to assure her sister that her letters and phone calls were very special to her and provided her with help that no one else could provide. This face-to-face meeting allowed for expressions of support that probably could not have taken place otherwise.

Despite the planning the therapist does before the family meeting, he or she should be prepared for surprises. Some family members use the forum to reveal information that greatly changes the situation, as in the next example.

Surprises at a Family Meeting

Two daughters, Joyce and Tina, were overseeing the care of their mother, who had severe AD. Their mother lived in her own apartment, assisted by a live-in housekeeper, but with both daughters spending considerable time helping their mother. Joyce and Tina were close to one another, but both had secrets that they revealed during the meeting. Joyce revealed that she and her husband were trying to have a baby and that if she got pregnant, she would be unable to do as much as she was doing now for her mother. Tina revealed that she was about to change jobs and could also do less for their mother. They each had been reluctant to talk openly about these issues before, believing that they were letting the other down. By discussing openly what they had been hiding from each other, they realized that they had reached the limit of what they could do for their mother and decided it was necessary to plan for nursing home care. Though they felt sad that they could not continue to keep their mother at home, they believed they had made the right decision. Subsequently, the placement went smoothly, the sisters remained close, and Joyce became pregnant.

I have also made interventions short of a full-scale meeting that accomplished the same goals. Phone conversations may be held with key family members, for example, a child of the caregiver, or we may have joint office sessions that involve one or two other family members. For some families, these more informal arrangements are preferable. The gains that can be made from face-to-face family meetings, however, should not be overlooked, especially the benefit of having everyone in the room together hearing the same information and being given the opportunity to contribute to a plan for support.

SUPPORT GROUPS

Support groups for caregivers, particularly those who are assisting someone with AD or another dementing illness, have become immensely popular. Part of a grassroots movement that began in the late 1970s to assist caregivers and build support among the general public for treatment of AD, support groups have flourished and led to the development of advocacy organizations such as the Alzheimer's Association. Research on support groups suggests that they are not as effective as one-to-one counseling or a combination of counseling and family meetings in reducing stress on caregivers but that they can provide long-term support to caregivers after a more intense period of treatment (Mittelman et al., 1996; Toseland, Rossiter, Peak, & Smith, 1990; Whitlatch et al., 1991).

Support groups have therapeutic processes that are not found in individual counseling or family meetings. These special properties of support groups enhance the three treatment techniques I use with caregivers—information, problem solving, and support.

Groups are an effective way of disseminating information. Caregivers share their firsthand experience with various community helpers and resources; they discuss which physicians are helpful, which attorneys to consult, and how to find good home helpers to assist the patient. They also share information about treatments, such as which drugs help patients, something that should be closely monitored by the group leader but that can be productive.

Groups also provide a special kind of support that is not available else-where, that of sharing experiences with people who are in the same situation. Caregivers feel less isolated after attending groups. Hearing how other people respond to similar situations can normalize a caregiver's experience. It helps caregivers understand that the strong emotions they feel are an expected part of the stress of caregiving, not something that is wrong with them. As an example, a man who was a member of a new support group in which people did not yet know each other well burst out that he had gotten so angry at his wife (who had dementia) that he had put his fist through the wall. The group sat for a minute in stunned silence, and then everyone began talking, saying that they felt angry and frustrated, too, but had been ashamed of those feel-ings. By acknowledging their anger to one another, group members felt less isolated and could now identify their anger as something to work on rather than hide.

In a similar way, caregivers are able to draw on one another's experiences to overcome their reluctance to accept help. They learn firsthand about the benefits of getting help and realize that it is not shameful or a sign of weakness to accept help. By giving as well as receiving support, group members gain a sense of their own competence and feel more positive about their involvement.

Problem solving takes on a new dimension in support groups. Caregivers often come up with original solutions that we would not have imagined. They also are more willing to try solutions when a peer suggests them.

PROBLEM SOLVING IN A GROUP

Harriet told a story in a group about how she had been trying to cross a busy intersection with her husband, who was suffering from dementia. Her husband had become frightened and would not cross the street when the light was green. Harriet caught her breath and realized that forcing him to cross would not work. Instead, when the light turned green, she took his arm gently and in her softest voice said, "Honey, it's time to cross." He walked readily with her. The other group members were struck by this example of using affection rather than con-frontation and tried this approach during the following week, with considerable success. Over the years, we have suggested using affection to deal with many dif-ferent kinds of problem behaviors, a solution that first emerged from caregivers themselves.

One thing that groups do particularly well is to encourage caregivers to take better care of themselves. The group can promote using respite services such as adult day care or taking breaks from caregiving. When some group members share their experiences of using help, it makes it possible for others in the group to put aside their fears or guilt and arrange to get some help.

Taking Care of Oneself

Probably the most dramatic example of caregivers encouraging one another to take better care of themselves occurred when Nate, a long-standing member of a group, complained that he had been having chest pains and that his doctor wanted him to have a thorough examination. Nate was ambivalent about going to the hospital because he was concerned about what would happen to his wife in the meantime. He had actually made arrangements for his daughter to care for his wife, but he told the group that he had changed his mind and was going to go home rather than keep his doctor's appointment, which had been scheduled after the group meeting. The group insisted that Nate go to the doctor. After examining him, Nate's doctor hospitalized him immediately, and he had successful heart bypass surgery the next day. Without the intervention of the group, Nate would not have had the immediate treatment he needed.

Groups, of course, are not inherently helpful. Therapeutic processes emerge or fail to emerge from the interactions in the group. A group that is dominated by an opinionated, self-centered person will not be helpful and may even become harmful. A major role of the support group leader is to create a therapeutic environment in which everyone's opinion is heard and respected, no one dominates the group, and no one is ignored. There needs to be both a sense of universality—that everyone is in the same boat—and a sense of differences—that it is all right to have different responses and feelings. As we do in the other treatments, we also do not advocate a position (e.g., that caregivers should or should not place a relative in a nursing home) but help caregivers explore issues in a nonjudgmental framework so that they can make the decisions that best reflect their values. In some mature groups (that is, groups with long-standing members), participants often create this therapeutic environment themselves, telling new members how much they have gained from the group and stressing that everyone's experience is different and that there is no single best way to do things.

Support groups are organized in many different ways. Some are led by clinicians and others by nonclinicians. Although a nonclinician can be an effective leader, we believe that any leader should have training in group process so that he or she can step in when necessary to maintain a therapeutic or supportive environment. The frequency with which groups meet also varies. Most community groups meet monthly. Research protocols have sometimes used weekly meetings, which may be especially helpful when caregivers first seek help. Finally, groups differ in terms of how they operate. Some groups emphasize information almost exclusively; they invite speakers and focus on specific topics. Other groups focus more on sharing feelings and experiences.

As we have stressed throughout, it is important to create an atmosphere in the group in which caregivers feel they can express their feelings but are not encouraged to dwell on them. Participants can be encouraged to identify the features of the situation they can change and not remain stuck on the things they cannot change.

Placement and Beyond

As we have emphasized, this decision should be the family's, not the clinician's. The clinician should not dogmatically state that a family ought to place an older relative in a home or that there is a right time to do so. Instead, clinicians should make sure families feel comfortable talking about the issue and viewing it as an option. If a family has not brought up the subject, the clinician can make a general statement to introduce the topic, such as, "Many people in your situation have thought about placing their relative in a nursing home. Have you thought about that?" When families bring the topic up themselves, the clinician should assure them that it is an appropriate option and that there is no shame in placing someone in a nursing home.

The clinician's involvement should not end with placement. Caregivers often need a variety of help following nursing home placement. Spousal caregivers, in particular, feel guilty and lonely. Caregivers also need to work out how often they will visit and how to interact with staff members in productive ways. We talk about working with families in institutional settings in Chapter 14.

Bereavement

The final transition, bereavement, does not necessarily bring resolution to the caregiver. Following the death of a relative with dementia, many caregivers continue to experience distress for some period of time (Aneshensel et al., 1995). Although grief and depression gradually decrease, some caregivers remain depressed for a sustained period of time. The intensity of ties during caregiving may paradoxically create this vulnerability.

CONCLUSIONS

Caring for a disabled older relative can be a stressful experience. Family caregivers may find themselves providing around-the-clock help with few breaks and little assistance from anyone else. Although an older person's disabilities may be irreversible, the caregiver may be able to change some features of the situation to lower her or his own stress. We have looked at the onset of caregiving, the stresses of providing care in the patient's home and community, and transitions to institutional care and bereavement. We emphasize a model of intervention for caregivers assisting a relative in the community that is composed of three treatment techniques—information, problem solving, and support—and three treatment modalities—one-to-one counseling, family meetings, and support groups. Each technique and modality provides a different resource for families and can be useful in lowering stress. In the end, the goal is to help families clarify their preferences and assist them as much as possible in providing care in a way consistent with their values and beliefs. Clinicians can provide technical expertise and support that helps families to do the best they can and to minimize the physical and emotional costs to themselves.

CHAPTER 14

Consultation in Institutional Settings

One of the most important roles for mental health professionals is consultation and treatment in nursing homes and other residential settings. The consultant role requires specialized skills and knowledge that are not typically part of general clinical training. Staff members must handle a wide range of behavioral, emotional, and cognitive problems of older clients and may not have the time or training to do so effectively. A mental health consultant can assess the possible causes of the problems and intervene with patients, staff, and family members to maximize the patient's functioning and reduce strain on an already overburdened staff.

Our approach combines basic consultation principles with an understanding of the tenets of geriatric mental health practice and the unique features of the nursing home setting. Besides bringing expertise on geropsychiatric problems, the consultant has the time to spend with patients to figure out what is going on. Staff members on the nursing units are busily caught up in daily routines and do not have enough time to get to the root of complex problems. Therapeutic staff members, such as occupational, physical, or speech therapists, spend a lot of time with patients, but they are task oriented and may not have the opportunity to see the bigger picture. Patients often recognize this and say to us, "You're the first person to take time to listen to me."

TYPES OF INSTITUTIONAL SETTINGS

Nursing homes are the best known institutional setting, and, given the complex health and mental problems that many residents have, it is the type of facility in which consultation is most likely to take place. Increasingly, however, other settings, such as assisted living, board and care, and residential care, provide an alternative to nursing homes. Unlike nursing homes, these programs are not regulated as medical facilities and so have more latitude in how they are organized. This difference creates opportunities for innovative ways of addressing quality of life (e.g., Zimmerman, Sloane, Heck, Maslow, & Schulz, 2005). Some assisted living facilities serve only older people, including those with dementia. Others serve old and young people with physical disabilities. "Board and care" is a designation for a facility that has historically served the chronically medically ill. Some board-and-care homes take only older residents, but some mix younger people with mental illness or substance abusers with older patients. That type of program can be frightening to older residents. Finally, a program may be licensed by the state as a residential care facility or may be unlicensed. Small, unlicensed facilities are often hidden from public view, but they sometimes provide a high quality of care (Morgan, Eckert, & Lyon, 1995).

Paralleling the growth of alternate institutions such as assisted living, nursing homes have also become more varied in their structure, adopting new models as providers that recognize the limitations of traditional care. One such approach is the subacute medical care unit, which can be found in many nursing homes and in some hospitals. Since the early 1980s, Medicare has provided incentives to hospitals to limit the length of inpatient stays. The result is that many older patients are discharged "sicker and quicker" and may require ongoing medical and nursing care. Sometimes care can be provided at home, with visits from home nursing personnel or by coordinating home care with outpatient services such as physical therapy. In other instances, patients are discharged from the hospital to a nursing home subacute unit. These units offer a higher level of medical services and more skilled personnel than chronic care units. A subacute program is often located in a wing of a traditional nursing home that offers chronic care in other parts of the building. The emphasis in subacute units is on providing rehabilitation services so that the patient can return to the community. In contrast to chronic care, a stay in a subacute unit that follows a hospitalization is covered by Medicare for up to 120 days.

Nursing homes have always included a small number of short-term patients, but this group of residents is now growing rapidly, for financial reasons. The stable and high reimbursement provided by Medicare has made subacute units an essential part of a nursing home's financial foundation. One of the ironies of shorter hospital stays is that they appear to lead to greater use of nursing homes. Thus it is not clear whether shorter stays are actually producing cost savings or are merely shifting costs from one source to another.

For the consultant, the main effect of subacute care is that some nursing home consultations involve issues of transition back to the community. In contrast to hospital settings, where the patient's stay is increasingly brief, the subacute unit provides consultants with the opportunity to implement treatment for issues such as depression or family conflict that can improve rehabilitation and ease the move back home.

Despite the growth in subacute care, nursing homes still predominantly provide chronic care. It is within chronic care that we see the second major development in nursing homes, the formation of separate units for care of people with dementia. These programs are typically identified as Alzheimer's or special care units. The number of these special care programs has grown rapidly in the past 25 years. There is as yet no consensus as to what constitutes special care (Holmes et al., 1994; Maslow, 1994; Zimmerman & Sloane, 1999), nor are there licensing rules that require specific features (e.g., staff–patient ratios) to qualify as a special care facility. The one consistent feature that marks most dementia programs is that the unit is locked. Other than that, facilities may offer a variety of special environmental features, such as indoor and outdoor areas in which residents can wander, orienting information to help residents identify their own rooms or other facilities on the unit, and more homelike furnishings and decorations. Activities are geared for patients with dementia who benefit from a high level of activity.

Part of the impetus for development of Alzheimer's units has been the recognition that the traditional medical model of nursing homes is not appropriate for these patients, who primarily require supervision and structured activities (e.g., Sloane & Mathew, 1991). Many creative programs for dementia have also been developed in assisted living facilities (Zimmerman & Sloane, 1999; Zimmerman, Sloane, Heck, et al., 2005). A similar shift has taken place in dementia care in Europe, from medically oriented facilities to more homelike settings (e.g., Malmberg, 1999; Malmberg & Zarit, 1993).

THE NEED FOR CONSULTATION IN LONG-TERM CARE

The need for mental health services in nursing homes and other long-term care facilities is considerable. As Smyer (1989) first noted, nursing homes have become the mental hospitals of our era. Estimates of the prevalence of residents with significant mental disorders in nursing homes have ranged from 50 to over 90% (e.g., German et al., 1986; Payne et al., 2002; Rovner, Kafonek, Filipp, Lucas, & Folstein, 1986). High rates of mental health problems have also been reported in assisted living and similar care facilities (Gruber-Baldini, Boustani, Sloane, & Zimmerman, 2004; Watson, Garrett, Sloane, Gruber-Baldini, & Zimmerman, 2003) Despite these high rates, most patients do not receive treatment for their mental health problems or at most receive only medications (Burns et al., 1993; Gruber-Baldini et al., 2004; Shea et al., 1994).

The most frequent disorders are those that are prevalent in the general population of elderly—dementia, delirium, depression, and anxiety. The clinician may, however, encounter the full range of psychiatric diagnoses in these settings. Consultations involve diagnostic questions, but usually the most important work is developing and implementing a multifaceted treatment plan that addresses the pertinent medical, psychological, interpersonal, and environmental dimensions of functioning.

Regulations in nursing homes emphasize the use of behavioral and other nonpharmacological interventions as the first choice for management of behavior problems. Nursing homes are restricted in their use of antipsychotic medications and physical restraints to control behavior. Use of these approaches must be carefully justified. This regulation grew out of recognition that antipsychotic medications were not consistently effective with agitated behavior (see Chapter 12) and that medication and restraints were used excessively without first trying behavioral approaches. A consultant can help staff develop behavioral treatments for patients who are agitated, depressed, or anxious.

THE ORGANIZATION OF CONSULTATION SERVICES

Mental health services in long-term care settings can be organized in different ways. The clinician can be a salaried employee of a facility, an arrangement found in some larger nursing homes. The more common arrangement is for clinicians to serve as consultants who are called in as needed. We find that there is an advantage to being a consultant rather than a member of the staff. In that role, we can provide more reassurance to patients and sometimes to staff about confidentiality. Even though confidentiality applies in both types of arrangements, we have more credibility when we are independent consultants. We are also freer to represent the patient's interests, not the institution's. Many patients, especially those on Medicaid in the United States, may feel vulnerable or that they have no choice about where they are living. A mental health professional who is a caring outsider can be a better advocate for patients.

Many nursing homes contract with private companies for mental health services. In our experience, however, the quality is usually not good. The clinicians who are sent in may have had little or no prior training in geropsychology, and the company is often more concerned with producing billable hours than with giving high-quality care. This situation wastes money and deprives patients, staff, and family of proper treatment. Good care costs no more to the facility or family than inadequate care, but it requires clinicians with the appropriate competencies.

PRINCIPLES OF CONSULTATION IN NURSING HOMES

This section describes how we approach consultation and the specific issues mental health professionals must address in nursing homes.

Foundations of Consultation

Consultations are intellectually challenging because of the variety and complexity of problems presented. As in solving a puzzle or mystery, the clinician must sort through several levels of data to identify likely contributing factors and possible avenues for intervention. Consultations are also satisfying because results can generally be seen immediately. Despite the age and disability of patients in nursing homes, interventions can be successful in alleviating the presenting problem and making the situation better for everyone involved—patients, their families, and staff.

An essential part of the puzzle is that consultations need to focus both on the patient and the care system. In his classic text, Caplan (1970) differentiated between four primary types of mental health consultation: (1) client-centered case consultation, (2) consultee-centered case consultation, (3) program-centered administrative consultation, and (4) consultee-centered administrative consultation. Because of the nature of the nursing home setting and the population of residents and staff, the consultation may involve elements of each of these approaches. Although the consultation is often client centered, the optimal solution may involve working with the consultee and, in some cases, with program or administrative systems. Nursing homes are not resource rich, and staff may have little training or experience in handling mental health problems. Thus a lot of what we do is to build the staff's capabilities. The cognitive impairments of many residents limit their ability to change, so interventions with staff may be the best avenue for treating a problem. When a consultant encounters repeated similar problems related to administrative or program policies, then intervention at that level may be appropriate. The opportunities for intervention at different levels of the nursing home community is another reason we find this work satisfying.

Another issue that we grapple with continually is the extent to which residents might be able to function independently or might need assistance. Parmalee and Lawton (1990) have described care in nursing homes as organized by the autonomy–security dialectic. Autonomy represents the patient's preferences for independence and control over his or her personal environment, whereas the institution, sometimes in conjunction with the family, stresses the need for keeping patients safe and secure.

There are many threats to autonomy in nursing homes, including the lack of privacy due to shared rooms and the tendency for nursing and medical staff members to make decisions for patients about their care or to provide too much care. A series of compelling studies by Margaret Baltes and her colleagues (Baltes, 1994; Baltes et al., 1987) documented that staff members reinforce dependent behavior and ignore or punish independent behavior. At the same time, there are legitimate needs for safety, especially for patients who are not competent to evaluate the risks of their own actions.

We emphasize supporting autonomy when possible, that is, when it does not compromise the resident's safety or that of other residents or staff. When patients or their families indicate their preference for autonomy, whether in making decisions about the type of care provided or regarding use of safety measures to prevent falls or other accidents, we believe it is important to find ways to support this preference. Often minor modifications in the usual way of doing things in the nursing home can set a balance between autonomy and security that is acceptable to everyone. Several examples later in the chapter address this issue.

Understand the Setting

The first principle of consultation is to understand the particular setting in which you are working and how it is structured. Although nursing homes can vary, some common features characterize most facilities.

Nursing homes will have specialized units or levels of care that serve different patients and functions. As we noted earlier, they may offer subacute care or special Alzheimer's care, in addition to traditional long-term chronic care. The consultant needs to be familiar with the levels of care offered in a particular nursing home. Solutions may sometimes involve moving patients from one unit to another in which a particular kind of care is more likely to be provided or to be appropriate.

Nursing home staff is organized in a hierarchy. Smyer, Cohn, and Brannon (1988) describe the hierarchy as a pyramid, with a few administrative and supervisory personnel at the top and nursing assistants at the bottom. Supervisors have the most influence over the program and policy but the least impact on day-to-day care. Although they have the least training and influence in the hierarchy, nursing assistants have the most contact with residents.

The director of nursing (DON) is usually the most influential person on patient care in the hierarchy. The DON oversees the clinical operation of the facility and is in charge of whatever happens clinically. The consultant should develop a good working relationship with the DON, establishing procedures for conducting consultations and getting support for the types of interventions the consultant makes. A helpful way of working with the DON is to set up regular (e.g., monthly) meetings to review the cases the consultant has seen.

In contrast to the DON, consultants spend little time with the nursing home administrator (NHA). Although technically in charge of all aspects of the facility, administrators are typically involved in paperwork and details related to business practices and regulations. Although exceptions do exist, administrators do not get involved in clinical activities and may not even have clinical backgrounds.

The next level of the hierarchy is the nursing supervisors. Nursing supervisors are registered nurses (RNs) who oversee clinical operations. Depending on the size of the facility, only one or two nursing supervisors may be on duty per shift. They are often the key people in making referrals to the consultant and in implementing changes.

Licensed practical nurses (LPNs) head units of the home. They oversee provision of regular nursing services to patients. Despite limited training, they have considerable responsibility for management of patients, and their work can be very stressful.

Finally, nursing aides or nursing assistants provide most of the ongoing care and spend the most time with patients. They may have little formal training or preparation for their work except for a small amount of mandated in-service training. The extent and depth of this training varies, as do opportunities for continuing education. Some aides have many years of experience and are highly skilled. Others have little or no background and may simply go through the motions of doing their jobs.

The consultant must also learn how to work with the different shifts. Information given to one shift needs to be conveyed to the other two shifts.

The medical staff is a critical part of the hierarchy. The medical staff can be organized in different ways. Some nursing homes have a physician on staff who sees all residents. Other nursing homes have a few physicians who regularly see patients at the facility. In most homes, residents can see their own physicians if the doctors are willing to come to the facility or if the patients can get transportation to the doctors' offices. Physicians who regularly visit the home have varying degrees of involvement; some do little more than review charts, and others spend considerable time with patients and staff.

Mental health consultants need to develop a relationship with staff physicians or other physicians who regularly see patients in the facility. This can be done by establishing credibility with the physicians when consulting on cases. Credibility can be gained through the way the consultant presents information. Both written reports and verbal communications need to be succinct and free of psychological jargon. Physicians tend to dismiss jargon as "psychobabble," even if the recommendations are sound. A report that speculates at length about the psychodynamics of a patient might be appropriate in a mental health facility but will not be helpful in a nursing home. Instead, the consultant needs to get to the point, summarizing the results of an assessment or providing a recommendation in a clear, concise way.

Another way to establish credibility is to become knowledgeable about common medical problems and about the medications used in nursing homes. Not only does this knowledge facilitate communication with physicians, but it is also critical in determining whether current medications or illnesses are contributing to the resident's behavior, emotions, or cognitive status. The following example illustrates the value of medical knowledge when working with physicians.

WORKING WITH PHYSICIANS

I was asked by the physician at a nursing home to consult in the case of an 80-year-old woman. The physician was someone I had not worked with much previously. She wanted to know whether the patient, who was suffering from PD, had a normal end-of-life depression or whether her depressive symptoms warranted more aggressive treatment. In evaluating the patient, I noted (as I usually do) the current medications. Included was the antidepressant Sinequan, which has anticholinergic effects and is not the best choice for someone suffering from PD, as it tends to worsen the movement disorder. When I provided feedback to the physician, she did not recognize the name of the antidepressant. I told her it was doxepin. She recognized doxepin as a tricyclic antidepressant and decided to change it. By being able to provide the physician with the generic name, as well as other pertinent information as part of the consultation, I established my credibility with her, and we have collaborated successfully on several cases since.

Gaining credibility with physicians and nurses also depends on familiarity with the common illnesses encountered in nursing homes. The consultant should have a good background in dementia, cardiovascular diseases, PD, stroke, chronic obstructive pulmonary disease (COPD), and diabetes. It is important to understand the behavioral and cognitive implications of these disorders. A useful resource is Morrison's (1997) *When Psychological Problems Mask Medical Disorders.*

A common referral is any patient who cries a lot. The first question to determine is whether the patient has suffered a stroke. If the patient has had a stroke, crying can be part of a depressive reaction, but in some instances the crying is not meaning based (i.e., there is no depressive content). Whether related to depression or not, crying can be treated with SSRIs, with behavioral approaches (providing attention when the patient is not crying), and by increasing activity levels.

Besides a familiarity with common illnesses and their features, clinicians should learn to recognize the terminal phases of disease. Terminal decline is frequently accompanied by anxiety and depression, which should be treated differently from typical affective disorders. Care in the terminal phase of an illness should emphasize making the patient comfortable and addressing any specific concerns or unfinished business. It may be useful to help family, and sometimes also staff members, to let go of the dying patient; that is, to stop trying to intervene actively or talking about recovery. In turn, families and staff may need support prior to and after the patient's death. Again, by having the time to talk with everyone involved, the mental health professional can play a very important role in the care of dying patients. The consultant, of course, needs to be comfortable dealing with the dying process and able to separate his or her own beliefs from the preferences of the patient and family.

Start with the Person Who Requested the Consultation

The second principle of consultation is to talk first with the person who requested the consultation. This point may seem elementary, but in a busy nursing home with its focus on patient problems, the easiest course is to see the patient first. We think it is beneficial to start with the staff member who requested the consultation to get an idea about the reasons for the consultation. A brief note or verbal request may not contain all the relevant information. A face-to-face discussion (or a telephone call, if the consultant has a good relationship with the person making the referral) can provide valuable information that will guide the consultation and may also contribute to the solution.

By going to this person first, the consultant also supports the hierarchy in the nursing home. Starting the consultation with the person who requested it recognizes that person's role and engages him or her in the process. That person may turn out to be peripherally involved, such as when a DON or nursing supervisor requests help with a patient on behalf of staff nurses or nursing assistants but is not involved in care. By going to the supervisor first, the consultant can gain support for the interventions that will be made. Changes that will benefit the patient have to be made within that structure, so the consultant needs the support of the people who can effect change.

Another reason to start with the person who made the request is that consultation addresses an interaction between staff and patient, staff and family, or sometimes all three. It is usually the staff or the family who can change, not the patient. As the consultant clarifies the situation, the real issue may turn out to be the staff members' well-being, not the patient's.

Read the Whole Medical Chart

The third fundamental part of consultation, but one that inexperienced clinicians omit, is to read the whole medical chart. The chart contains useful information about the patient's typical functioning and about ongoing medical and nursing care and medications. We review the chart for information about the patient's history and physical examinations, physicians' progress notes, medications list, information about other consultations, and notes from therapists who see the patient (e.g., physical or speech therapists).

There are two key points for the consultant when reading the medical chart. The first is to look for discrepancies. Do the observations of the patient's behaviors, moods, or functional capacities seem to vary? Do these variations follow any pattern, such as changing with different shifts? Do different staff members have varying impressions of the patient's behavior or capabilities? Another type of discrepancy is between how medications are supposed to be given and how they are actually administered. We have seen instances, for example, in which antidepressants are given as needed rather than on a regular basis. That pattern of administration is not adequate to build up to a therapeutic level of the medication.

The second point about chart information is that consultants should retain their objectivity. It is possible that some of the data in the chart are inaccurate or outdated, especially when the patient's condition has changed. This is often the case when the first person making a note in the chart writes that the patient is disoriented or confused. Everyone who follows may make similar notes without evaluating specifically what the patient's cognitive problems are or whether the patient's functioning has changed. On occasion, it may turn out that the problem is different from dementia or delirium.

Gather Information from All Relevant Sources

The fourth principle is to gather information from all relevant sources, including the staff members who actually spend time with the patient. A nursing supervisor may not have all the relevant information about the problem or how staff has tried to deal with it.

The family or other involved caregivers can be a valuable source of information. The consultant needs to identify the main family members involved in the patient's care. Many family members visit their relatives frequently, so the consultant may meet them in the course of talking to staff and patients. Or it may be necessary to telephone them, particularly adult children who are employed and do not come to the nursing home during daytime hours. In any case, it is essential to have a conversation with the family early in the consultation process in order to obtain a history of the patient and the family's view of current problems.

When patients are competent, it is necessary to get their permission before talking with the family. The patient has a legal right to confidentiality (see Chapter 15). The clinician should build the patient's trust that he or she will act in the patient's best interests. When patients are not capable of giving consent, the family should be involved, because they have legal and financial responsibility. At one home where I work, the social services agency informs the family that a consultation has been arranged. That way it is not a surprise when I call them. If competence has not been established (and establishment of competence may, in fact, be the reason for the consultation), the consultant should assume that the patient is competent until evidence suggests differently.

Respond in a Rapid and Relevant Way

The consultant needs to respond in a rapid and relevant way. The pace in nursing homes is quick, and decisions about problem patients need to be made in a timely way. Staff members become impatient with a consultant who dallies before conducting the consultation or who is slow in reporting the result. The sluggish consultant may find that recommendations have become irrelevant and that staff members have taken steps on their own to manage the situation.

The consultant makes a response at several levels. One response is a note in the medical chart. This is a necessary and legally required step. The note should be clear and brief and should provide the necessary information for the physician and staff to understand the problem and to take steps to correct it. As we have stressed previously, the consultant needs to use jargon-free language. The note also should be written at a level that is comprehensible to anyone reading it. Many of the nursing assistants and even some of the RNs have limited educational backgrounds, yet these are the staff members who will implement the consultant's recommendations. The note should be written so that they can easily understand what the consultant is proposing. The note should not detail all the steps in the consultant's reasoning; rather, it should briefly summarize conclusions and recommendations. As an example, a consultant may discover that a patient gets upset when she cannot hear what people are saying to her. Her hearing is somewhat better in her right ear. The consultant notes in the chart: "When speaking to her, be sure to be on her right side."

The consultant should be aware that a note in the patient's chart can be read by any staff member. For that reason, the note should not contain any confidential information that the patient or anyone else reveals (see Chapter 15). That information should be kept in a separate, locked case file, which the consultant maintains with the confidentiality of a therapy file.

The note in the chart can clarify how staff members can respond to an ongoing, difficult situation. We are often asked to consult when staff members have difficulty involving patients in activities. Sometimes we find that a person is reluctant to participate but can be encouraged. In these situations, our note reads something like "When trying to get Mrs. Q. involved in activities, don't take an initial 'no' for an answer." Other patients, however, may be competent to choose not to get out of bed or become involved in activities, as in the next example.

CONSULTATION ON A PATIENT UNWILLING TO BECOME MORE ACTIVE

Doreen went to a nursing home following a hip fracture. She had been an artist and had always led a somewhat reclusive life. Prior to the fracture, Doreen had already suffered from painful arthritis and never regained the ability to bear weight on her hip. In the nursing home, she refused to do more for herself or to get involved in more therapy. The staff of nursing homes often has difficulty dealing with patients like Doreen who could function at a higher level but refuse to do so. The staff asked for a consultation to determine whether Doreen was competent to make this decision or whether her refusal reflected depression. The evaluation revealed that Doreen fully understood the decisions she was making and their implications. She was also not depressed.

The progress note in a case such as this has to explicitly address the patient's mood and her competence to make the decision, along with recommendations to the staff on how to handle her. The note could state:

> The patient's mood was evaluated, and she was found to be at the most mildly depressed. She is fully competent to make decisions regarding her person and clearly states that she understands both the short- and long-term consequences of her activity. Staff can best respect her decision by asking her once if she wants to perform an activity and accepting her response without comment.

In addition to the note, the consultant should respond to all the relevant people involved in the case: the referral source, physician, nurses, nursing assistants, family, and patient. In some cases, the intervention is developed with key people on the staff. In other cases, the consultant explains the recommendations and enlists support in implementing them with the patient.

Follow-Through

Another critical part of a consultation in a nursing home is follow-through. Follow-through typically needs to be conducted with all the involved parties— patient, staff, and family—to see how the proposed actions have worked out. Mental health professionals who consult in settings such as rehabilitation or psychiatric hospitals are accustomed to conducting their evaluations and then writing detailed reports. A psychologist in one of those settings may test the patient and then write a report on the results that addresses the reason for consultation. The psychologist is unlikely to have any further contact with the patient or any follow-up with the staff. The difference between that kind of consultation and one in a nursing home is that the problems in nursing homes typically involve long-term adjustment to the facility. Patients in other inpatient settings leave relatively quickly, so consultations in those settings involve diagnostic questions or address short-term problems. The nursing home patient often is not going anywhere else. Although the consultation may involve diagnostic questions, there is almost always a component dealing with management of behavior. In order to be most effective, the consultant should follow up to see how well the recommendations have been implemented and to provide additional support or make changes if the plan is not working. A longer term involvement may be needed in some instances just to figure out what may be triggering or reinforcing problem behaviors.

Another reason for follow-up is that the staff members of nursing homes do not have much background in mental health problems or behavioral management. The consultant provides that expertise in a tactful and respectful way. But it is usually not sufficient to lay out a plan, even in clear and concise language, and expect that staff members will carry it out as planned. The staff may not fully understand the plan or may be too preoccupied with other problems to give it their full attention.

PUTTING THE PIECES OF THE PUZZLE TOGETHER: EFFECTIVE CONSULTING

The typical outcome of a consultation is recommendations that focus on improving the care or living situation of a patient, but the concerns of the family and staff also need to be taken into consideration. Staff and sometimes family as well must be involved in the treatment plan to some degree. At the minimum, they must consent to the recommendations and not disagree with or actively subvert them. More often, the consultant recommends ways in which they can change their interactions with the patient. The consultant can also focus on ways to alter the communications between family and staff. In a way, the consultant is often being asked to consider the well-being of the family and staff, as well as that of the patient. In doing so, the consultant must make sure that each person's interests are balanced. It is essential not to lose sight of the patient or the patient's interests, but many consultations concern problems that staff or family are having with the patient or with each other. Although the patient may be the overt reason for the consultation, solutions often lie in interventions with family and staff.

Helping Families Get What They Want

Another key role for consultants is empowering families. Families need to feel that they can have an impact on the care their relative is receiving, while appreciating the limitations of the situation and the fact that the care will not be as consistent or as personal as they would like or as they might give themselves. A starting point in building a relationship with the family is to empathize with their complaints. The consultant should not become defensive or move too quickly to propose solutions but should instead listen and reflect the family's feelings.

Families are most likely to raise concerns about the kind of care the patients receive. They wonder whether their relatives are receiving appropriate and sufficient care. They may be feeling guilty about placement and may even be wondering whether they should move their relatives back home. The family may also be having difficulty communicating with staff. The most frequent complaints they make are about the personal care the home provides the patient— whether the patient is bathed carefully enough or taken to the toilet frequently enough and whether the staff members speak respectfully to the patient and family or make the family feel guilty.

Sometimes the staff and the family have different goals that lead to misunderstandings, as illustrated in the following example.

WHEN GOALS OF STAFF AND FAMILY DIFFER

A consultation was requested for Max, who had suffered a severe stroke and had been moved to the nursing home after a stay in an acute hospital. He had rallied somewhat in the nursing home and wanted to go home. The staff was telling Max that when he got better, he could go home. This made his wife, Shelly, feel terrible. Despite his recovery, Max was still was too disabled for her to manage. In addition to the disabilities from his stroke, he weighed more than 200 pounds (90 kg) and was cognitively impaired, both of which contributed to Shelly's reluctance to take him home again. She felt bad about not wanting to take him home, and so she did not indicate her wishes directly to the staff. Compounding the situation was the fact that one of the nurses was caring at home for her own husband, who had suffered a stroke. I suggested that Shelly tell the staff that she could never give her husband the kind of care they did. This intervention helped the staff understand that Max could not go home, and it helped Shelly feel better about her decision. I also took the opportunity of a care planning meeting to change the focus of his care from short term to long term. During the meeting, Shelly did not say directly that she did not want to take him home, so I brought the issue up and worked with her and the staff to develop a new plan for Max to stay in the facility.

We should note that the nursing homes in which we have been consulting are better than average in quality of care. Families are likely to have other concerns if the care is really substandard. A consultant in a substandard nursing home needs to take an activist role with the administrator and director of nursing. The bottom line is that it does not cost more to give good care.

Teaching the Family How the System Works

Nursing homes are complex organizations with their own rules and procedures for doing things. Families usually do not have any idea how this system works, and they often become frustrated because they do not know who to approach about a problem or to make a request.

I coach families on how nursing homes work. I tell them who to talk to about which problems. When families see something they do not like about the care their relatives are receiving, they may walk up to the first staff person they see and mention it. They are then surprised and angry when no changes are made in the patient's care. The consultant should know enough about how a particular home works to advise the family on who to talk to. Typically, that would be the LPN who consistently cares for the patient. In some nursing homes, however, it is better to ask the nursing supervisor. We also encourage families to develop a relationship with staff members who they notice are kind or go out of their way to help patients.

When a family is very demanding and makes a lot of complaints, or when a patient's condition is very complicated and the family wants frequent updates, it can be helpful to designate a spokesperson to talk with them. That way the family knows there is one person who is knowledgeable about their relative and whom they will be able to reach.

The family needs to feel that the staff cares about the patient. When the patient has a pleasant personality, staff members often become attached to the patient and go out of their way to do extra things. (When one of these patients dies, the staff members grieve and may need extra support.) By contrast, when the patient is a difficult person, the family may mainly hear complaints from the staff. In part, these complaints are a function of the regulations in nursing homes. The staff is obligated to report all incidents to the family, such as a patient injuring himself or touching someone else. If the family is hearing about only these incidents, they may feel depressed or criticized by the staff because their relative is so difficult. In this type of situation, I try to get the staff to be more balanced in their communications. When staff members report an incident to the family about a problem patient, I encourage them to make sure to mention the good days the patient is having or any other positive behaviors.

In a parallel way, some families need to learn how to soften their complaints and give the staff compliments, as well as suggestions. I have known caregivers who voice a lot of complaints about staff members to me but maintain easy and friendly relationships with them. In the end, their relatives get better care because the staff members like the family and want to do more for them. When the family complains excessively or does not show respect for the staff, the care their relative receives suffers. The consultant needs to teach complaining families to use better strategies to get what they want, which is better care for their relative.

The book *Promoting Family Involvement in Long-Term Care Settings* (Gaugler, 2005) offers examples of innovative programs that create partnerships between programs and families.

Limitations of Group Treatment in Nursing Homes

Spayd and Smyer (1996) provide a concise description of the uses of therapy groups in nursing homes. We do not, however, think that therapy groups for patients are generally a good idea. We believe that several factors limit the effectiveness of therapy groups in this setting. First, patients live with each other on a 24-hour basis, and that is a deterrent to their talking about personal issues. There is so little privacy already in a nursing home that pressure in a group to reveal personal matters would be perceived as another privacy threat. Second, patients are often hesitant about getting attached to one another and find it hard to reach out and form friendships. Residents move out, go downhill, or die, and this imminent prospect of loss probably dampens interest in reaching out to others. There is not a lot of socialization among residents even at meals or social events. This is in contrast to personal care homes or retirement homes, where residents pair off and form friendships. In those facilities, the residents function better and are able to form social relationships. The main social relationships patients in nursing homes have are with family or old friends. We should facilitate those relationships as much as possible. The goal for patients to socialize more with one another or to share personal experiences usually comes from staff members and families, not from patients themselves.

One type of treatment that can be effective is a reminiscence or socializing group (Woods, 1996). These groups can be run by recreational therapists (RTs) or other staff members. They do not need a mental health professional and usually do not have an explicit mental health focus. The mental health consultant can work with the RT to decide what kind of group is appropriate. The RT should not try to conduct a therapy group and should be given guidelines on identifying problems (e.g., someone who is depressed) for referral to the consultant.

Support groups for relatives of nursing home residents can be also helpful, but we prefer that these groups are run outside the facility. Families can talk more freely about the problems and concerns they have when the group is not connected with the facility. Just as a consultant who is not employed by the facility can give the family an independent perspective on their concerns, so can groups that are run in the community, not in the nursing home.

Individual Therapy with Patients

In contrast to groups, we find that individual therapy is helpful with some patients. People who are depressed or who are dealing with the implications of their illness or placement can benefit from therapy. We have briefer sessions (e.g., 30 minutes) with nursing home patients if they do not have the stamina for a longer session. These sessions can reduce feelings of depression and isolation. Sessions can also identify ways in which the resident can ensure that his or her needs are met by the nursing home staff or by family and friends. Interventions are usually short term, though in rare instances we have treated a patient for a sustained period of time, usually for chronic depression.

Spayd and Smyer (1996) describe other uses of individual psychotherapy in nursing homes.

Confidentiality is a necessary condition for psychotherapy in any setting, and more so in nursing homes. The therapist and client must be able to meet in private, where they will not be overheard or interrupted. Residents often share double rooms and so do not have their own private place to go. Nursing homes will have examining rooms or offices that can be used for this purpose. As in any therapy situation, the therapist cannot reveal what the patient says to anyone else without specific consent. The therapist should make a note in the patient's chart that the session occurred and may include information that would be helpful to the staff, such as suggestions for their interactions with the patient. Confidences that have been shared by the patient during a session do not belong in an open chart, but they can be recorded in confidential files that the consultant maintains in his or her office. On occasion, patients have asked for more complete confidentiality. In that case, a notation that meets Medicare regulations is made in the medical chart (date, time, length and type of service, plus the consultant's signature), with the notation, "Notes are in confidential files in the doctor's office."

Empowering and Training Staff

Much of the work of the consultant is to enhance the capability of staff members to manage problems. In both overt and subtle ways, the clinician can help staff members learn how to deal more effectively with patients and their families and to handle the many hassles in their daily routine.

An effective approach for dealing with a problem patient is to identify the staff members who are working with that patient and then do a short in-service program that focuses on practical issues for managing the problem. The clinician should model problem solving (see Chapter 12) and give the staff solutions. Solutions should be concrete and behavioral; that is, they should direct the staff to respond in a specific way. It is important to follow up with the staff, determining how well the solution worked and continuing to use problem solving if needed to resolve the problem.

PROBLEM-FOCUSED IN-SERVICE PROGRAM

Janet was a narcissistic woman who was heavy and required two people to assist her with transfers. She would periodically go limp during the transfers, which resulted in staff members being injured. The nursing supervisor was furious with Janet for causing injuries to her staff, and the staff, not surprisingly, did not particularly like Janet.

The intervention developed in the in-service program was complex. The key was to help the staff think about solutions rather than focusing on their anger. I reframed the nursing supervisor's presentation of the problem from "I can't let the patient continue to do this to my staff" to "How can we solve the problem?" Doing that led to the suggestion of two solutions. One solution was to have a third person stand by during transfers to help out if the patient went limp. That took staff time but also prevented injuries. Another solution was proposed by a social worker on the team. She observed that Janet was poorly socialized, so no roommate had been able to stand her. She had little contact with anyone and was very angry, which she expressed by going limp. In the past, because of her own bad behavior, she had been placed with roommates who had poor functioning. The social worker proposed a different strategy—moving Janet in with a psychologically healthy patient in the hope that she would be stimulated to behave more appropriately. That is exactly what happened. The new roommate told Janet she needed to get up, get dressed, and go to the dining room. Janet responded to this challenge and started doing more for herself. She also stopped going limp during transfers.

This solution is contrary to the usual procedure in many nursing homes, which is to put problem people together. It is, of course, not something that works every time, and it can be unfair to the high-functioning individual to be paired with someone with pronounced social and emotional problems. In this instance, however, the psychologically healthy resident had a positive effect on the problem resident without suffering from having to share a room with her.

We want to stress that a mini-in-service program is just that, a small working group focused on a specific problem. This type of approach should not be used for providing ongoing in-service training to the whole staff. When a number of common problems emerge from different patients and units, however, then the consultant can organize an in-service program on that topic for the whole staff.

Another role the consultant can play is to validate the staff's feelings in dealing with difficult families. Families can place excessive or unrealistic demands on staff members or treat them disrespectfully (Looman, Noelker, Schur, Whitlatch, & Ejaz, 2002). The consultant needs to support staff members in these situations and help them develop strategies to deal more effectively with these families. Helping staff members be more assertive about what they can and cannot do is also useful. As noted, appointing one staff person to talk with a problem family can take the pressure off the other members. If a family is verbally abusive with staff members or physically threatening, the consultant needs to work with the leadership in the home to set clear guidelines for the family's behavior.

When dealing with complaining families, the consultant continually has to consider which of their complaints has a basis in reality. Even in the best nursing homes, staff members face too many demands and have too little time to respond to them. Patients sometimes have to wait too long for someone to assist them, and staff members may not always do the best job bathing or dressing a difficult patient. The consultant must walk the difficult path of encouraging staff to do the best they can within the constraints put on them and helping families learn to make more realistic and appropriate demands.

ENVIRONMENTAL AND PROGRAMMATIC INTERVENTIONS WITH PATIENTS WITH DEMENTIA

It has long been recognized that features of the environment in long-term care settings influence behavior and that modifications in the environment can be used to enhance an individual's capabilities. The work of M. Powell Lawton (e.g., Lawton, 1986; Lawton & Nahemow, 1973) has provided a framework for understanding the influences of the setting on individual behavior and competence. Central to this framework is the concept of the person–environment fit. In an optimal situation, the demands of the environment do not exceed the individual's capability for responding. People with higher levels of competence function best in settings that provide adequate challenges, whereas individuals with more limited abilities need appropriate amounts of support and assistance. Settings that provide more challenges than an individual can manage are experienced as frustrating and overwhelming and sometimes lead to catastrophic responses. In turn, settings that are understimulating are experienced as boring and may lead to deterioration in adaptive behavior, as the individual no longer has opportunities to engage in certain skills or activities.

Probably the most important use of environmental design in nursing homes and other residential care settings has been the creation of special units for patients with dementia. As noted, no consensus yet exists on what special environmental features might be therapeutic for dementia. Drawing on our observations of special care units (e.g., Zarit, Dolan, & Leitsch, 1998; Zarit, Zarit, & Rosenberg-Thompson, 1990), as well as on a growing literature (e.g., Calkins, 2001; Malmberg, 1999; Zgola, 1999; Zimmerman & Sloane, 1999; Zimmerman, Sloane, Ekert, et al., 2005; Zimmerman, Sloane, Heck, et al., 2005), we present several key components that are fundamental to special care for patients with dementia.

Locked Units and Freedom of Movement

When the dementia unit is locked, staff does not have to worry about residents leaving the facility. Residents can wander freely within the unit. This freedom enhances their autonomy and avoids power struggles with staff. Some patients with dementia walk a great deal during the day. Encouraging this activity is helpful, because it gives patients something to do and also tires them out, reducing behavior problems during the day and sleep problems at night.

Even in a locked unit, struggles can occur around the entrance, with residents trying to force the door or waiting for someone to come in so they can scoot out. Some units have been designed so that the main entrance is hidden from view. Other units use the floor plan to divert residents away from the entrance. Facilities can be designed to reduce residents' feelings of confinement in other ways. Many special units have a secured outdoor walking area that patients can freely use. In our experience, only a few residents use these outdoor areas consistently, but knowing that they can go out on their own may be important to some residents. Design can also include indoor walking areas. In one such design, the unit is constructed in a circle so that residents can walk without coming to a barrier or exit. The main goal of all these approaches is to offer residents freedom of movement with little need for ongoing staff supervision.

Some risks are associated with free movement. Residents can fall and suffer serious injuries, such as a fractured hip. Some special care units inform families of this risk at the outset (e.g., Zarit et al., 1990). The alternative is to restrain patients, which reduces quality of life and also can lead to other complications, such as a more rapid decline in functional competence. Another risk of unrestricted movement is that residents can get into altercations with one another or with staff members. Using a behavior management framework, the consultant may be able to identify the triggering events for these altercations and work with staff to prevent or reduce their occurrence.

Environmental Cues

Special care facilities typically use environmental cues to help residents identify their own rooms. A variety of solutions are used for this problem. Sometimes rooms or doors to rooms are painted different colors. Placing patients' names on the doors is not usually helpful because some patients no longer read. A more effective strategy is to place a photograph of the patient outside the room, especially a picture taken several years earlier. Patients may not recognize their current appearance, but they remember how they looked in the past. Another strategy is to have a window box at each door that contains objects that residents associate with themselves. In a facility that used this approach, one resident who had been a hunter had a bow (but not an arrow) in his window box, whereas another resident who was an avid bingo player had a bingo card in hers.

Signs and cues are frequently used to denote other facilities on the unit, such as dining and social areas. It is probably useful to use visual cues when possible, but there is no consensus on what type of approach works best.

Some facilities allow residents to bring in their own furniture or other possessions. Having their own furniture may help residents recognize their own rooms and also feel more comfortable in the setting. The main risk is that valuables might be taken by another resident or by staff members. This vulnerability is at the heart of the dilemma facing institutions that want to provide a home-like atmosphere but cannot guarantee enough security to make it feasible.

Most nursing homes, whether they provide special dementia care or not, present basic orienting information, such as the date and the weather. Some facilities hold orientation classes, which drill patients in this information. We believe that orientation classes have little value and that staff efforts are better directed to other activities that are more likely to be rewarding for residents. Some orienting information posted in the unit is probably helpful to some patients. But most patients with dementia cannot stay oriented, no matter how much support is provided. Rather than emphasizing cognitive functioning, we think that special units need to find other ways of enhancing residents' quality of life.

Sensory Stimulation

One of the most important but often neglected design issues is the amount of sensory stimulation that exists in patients' environments—in particular, light and noise. Exposure to light can contribute to maintaining good sleep patterns (Calkins, 2001; Dowling, 1996). A typical nursing home unit offers little exposure to daylight, whereas at night lights in the corridor and other locations in the unit remain on. Because exposure to light regulates biorhythms and the sleep–wake cycle, it should not be surprising that some residents of nursing homes mix up day and night. Dementia may predispose people to sleep problems (e.g., Bliwise, 1994), but environmental factors potentiate them.

Research suggests that regular exposure to daylight both reduces sleep problems at night and decreases sundowner's syndrome, the pattern of increased confusion in late afternoon and early evening (see Dowling, 1996, for a review). As an example of this relation between exposure to light and sleep patterns, an assisted living residence for dementia has a sitting area with large windows in which residents typically gather during the daytime. Initially, staff members were concerned that residents would be upset by looking out the windows, so they darkened the windows with shades. Staff members then observed a marked increase in disturbed behavior in early evening. When the windows were opened again so that residents were fully exposed to daylight, the amount of "sundowning" behavior decreased.

In the same manner, exposure to bright lights in the middle of the night can alter residents' sleep–wake cycle, making it more difficult for them to go back to sleep. When it is necessary to assist a resident at night, staff members should keep lights as dim as possible, providing the resident (and any others who are wakeful) with the cue that it is, indeed, nighttime.

Noise levels are a significant irritant in nursing home environments. Restricting noise levels is considered an important part of overall sleep hygiene. The role of noise, however, has received little attention in studies of sleep disturbances among elderly people in nursing homes. In our visits to facilities in other countries, particularly Sweden, we have been struck by how much less agitated patients with dementia are. Certainly many factors are involved, including cultural differences and greater autonomy for residents. But one of the most remarkable differences is how much quieter Swedish nursing homes and group homes for dementia are compared with facilities in the United States. Facilities in the United States typically have paging systems throughout the building. Television sets may be blaring, staff members talking loudly, dishes on food carts rattling, and so on. Noise levels can remain high even at night. In contrast, Swedish facilities do not have paging systems and greatly limit the noise from other sources. This type of random noise may be a contributing factor to increased agitation and problems sleeping at night among the patients.

A study by Burgio, Schilley, Hardin, Hsu, and Yancey (1996) suggests that the type of noise in a residential setting may be related to agitation. Using the observation that residents' agitation decreased when they were exposed to white noise (while sitting under a hair dryer in the beauty salon of the facility), the researchers designed a trial in which agitated residents wore earphones that played pleasant environmental sounds (mountain stream or ocean sounds). Reductions in verbal agitation were found both in a laboratory trial and in the nursing home unit. The researchers speculate that white noise may reduce agitation by presenting calming audio input. An alternative explanation is that the headphones block out the typical random clatter in nursing homes. In any case, level and type of noise may be an important and potentially modifiable environmental feature associated with agitated behavior.

The amount and type of visual stimulation is also an important consideration. Questions such as whether there should be a lot of variety or limited amounts of visual stimulation and the role of familiar objects remain to be resolved. Our recommendation is an overall design that is calm and orderly and that emphasizes familiar furnishings rather than looking like a clinic or hospital.

Structured Activities

A well-designed special care program can engage residents in activities that allow them to use their remaining abilities. Traditional nursing homes have long provided programs in arts and crafts, as well as social programs. With dementia, it may be better to build on past abilities to the extent possible rather than trying to teach new skills. Swedish group homes, for example, structure the day around familiar household activities. Some U.S. nursing homes have used exercise equipment, which benefits some patients with dementia (Fisher, Pendergast, & Calkins, 1991). Walking has been found to improve communication (Friedman & Tappen, 1991). Videotapes recorded by the residents' families have been used to provide reassurance when the families cannot be there (Lund, Hill, Caserta, & Wright, 1995). In most settings, activities are available only during the daytime, but structured programs during the evening and on weekends may be helpful. An activities specialist who is familiar with the emerging literature on working with patients with dementia is a key part of the program. Zgola (1987, 1999) and Buettner and Fitzsimmons (2002) present useful suggestions for involving patients with dementia in activities.

Behavioral Management

Behavioral management can play a central role in special care. We use the problem-solving approach described in Chapter 12 to identify antecedents (triggers) and consequences (reinforcers) of behaviors and to design and implement interventions in nursing homes. As with situations in the home, each problem involves a unique set of triggering or reinforcing events. Based on observations of these events, we develop a hypothesis about what the role of the behavior is in that setting. An intervention is then designed to disrupt the current pattern of triggering events and reinforcers.

Staff members often have difficulty managing behavior problems that occur while they are assisting residents in activities of daily living, such as dressing or bathing. Again, each situation is unique, and it is important to examine the unique causes for each case. The best choice is to allow residents as much autonomy as possible, letting them do activities their own way as long as that is feasible. It is better to have a resident make idiosyncratic choices in clothing, for example, than to struggle over dressing. Staff members may, however, have to work with families on this issue so that family members do not assume that the patient is being neglected.

Bathing is often a difficult problem. Patients with dementia frequently become agitated when staff members try to bathe or shower them. In some cases, their fear seems to come from being undressed. Both the attitude and the gender of the staff member may be problems (e.g., Somboontanount et al., 2004). With some difficult patients, the struggle over bathing can be solved by allowing them to keep their underwear on, changing it after the bath or shower. The temperature in the bathroom can also be a problem. Patients with dementia appear to have difficulty regulating body temperature, and they chill easily. A bathroom that is too cold can be unpleasant to them. Increasing the temperature or allowing residents to keep themselves covered with a towel may be helpful. Other useful strategies include using no-rinse soap, using bath products suggested by family, modifying the shower spray, and giving patients food or other distractions (Sloane et al., 2004). A lot of verbal reassurance, as well as making bathrooms more home-like, can reduce problems. Finally, some older residents may never have bathed frequently, and so increasing the interval between baths could reduce problems.

One area in which considerable research has been done is management of incontinence. The method of prompted voiding—in effect, placing patients on a schedule and reminding them to go to the bathroom—has been found to be very effective in reducing incontinence in nursing home residents, including patients with dementia (e.g., Burgio et al., 1990; Schnelle, Newman, & Fogarty, 1990; Schnelle et al., 1989).

Activities play an important role in preventing or reducing behavior problems. Sleeping in the daytime and inactivity are frequent antecedents of sleep problems at night. Although the literature is not conclusive, at least some evidence suggests that increasing daytime activities improves sleep at night in patients with dementia (see Dowling, 1996, for a review). In a similar way, inactivity and napping are frequent antecedents of agitation or other problem behavior in the daytime. An effective strategy is to involve patients in activities in advance of periods of agitation, or other problems. Activities can head off agitation as well as the reinforcement of inappropriate behaviors that occurs when staff respond mainly to problems.

Sloane and his colleagues (Sloane et al., 1997) suggest strategies for managing one of the most disturbing behavior problems in nursing homes: disruptive vocalizations, such as repetitive speech, screaming, and moaning. They suggest that these vocalizations are linked to specific antecedents, such as over- and understimulation, pain and discomfort, restricted mobility, delusions or other psychiatric symptoms, depression, and fatigue. Interventions can be designed that address the antecedents through changes in the environment, in the patient's or staff's routines, or behavioral intervention.

ANTECEDENTS OF DISRUPTIVE VOCALIZATIONS

Bob was repeatedly calling out to staff members, "I want to die." Staff members ignored him and went on with their business. Called in to consult on this case, I talked with Bob and asked if he wanted to die. He said no but stated that he was in pain and would like to get relief from his pain. I then talked with the staff, who decided to treat him with a pain patch for his knee, which was the main source of his pain. The treatment calmed Bob down and led to more appropriate communication with staff.

Two processes in this example contributed to the lack of communication. The patient had some cognitive impairment, and so his requests for help did not indicate his real need, although he was able to state that he was in pain when we took the time to talk with him. This case also illustrates how a busy staff becomes insensitive to repetitive vocalizations, especially those that they consider irrational. As a result, they are not able to identify antecedents or possible interventions.

Autonomy

An overriding issue in interventions is striking the right balance between autonomy and security. Autonomy is at the heart of so much that is involved in special Alzheimer's care, as well as care of residents who do not have cognitive deficits (Hofland, 1995).

Working with patients with dementia can be challenging because they often try to maintain control without recognizing their limitations. It is easy to fall into struggles with them over bathing, dressing, following routines, and a whole host of safety issues. As we noted earlier, a locked unit removes one source of struggle, but there are many other ways in which staff members try to limit a resident's autonomy. The key is to do as little limiting as necessary, consistent with the safety of residents.

Group homes for dementia in Sweden offer residents much more autonomy than typical facilities in the United States or in many other countries, for that matter (Malmberg & Zarit, 1993). Residents sign a lease to an apartment when they enter the group home. Their apartments, which contain kitchenettes and private bathrooms with appropriate safety features, belong to them. They have keys to the apartments and do not share them with anyone else. They are, in fact, encouraged to lock the doors so that other residents do not wander in. Apartments are furnished with their own possessions and are home-like, not institutional, in appearance. The risk that someone might steal valued possessions is minimized because residents do not share their rooms with anyone and they can keep their doors locked.

Group homes have been found to be a viable living environment for all but the most agitated patients with dementia (Malmberg & Zarit, 1993). They are remarkable for their low rates of behavioral disturbance, compared with U.S. facilities. Many factors undoubtedly contribute to their success, such as the low level of noise in them and the amount of training staff receives. But residents' autonomy may be the crucial dimension. Having one's own apartment automatically eliminates the problems that come with having roommates, which are endemic in U.S. facilities. Double rooms are an anachronism based on a medical model of care. Although they make sense in a hospital, where people stay for only a few days, shared rooms are not appropriate in a long-term residence. Beyond shared rooms, however, the attitude conveyed in group homes by allowing residents keys and locks supports their autonomy and may reduce fears and struggles that are commonplace in more typical care facilities.

One Special Unit or Many?

Finally, there may be good reason to consider whether different types of special care units are needed. Special units have usually been designed with a prototypical patient with AD in mind, that is, someone who wanders, who may become agitated at intermittent intervals, and who benefits from activities and environmental reminders. The typical patterns of behavior found in other types of dementia, however, may be better suited to different types of environment.

We propose creating special units to meet the needs of the diversity of problems in dementia. Although we identify some of these units by diagnostic category, how patients actually function should be the main consideration in matching them to a special program. These programs are:

A Special Unit for Frontotemporal Dementia

Patients with FTD or with frontal damage associated with vascular disease or injury are often very difficult to manage. Their high levels of activity, impulsiveness, and lack of empathy for others may prove too difficult for most special units. They can become threatening to other residents and staff.

Special units for FTD have been developed in the Scandinavian countries, although there are relatively few programs. We have visited one special frontal unit. Features of the unit included a higher staff-to-patient ratio than found in other dementia care (which in Sweden is already higher than in most other places), and staff members who were specially selected and trained for their ability to manage these types of behaviors. There appeared to be no special environmental features, though as in other Swedish facilities, residents had their own rooms. Staff members described their work days as stressful, but they also gained a sense of accomplishment from being able to deal with these very challenging residents.

A Special Unit for Dementia with Lewy Bodies

Patients with DLB are likely to have increasing difficulties with walking and balance and will be more prone to falls than other people with dementia. They may be put at risk on an ordinary dementia unit filled with active, mobile patients with AD. Environmental modifications might include attention to the hardness of surfaces and less complex visual stimuli. The program could also address their more common hallucinations and delusions by trying different environmental features that might reduce these problems. Patients with comorbid AD and PD might also do well on this kind of unit.

A Special Unit for Late-Stage Dementia

As their disease progresses, people with dementia grow weaker and eventually lose the ability to walk. They spend increasing amounts of time in bed. Many special units move these patients to a regular nursing unit because the staff feels they no longer need the special features and resources of the dementia unit. We have found that this move is upsetting to families, who are concerned that their relatives will no longer get the special attention for their problems that they had on the dementia unit. Families also lose the sense of community that develops in good special care units.

People with late-stage dementia need a different kind of special care, a palliative approach based on hospice principles that keeps them as comfortable as possible and that allows them to die as peacefully as possible. Certainly many nursing homes manage this kind of care well, but our experience is that late-stage care is uneven. Some nurses and physicians want to continue treating patients aggressively, despite the wishes of family or the intentions that the patient may have expressed in the past. Care can also become perfunctory, because less and less reinforcement is provided to staff by increasingly unresponsive residents. A special unit could provide a more consistent setting for late-stage care.

Care for the "Pleasantly Demented"

We use the term "pleasantly demented" in a descriptive, and not pejorative, way. We have worked with many people who have progressive cognitive decline, but who remain pleasant and sociable and never get agitated or disruptive. These individuals do not need a special care unit that places them with patients who are frequently upset and agitated. We have found that this type of person often does well in an ordinary assisted living facility. The person responds positively to the normal surroundings and opportunities for social interaction with other residents. Staff, of course, needs to be understanding and supportive and to occasionally look out for dementia-related problems, such as wandering out the front door. As long as those problems remain infrequent, however, the person should be able to do well in assisted living until late in the disease.

We end this chapter with two case examples that illustrate the consultation process and the principles we have presented.

An Issue of Capacity

During a hospitalization, Bernice's condition deteriorated rapidly, and it was assumed that she was terminally ill. Hospice was ordered, and she was moved to a nursing home. In fact, Bernice had probably suffered from a bad reaction to a cardiac medication, and she actually began to clear up mentally and improve physically in the nursing home. When she began insisting on going home, the staff asked for a consultation.

Normally, Bernice's improvement would not have posed a problem. The complicating factor was that Bernice's daughter was a physician, and she was the person who had ordered hospice. The attending physician approached me about doing a consultation, stating that she felt that Bernice was probably capable of making the decision to go home. I replied that it would be important to carry out a careful evaluation of capacity, given the circumstances and the need to deal with Bernice's daughter in a tactful way.

In a capacity evaluation, it is important to decide first what question is being asked. In this case, the question was "Does the patient understand how to make decisions about her health?" Answering this question required two steps. First, I determined the quality of her thinking using the Comprehension and Similarities subtests of the WAIS-Ill (Wechsler, 1997a). The Comprehension subtest evaluates a patient's ability to understand common situations, and the Similarities subtest assesses abstracting ability. I also administered the MMSE (Folstein et al., 1975). I then talked with Bernice about the decision she was making, asking practical questions such as "Where would you go if you left the nursing home?" "What kind of care would you need?" and "What do you think would happen if you left?" I evaluated the quality of her thinking and the degree to which she indicated an awareness of the risks and problems she might encounter.

The evidence from the evaluation indicated that Bernice was capable of making this decision. The challenge, then, was to approach her daughter tactfully and to help her reevaluate her view of her mother's situation. With Bernice's permission, I met with her daughter and went over the results of the testing in a way that helped her understand her mother's competence without making her defensive. With the daughter now aware of the changed circumstances, she agreed to allowing Bernice to move back home.

Don't Fix What Isn't Broken

When a patient is functioning adequately, it is important to avoid destabilizing the situation with unnecessary change. The following case was referred by a new and relatively inexperienced physician. Lois was an older woman who had been taking a major tranquilizer. Concerned about the amount of sedation and mild parkinsonian side effects, the new physician decided to switch Lois to another medication with potentially fewer side effects but also less sedation. In the process of being withdrawn from the first medication and put on the second, Lois became extremely agitated and difficult to deal with, using profane language and occasionally acting abusively. A consultation was requested. I reviewed the available information on Lois, which indicated that she had been a long-term psychiatric patient at a state hospital with a diagnosis of chronic schizophrenia. The original medication was, in fact, controlling her symptoms despite the side effects. I decided to talk with the doctor about the medication change. It turned out that he did not know why Lois had been placed on a powerful antipsychotic medication in the first place. Now that he had a better understanding of Lois's history, he put her back on the original medication and took steps to control its side effects.

CONCLUSIONS

Working in nursing homes and other institutional settings can be one of the most rewarding activities for a mental health professional. The consultation process offers a variety of challenges, ranging from interesting diagnostic issues to complex interventions that involve staff, resident, and family alike. The consultant sometimes provides treatment and in other cases serves as a resource for staff and families to learn new approaches to what is a very stressful situation for everyone involved. Problems arise when family and staff members see their interests as diverging, but the consultant can reframe and redirect their viewpoints so that everyone agrees on the best approach to a problem.

A successful consultant needs a strong foundation in geropsychological knowledge and skills, as well as an appreciation of how to function within a complex system. The ability to work with people from many different social backgrounds—from physicians to nursing assistants—is another important component. Nursing homes do not have the resources they need to manage all the complex problems of residents and their families. The consultant brings expertise on the behavioral, emotional, and interpersonal problems of residents and their families and helps to increase the staff's competence in dealing with these problems.

CHAPTER 15

Ethical Issues in Geriatric Psychology

Ethical issues are always a part of clinical practice, but they can take on added dimensions with older clients. As they do when working with younger clients, clinicians need to place practice with older people within the framework of ethical principles and the code of conduct that has been developed to guide their profession. In this chapter, we examine how established ethical standards can be applied to practice with older clients.

As psychologists, we draw on a set of principles developed by the American Psychological Association (2002; www.apa.org/ethics/), "Ethical Principles of Psychologists and Code of Conduct." These standards are built on a foundation of six general principles: (1) competence, (2) integrity, (3) professional and scientific responsibility, (4) respect for people's rights and dignity, (5) concern for others' welfare, and (6) social responsibility. We encourage readers who are not psychologists to become familiar with the ethical guidelines developed by their professions.

As we have stressed throughout this book, clinical practice with older adults requires specialized knowledge and training, and that applies as well to issues related to ethical practice. For this chapter, we have chosen the three most frequent ethical dilemmas in a geriatric practice: competence of the clinician, confidentiality, and end-of-life issues.

COMPETENCE OF THE CLINICIAN

A basic tenet of ethical conduct is not to practice beyond one's competence and training. The need for mental health professionals to work with the

---

Parts of this chapter appeared in Zarit and Zarit (1996). Copyright 1996 by the American Psychological Association. Adapted by permission.

elderly has always been greater than the number of trained people who could potentially provide services (Shea, 2003). As the older population has grown and the demand for services increased, many people who do not meet minimum requirements for training and experience in geropsychology have been pressed into providing services. Many learn on the job, utilizing input from experienced colleagues and continuing education. The problem of undertrained professionals, however, remains, and may be greatest in nursing home settings. Although unbiased data are difficult to come by, reports by clinicians across the country suggest that a lot of practice in nursing homes is carried out without much knowledge of clinical issues in later life. We have reviewed case notes and other documents in nursing homes that were prepared by clinicians who had little or no background in geriatrics and have found their lack of competence to be startling. In other settings as well, clinicians will take on older clients without understanding basic assessment issues or when and how to vary treatment to address age-related questions.

One response to this growing concern is the development of standards for training in geriatric mental health. The American Psychiatric Association (2004) has had a formal specialization in geriatric psychiatry for several years. As noted (Chapter 1), the American Psychological Association has issued guidelines for psychological practice with older adults that outline the knowledge and skills that form the foundation of competent practice. The group Psychologists in Long-Term Care has prepared guidelines for practice specifically in institutional settings (Lichtenberg et al., 1998). Not everyone who works with older people needs to be a specialist. However, the minimum ethical standard states that they should have some prior exposure and training.

A major factor contributing to the dearth of trained professionals is that very few graduate and professional programs include geriatrics as part of their curricula or clinical experiences. Despite continued efforts of a committed core of professionals, the situation has not changed much in the United States over the last decade. As a consequence, most professionals (including physicians) emerge from training without a sufficient foundation in geriatrics to practice effectively. A different model is found in the United Kingdom, where geriatrics has become a mandated part of graduate training in clinical psychology. Given the continued growth in the older population and the ongoing ageist bias in professional education, mandatory training may be a necessary step.

CONFIDENTIALITY

Confidentiality is a basic ethical principle in clinical practice, but it takes on some new aspects in a geriatric practice. Confidentiality can be differentially affected by the client's living situation (independent community dwelling, assisted living, nursing home, hospital), by the nature of the psychological problem (functional vs. organic), and by whether or not family members are involved in treatment. Because older clients are likely to be receiving concurrent medical treatment, there is often a need for consultation between the mental health specialist and a variety of physicians. Important differences exist in the kind of confidentiality issues that arise, depending on the setting in which the older person lives. We have organized our discussion according to place of residence. The section ends with an examination of situations in which mental health professionals must break confidentiality.

Community Living

For older adults who live independently in the community and do not suffer from dementia or similar problems, confidentiality issues are generally the same as they would be for a younger client. In other words, an older person is entitled to the same confidentiality as any other client. For example, if a concerned son or daughter calls about his or her mother, who is in treatment, the client must sign a release before a conversation with her children can take place. The therapist and the client should also discuss whether or not to confine the communication to specific domains.

Family members are more likely to contact therapists about elderly clients than about younger ones, as are neighbors and other involved service providers, so a well-thought-out response to calls is essential. When an unexpected call occurs, the best response is to listen to the information being given without divulging whether or not the person is in your care, then advise the caller that he or she may wish to raise this concern with the person and that any professional who is involved with that person will need a signed release to communicate with the caller directly. This tactic allows the clinician to assess whether a dangerous situation exists without compromising the client's confidentiality.

The dilemma then becomes how to use the caller's information. Of course, if the situation involves imminent danger to a client or other people, clinicians need to take appropriate steps to protect the people involved, even if that means breaking confidentiality. In other situations, it may be in the client's best interest for the therapist to talk with the caller, which can be done if the client signs a release. The "Ethical Principles of Psychologists and Code of Conduct" (American Psychological Association, 2002; www.apa.org/ethics) contains specific tenets regarding confidentiality that can be used to guide decision making.

The situation is slightly different when the client has been referred by a physician for a specific purpose, for example, for evaluation for cognitive problems. With a physician referral, it is usually necessary to coordinate assessment and treatment with the physician and to exchange information that can clarify the diagnosis. A client who is competent can sign a release at the outset. If a power of attorney (POA) for health care is in effect, releases to obtain information from or to send reports to physicians or other professionals must be signed by the person who holds the POA. In situations in which it is not clear whether the client is competent or not—including referrals for the purpose of establishing competence—we would get consent from the client first. Until it is determined that a client is not competent to give consent, that person would still legally be presumed able to do so.

Clinicians need to be aware of the legal mechanisms for granting decision-making powers to another person. In the United States, a POA is the most typical way consent is handled, though the specifics vary from state to state. POAs are executed by lawyers and are a straightforward and inexpensive procedure. Many people get a POA at the time that they make a will. The POA specifies who can give a substituted judgment in the event that the person can no longer make his or her own decisions and for what types of decisions. A POA can be granted for health care, financial matters, or both. Another procedure, guardianship, is used rarely for older people with compromised intellectual functioning. Guardianship involves review by a judge and assignment of a guardian. Unless there are significant disputes about a case, a POA is sufficient to give consent for treatment and for release of information.

Most clients quite willingly sign releases to allow the mental health specialist to talk with their physicians when the specific purpose is explained to them. Others may not be willing to sign releases at all. If a client is reluctant to sign a release to his or her primary physician on an initial visit, it may be possible to reintroduce the issue in a subsequent session after some trust has been established.

One way to address this problem is to include a form for release of information at intake. Medicare, in fact, requires that psychologists offer to consult with the primary physician at the onset of treatment. An example of this type of release is shown in Figure 15.1. This release, of course, does not resolve the problem of sharing information with the family, which can be done only with the client's consent. In almost all cases, however, clients give permission to talk with their families. We share information with the family only when it is relevant and in the client's best interests—for example, when the family is providing care for the client and the results of the assessment will help them plan more effective care.

Questions can be raised about whether a release signed by someone who is believed to lack the capacity to give consent is valid. From a legal perspective, until there has been a court evaluation of capacity, that person is considered competent. That does not, however, relieve clinicians of their obligation to weigh conflicting ethical concerns. The decision to obtain consent to release information from a client with questionable competence must be based on the evaluation that doing so is in the client's best interests. We should also add that a finding of dementia or other type of cognitive deficit does not necessarily mean that an individual is no longer legally competent (see Chapter 7). Rather, competence depends on understanding the specific issues involved; in

Medicare Consultation Release

It may be beneficial to you for me to contact your primary care physician regarding your psychological treatment or regarding any medical problems for which you are receiving treatment. In addition, Medicare requires that I notify your physician, by telephone or in writing, concerning services I provide unless you request that notification not be made.

Please check one of the following.

_____ I authorize you to contact my primary care physician, whose name and address are shown below, to discuss the treatment I am receiving under your care and to obtain information concerning my medical diagnosis and treatment.

_____ I do not authorize you to contact my primary care physician about the treatment I am receiving under your care or to obtain information concerning my medical diagnosis and treatment. I am providing you with the name and address of my primary care physician only for your records.

_____

Signature and date

FIGURE 15.1. Sample release of information form.

From *Mental Disorders in Older Adults* (2nd ed.) by Steven H. Zarit and Judy M. Zarit. Copyright 2007 by The Guilford Press. Permission to photocopy this figure is granted to purchasers of this book for personal use only (see copyright page for details).

this case, giving consent for release of information (American Bar Association & American Psychological Association, 2005). This problem fortunately occurs only rarely in practice. Many of the clients I see have signed POAs in the past.

CHALLENGES IN MAINTAINING CONFIDENTIALITY WHEN SEVERAL MEMBERS OF A FAMILY ARE INVOLVED

The initial contact was made by John, a 48-year-old attorney who had power of attorney for his father, Harry, who had developed cognitive impairment following open heart surgery. Although the main focus was on his father, John requested help for both his parents. He had observed that his mother, Mary, was not coping well with his father's impairments. The initial evaluation was done with the father. Mary (who also had POA for her husband) was present. Mary did not consider herself in need of any help but simply wanted her husband restored to his former self. From a practical perspective, beginning with an assessment of Harry would clarify the extent of his deficits and the kinds of problems his wife had to cope with. As often happens in caregiving situations, Mary could then be brought into treatment as the focus shifted from finding out what was wrong with Harry to identifying what the family could do to manage the problems effectively. Mary signed consent forms for information about Harry to be freely communicated with her son and all the physicians involved in Harry's care.

After a few visits, John called, wanting a summary of the treatment. Because his mother had signed a release to discuss his father, John was given a summary. In the course of the conversation, it became clear that John wanted to talk as much about his mother's functioning as about his father's. He expressed concern that she was becoming overwhelmed by having to care for Harry and that she was behaving oddly, for example, kicking Harry under the table if he said something she objected to. As it became apparent that the focus of the discussion was shifting from John's father to his mother, I felt I had to obtain a release from her before sharing any part of my impressions of her. Through the assessment of Harry, Mary had become engaged in trying to understand his difficulties and her reactions to them. At this point, she was eager for open communication among everyone and gave the release for me to talk with her son.

This step became important later when the decision was being made to place Harry in a nursing facility. That decision occurred only after many conversations with John about what would be in both Harry's and Mary's best interests.

In general, if a clinician anticipates the need to speak with family members, it is wise to obtain releases early in treatment. When dealing with a frail older person, questions about moving the person to a more protective setting are very common, and families naturally want to be involved in the decision making. The therapist can be helpful in this situation, because the family often turns to him or her for an expert opinion in choosing among the available options. The therapist can also ensure that the client's best interests are taken into account rather than those of the most forceful person in the family.

The previous example raises another issue—who is our client, Harry or Mary? As is often the case with dementia, we start out working with the person with dementia, but then the focus shifts to the caregiver. It is incumbent on the clinician in those situations to keep sight of the best interests of both persons, particularly in discussions of placement.

We have also noted throughout that there are other circumstances in which we bring in family members for a few sessions. There are special ethical considerations in that type of situation. We need to think about whether we can take a position that is in everyone's best interests. That may require being able to reconcile very different viewpoints about issues. We also must be sure not to reveal anything said to us in confidence by our primary client or by another family member. Although communications can become complicated, it remains preferable to channel everything through a single therapist than to add more specialists to a situation in which the family is already overburdened with doctors.

Assisted Living and Similar Residential Settings

When a client lives in an assisted living or similar facility (e.g., board and care, residential care), confidentiality issues can be rather tricky. Unlike nursing homes, these facilities are not licensed and regulated as medical facilities. In a nonmedical setting, the fact that a client is even seeing a mental health professional is confidential information. Even though some facilities keep a chart that resembles a nursing home or hospital chart, the clinician should not write in that chart, because that would violate the resident's confidentiality. With an appropriate release, however, the clinician can consult with staff on care issues. All confidential records should be kept in locked files in the therapist's office, as would be done with any other client.

Consistent with maintaining confidentiality, it is best to limit the transmission of information to the least number of people who need to know. A self-referred client should be asked whether he or she wants the primary physician kept informed, and a release should be either signed or denied. Beyond that, the only time the facility needs to know about therapy is in a situation involving danger for the client or other people or if the person's capacity becomes an issue.

When family initiates the request for treatment, an assessment should be made concerning the extent to which they should be involved in treatment and whether it is in the client's best interest for the therapist to stay in communication with them. Releases must be signed to allow free exchanges of information. Occasionally a physician refers a client who does not have any identified family members. Again, if the client is competent, the only release necessary is for the physician. But if the client is not competent, then it may be necessary to communicate with the facility to determine whether the client has or needs the involvement of a geriatric case manager or whether an appropriate public agency should assume guardianship to ensure that the person's best interests are being protected. Even in that case, a release from the patient to communicate freely with the facility would still be necessary.

Sometimes the clinician would like to share the findings of the evaluation with the facility, but the resident refuses to give consent. This problem can be especially troubling when the resident has dementia and is having obvious difficulties in the facility. We have often encountered older clients early in the dementia process who are aware of some of their deficits. Out of their anxiety and fear over what is happening to them, they refuse to allow any communication to occur between the therapist and the facility. Their right to confidentiality must be respected unless the situation is or becomes dangerous. Usually, if we continue to see them, they develop sufficient trust in us to sign a release so that we can communicate at least in a limited way with the facility. We would, of course, keep our client's best interests in mind, which could at times be at odds with what is best for the institution.

Nursing Home or Hospital

In these settings, Medicare requires that each visit be documented in a patient's chart with the date, type of service provided, length of service, some indication of the content of the service, and a signature. Because these records are open to all medical and ancillary personnel who have access to records, and because security of the records is light, it is preferable for the clinician to make only the entries necessary to ensure continuity of care in the facility and to keep extended notes in more secure confidential files in the clinician's own office. For example, if a client is depressed, the clinician would note that fact in the chart in the facility, along with any suggestions for how staff might assist the client or recommendations that the patient be evaluated for antidepressant medication. The clinician would keep the documentation of what the client said, what tests were used, and so on in his or her own files.

Patients in nursing homes and hospitals have usually signed a blanket release from confidentiality that pertains to all who treat them, allowing free communication among professional staff. It still is important to consider the client's privacy and best interests. Just because it is permissible to communicate with staff members does not mean that it is in the client's best interests to communicate everything. Care should be taken to share only what is necessary for the staff to know about a client without violating the client's privacy. Bear in mind that residents in nursing homes and patients in hospitals feel intruded on and powerless and that the mental health professional may be the only person they can confide those feelings to.

One of the most useful roles of a mental health professional in the nursing home is as a consultant to staff about behavior problems of patients, particularly patients with cognitive impairment but also those with other problems that put undue stress on the staff (see Chapter 14). The best way to protect client confidentiality in these situations is to make positive suggestions to staff members in very general terms, rather than discussing a particular patient. When the consultant talks about a class of patients, rather than an individual, it allows the staff members to think about applying suggestions across a variety of patients, which helps them stay oriented to the suggestions in a professional rather than a personal way.

Even if the patient or the person holding POA has authorized communication within the nursing home or hospital, it is still necessary to obtain a specific release before communicating with other family members. Although this step sounds obvious, it is not always possible to anticipate the particular family structure (or dysfunctions) that will be encountered. So a certain amount of vigilance is necessary when responding to family members who inquire about their relatives.

Confidentiality issues, then, can arise in a variety of different ways for older people, depending on the setting in which they live, the client's competence to give consent, the involvement of family, and the need to exchange information with other health care providers. Situations arise in which clinicians must weigh the competing demands of different ethical principles. The clinician's responsibilities to clients, particularly in protecting confidentiality, should guide all decisions about treatment and release of information.

Exceptions to Confidentiality

Clinicians are obligated to break confidentiality under some specified circumstances. Although the laws on exceptions to confidentiality vary, mental health professionals are generally required to take steps to prevent clients from committing suicide or from harming other people. This responsibility includes the duty to inform an intended victim of violence. Reporting child abuse is mandatory, especially abuse involving sexual activity. These statutes apply whether one's client is old or not.

The issue of suicide in late life is complex. Even though a client is old or suffering from a terminal illness, laws that require clinicians to intervene to prevent suicide still apply. When clients talk about suicide, we discuss with them our responsibilities, letting them know that we must intervene if we see an imminent risk. Of course, we also work with the client on the issues that are leading to the suicidal ideation.

A clinician might in principle support rational suicide—for instance, to forestall intolerable pain or inevitable deterioration—but encouraging a suicide or neglecting to intervene is a violation of professional ethics and legal statutes. Whether or not clients have the right to end their lives is an important social and ethical issue. There are many differences of opinion about how these issues are addressed by the legal system, but professionals must put aside their own preferences and work within that system. We continue discussion of this issue later, when we examine the decision to refuse treatment.

The other issue involving exceptions to confidentiality is elder abuse. Elder abuse laws are not as widespread as child abuse laws. In some jurisdictions, the duty to report elder abuse is voluntary. Elder abuse statutes also vary in their definitions. There tends to be a consensus that causing physical harm constitutes abuse, but there is less agreement on definitions of psychological abuse and neglect. Clinicians should also not forget about the possibility of sexual abuse, just because a client is old. Reports of sexual abuse in nursing homes are not uncommon (Teaster & Roberto, 2004). Most complaints involve residents abusing other residents, but staff members are sometimes implicated. Cases of sexual abuse of older people probably do not come to the attention of authorities as often as they might.

When reporting elder abuse is not mandated, the clinician can take into consideration how serious and chronic the abuse has been and whether psychological interventions are likely to be sufficient to prevent further abuse. We would not report, for example, a family caregiver who got so frustrated with a patient with dementia that she pushed him once in anger, even though that act might be covered under some interpretations of the legal statute. Instead, we would work with the caregiver to understand her anger and head off future outbursts. On the other hand, we would not hesitate in reporting a nursing home employee who was physically or sexually abusing patients.

END-OF-LIFE ISSUES

End-of-life decisions are difficult for everyone involved—the family, physicians, and nursing staff. As this example illustrates, communication can suffer even as everyone tries to do the right thing. The physician may ask the family to make a complex decision without giving a full explanation of what it means, leading the patient down a course that neither patient nor family wanted.

END-OF-LIFE DECISIONS

Bess was a 70-year-old woman with AD, who was being cared for by her 72-year-old husband of 45 years, Frank. In the course of the neuropsychological evaluation, it became apparent that Bess was acutely and painfully aware of her deficits and clinically depressed as a result. I began psychotherapy with her and continued the treatment until her memory deficits were sufficient to contraindicate talking therapy. As she declined, I shifted treatment to Frank, who had become increasingly depressed and angry about the deterioration he saw taking place in his wife. I saw them together and separately over a 5-year period, both in the office and later at home, when Bess was no longer able to leave the home because of degenerative arthritis and increased fear of falling outside the home. Eventually, she started falling helplessly to the floor at night, and Frank had to call the police and neighbors to help get her up. When he realized that he could no longer take care of her, he placed her in a nursing home.

Three months after she went to the facility, Frank asked that Bess be coded as DNR (do not resuscitate) and also that no extraordinary means be used to prolong her life. Bess was severely aphasic but was able to communicate her unhappiness about her situation, both through an anguished expression and very occasionally by asking plaintively, "Why me?" She also talked at great length about how unhappy she was with what had become of her. Bess did not want to be a burden to Frank and worried about his depression. While she was still able to, she granted Frank POA, including responsibility for health care decisions.

About 6 months after she entered the nursing home, Bess suddenly became ill. Tests showed that she had been bleeding internally, probably secondary to the nonsteroidal anti-inflammatory medication she had been taking for her arthritis. What followed was a series of ethical dilemmas about whether the situation should be defined as "end of life," which would then trigger the prohibition on using extraordinary means, and about the hidden consequences of decisions that physicians ask families to make about treatment.

The physician, Dr. Smith, explained the situation to Frank and very gingerly asked him whether he wanted Bess to have a transfusion. Frank responded by asking Dr. Smith what he would normally do, a response that the doctor interpreted as an indication that he wanted treatment started. Once the transfusion was started, Bess immediately had an allergic reaction, which is very rare. The physician stopped the transfusion. Bess was now running a temperature of 102°, and the physician asked Frank if he wanted an intravenous (IV) started to hydrate her. Frank replied, "Yes."

When Bess returned to the nursing home, some of the staff were upset that the IV had been started in light of Bess's "no extraordinary measures" status. Given her physical situation, they felt she was clearly in decline and would die soon. Without the IV, the process would take anywhere from 5 to 14 days, but with the IV, she could linger for much longer. Dr. Smith had not explained that to Frank. The nursing staff asked me to discuss the dilemma with Frank, given the length and nature of our relationship. Frank was distraught by the turn of events and did not want his wife's life needlessly prolonged. With Frank's consent, I called the physician, with whom I had worked well on previous cases, and asked what his intentions were. Dr. Smith said that when he had started the IV in the hospital he had explained to Frank that it would only be in place for 4 days, just to rehydrate Bess after the transfusion reaction, and that it would then be removed. And, indeed, on the 4th day, when the IV came loose, the nurses were instructed not to replace it. At that point, Bess was in a coma, nonresponsive, and dying. She lingered for another 5 days, being kept as comfortable as possible, and then expired peacefully.

My role in this situation was complex. Because of the nature and longevity of my relationship with Frank, I was thrust into the role of the person who could best lay out the choices that could be made. The physician was prepared to abide by Frank's wishes not to prolong Bess's life needlessly, but he did not make explicit exactly what each choice meant. Some physicians would, in fact, have been reluctant to remove the IV once it had been started. Frank was relying on the physician to make the decisions for him, including determining the point at which no further treatment should be given, but the physician was bouncing the decision making back to Frank. Frank was put in the position of determining whether or not the transfusion and then the IV were extraordinary steps. After I intervened, Frank was able to defer to the physician, who followed the original plan. Frank felt that a medical protocol had been followed, rather than that he had made a decision that might shorten his wife's life.

In this example, I found myself in the situation of advising the caregiver on the decisions. I had to remain neutral, not indicating a personal preference for one decision over another. The clinician's own personal biases must not enter into such a decision. As mental health professionals, we have tremendous power to influence our clients, and in a situation such as this one, we have to continuously assess whether our own values and biases are influencing the decision-making process.

Whether therapists ought to assume that role is a major question. Because of the nature of the psychotherapeutic relationship, which involves talking extensively to clients and getting to know their beliefs, attitudes, and values, mental health professionals may be in a unique position to address end-of-life issues. Physicians rarely have the time to spend with their patients or the patients' families to explore these issues in depth. Consequently, many geriatricians and family practice physicians are eager for help in this kind of decision making and even to defer some of the explanation of alternatives to the mental health professional. Occasionally, the physician may make a referral to a therapist specifically to determine what the individual's wishes are, particularly if there is a question about capacity or if depression or anxiety might be clouding the patient's decision-making abilities. The intervention with a patient can gradually include a widening circle of concerned family members, who can be involved individually or in a family session. On the other hand, mental health professionals have not been prepared specifically for this role, which can be emotionally demanding and includes knowing the explicit and implicit medical, legal, and ethical considerations for addressing end-of-life decisions.

A growing body of legal and ethical writing bears on end-of-life issues. The National Institutes of Health Consensus Development Program (2004) has developed a consensus statement on state-of-the-art end-of-life care, which is available at consensus.nih.gov/2004/2004EndOfLifeCareSOS024-html.htm, along with a literature review that gives background for the recommendations. Most writers on these issues make a distinction between active euthanasia and passive approaches that involve withholding procedures that might prolong life (Thomasma, 1992). Active approaches, such as that of Jack Kevorkian, are clearly more controversial. As we stressed earlier, whatever one's personal opinion of euthanasia, we have a legal and ethical obligation to prevent suicides, assisted or otherwise.

Legal and ethical issues concerning the decision to cease or withhold active treatment of terminally ill individuals are complex and evolving. Considerable debate has occurred over whether decisions should be made according to the principle of beneficence—appropriate people choosing what is in the patient's best interests—or the principle of autonomy—the patient or his or her proxy making the decision.

In the United States, the Cruzan case has had a large influence on legal standards for cessation of treatment (see White, 1992). Nancy Cruzan was a young woman who fell into a persistent vegetative state as a result of injuries suffered in a serious automobile accident and was kept alive on life supports. Her family sued to have her life supports removed. The courts eventually ruled in favor of the family, largely on the basis of testimony that the patient had stated in conversations before the accident that she preferred not to be kept alive in that kind of condition. In deciding for the family, the court endorsed the principle of autonomy.

The more recent case of Terri Schiavo shows, however, that these issues are far from settled (e.g., Preston & Kelly, 2006; Skene, 2005). As with many end-of-life controversies, the dispute was fueled by conflict in the family, in this case between Terri's husband and her parents. At the heart of the controversy was a difference in assessment of her condition. Her husband and her physicians believed her to be in a persistent vegetative state from which no improvement was possible, and so they wanted to discontinue use of a feeding tube. Her parents and their supporters held the view that there was still a potential for recovery and opposed ending life-supportive treatment (Ditto, 2006). There was also disagreement about Terri's own wishes and whether either her husband or her parents was an appropriate surrogate to act in a way consistent with her preferences.

Preston and Kelly (2006) provide an insightful analysis of the Schiavo case from a medical ethics perspective. They argue that the insertion of a feeding tube to keep Terri Schiavo alive was an artificial treatment that prolonged life without the possibility of recovery. They also agree with the predominant medical opinion that she was in a persistent vegetative state and that, based on the statements she had made in the past, she would not have chosen to live that way. From that perspective, the issue in the case was not between living and dying but being allowed to die in a manner consistent with her wishes. That decision was ultimately supported by the court.

The principle of autonomy in end-of-life decisions is supported in the Patient Self-Determination Act (1990). Under the provisions of this act, all

Medicare and Medicaid provider organizations, including hospitals and nursing homes, must obtain at the time of admission advance directives that indicate the patient's preferences about terminating treatment. When the patient is not able to respond, the closest family member indicates a preference, as in the DNR order in the previous example. A concurrent trend has developed as a result of the Cruzan case in which people execute advance directives (sometimes called living wills) that indicate their preferences concerning medical treatment in extreme situations.

Though these approaches offer people some degree of control over end-of-life decisions, many problems and questions remain. From a practical perspective, most people do not have advance directives (Moore et al., 1994). Complicating the situation is the fact that health care providers often do what they believe to be appropriate, regardless of an advance directive or POA. That happens especially if the family is divided over what the appropriate treatment should be (Moody, 1992). As the Schiavo case demonstrated, some people maintain that life should be always be extended, no matter what the patient's condition.

Some ethicists have raised serious objections to the principle of autonomy. Dresser (1992), for example, argues that the patient's prior choices should not influence current decisions, because the person may not have foreseen this particular situation and might now make a different choice. Proxy decisions by family members are criticized even more strongly, because, in the absence of an advance directive, the family cannot truly know what the patient wanted (Rhoden, 1988).

The importance and complexity of these issues have grown out of a long-standing trend in medicine whereby what were previously considered heroic or extraordinary measures are becoming standard procedures for care. An obvious example is the use of hydration and feeding tubes for patients with late-stage dementia. Are these procedures heroic measures, or have they become routine and expected care? Does hydration or a feeding tube contribute to the comfort of an end-stage patient, or do these procedures needlessly prolong suffering? In his powerful book, *How We Die*, Sherwin Nuland (1993) posed the question of whether we merely make people uncomfortable at the end of life with all our medical technology, rather than helping them die peacefully. Thomasma (1992) argues that we need to reverse current premises in end-of-life situations. Rather than assuming that everything must be done to prolong life, he proposes that the "default mode" of modern medicine should be to do nothing to extend life in a hopeless situation unless requested by the patient, by the family, or by an advance directive. While the debate among medical ethicists continues, medical technology is extending the boundaries of life-and-death decisions in new and unexpected ways, placing families in situations for which they are not prepared.

Beyond the ethical dimensions involved in these situations, clinicians need to be aware of the practical implications of medical decisions in life-threatening situations so that they can help patients and their families obtain the kind of care they prefer. As illustrated in the case example at the beginning of this section, medical personnel have developed a set of implicit rules in end-of-life situations, by which each decision has certain consequences. Families are asked to make decisions, but often without being aware of the long-term implications. Once procedures to manage an acute situation are started, physicians will usually feel obligated to continue them. It is very difficult to discontinue some procedures, such as feeding tubes and respirators, after they have been started if the patient cannot survive independently without them. In the case example, the physician could have argued for the need for continued hydration or might have encouraged the use of a feeding tube. Indeed, the decision to cease hydration would have been controversial in many medical settings. In some nursing homes and hospitals, staff members have actively opposed the removal of these treatments and have gone to court to prevent it. The result is that families who do not want to prolong suffering sometimes find themselves on an irreversible course of doing just that because they have made decisions without fully understanding what their choice meant.

For families, an awkward but necessary step is to determine whether physicians, hospitals, and nursing homes will support their relatives' preferences. Some physicians will not agree to follow advance directives or to implement a treatment plan proposed by the family; some facilities have their own guidelines. Once a terminal phase of care has begun, it may be impossible to reconcile these differences in beliefs. Families caring for someone with a predictable course of decline, such as dementia, should be encouraged to talk about terminal-stage care ahead of time with the patient's physicians to make sure that the patient's preferences are likely to be implemented. Topics should include use of feeding tubes, hydration, and antibiotics, as well as methods for reducing discomfort or pain.

One of the more problematic aspects of these situations is determining whether a patient has entered a terminal phase. Physicians may be reluctant to make this determination and, as in the case example, turn to the family for guidance about whether or not to continue treatment. In other instances, physicians insist on initiating treatment in situations that the family regards as terminal. As physicians' skills in prolonging life continue to improve, the decision that a situation is terminal may become increasingly social, not medical.

A further consideration is that older people and their families need to understand the implications of their decisions concerning use of different types of medical facilities. Specifically, the patient's preferences, as indicated by DNR orders, no-extraordinary-measures orders, or advanced directives, are all invalid in an emergency room and in situations in which emergency medical services have been called. In emergency situations, medical personnel need to be able to respond to the crisis immediately before them, and they may not honor advance directives or DNR orders. As a result, a severely impaired patient with dementia who has a significant medical event, such as a myocardial infarction or cardiovascular accident, may be taken to the emergency room and resuscitated, contrary to the wishes of the patient and family. Often the only physician who can honor advance directives is the primary care physician. Family members can consult with this doctor before making a trip to the emergency room. When the older person resides in a nursing home, the family can make similar arrangements with the staff. Some nonmedical programs, such as adult day care or assisted living facilities, feel obligated to call for emergency help, despite the presence of a DNR order.

It may fall to the mental health professional to make explicit to the family what the consequences will be of using emergency services and to help them discuss these issues with nursing home staff or other people involved in the patient's care. Again, we stress that it is not up to us to decide what is best for the patient or family. We should instead help families understand the implications of their decisions and help them make decisions that reflect their preferences and those of the patient. To be effective and helpful in the decision-making process, we need to be able to present the various choices in a nonjudgmental and clear manner, and to do so we must understand our own values and clearly differentiate them from our clients' values. As an example, my own personal belief is that patients deserve a natural death, unencumbered by technology, except to keep them as comfortable and free from pain as possible. Some patients and families may value prolonging life as long as possible, and I support their decision. Whatever the situation, the therapist's role is to help people articulate their values and then to make decisions in a manner consistent with those values.

CONCLUSIONS

Ethical issues in treatment of older people take on a different character than with other clients. Competence in assessment and treatment of older people is a necessary requirement. Confidentiality and end-of-life issues are complex and require thoughtful consideration. Professional codes of conduct and legal statutes provide a framework for addressing the dilemmas that are encountered. But because these principles are broad and abstract, clinicians often find themselves having to apply and extend the basic tenets in situations for which there are no specific precedents. It is important for clinicians to approach these decisions very carefully, getting input from colleagues and, if warranted, from attorneys. Most important, they need to examine their own biases and values so that they are able to differentiate what they would want for themselves from their clients' best interests. Ethical practice needs to be at the core of all the work we do with older people.

References

Aarsland, D., Andersen, K., Larsen, J. P., Lolk, A., & Kragh-Sorensen, P. (2003). Prevalence and characteristics of dementia in Parkinson disease. *Archives of Neurology, 60,* 387–392.

Abrams, R. C., & Horowitz, S. V. (1999). Personality disorders after age 50: A meta-analytic review of the literature. In E. Rosowsky, R. C. Abrams, & R. A. Zweig (Eds.), *Personality disorders in older adults: Emerging issues in diagnosis and treatment* (pp. 55–68). Mahwah, NJ: Erlbaum.

AD2000 Collaborative Group. (2004). Long-term donepezil treatment in 565 patients with Alzheimer's disease (AD2000): Randomized double-blind trial. *Lancet, 363,* 2105–2115.

Adams, W. L. (1995). Potential for adverse drug–alcohol interactions in elderly retirement community residents. *Journal of the American Geriatrics Society, 43,* 1021–1025.

Adams, W. L. (1997). Interactions between alcohol and other drugs. In A. M. Gurnack (Ed.), *Older adults' misuse of alcohol, medicines, and other drugs* (pp. 185–205). New York: Springer.

Adams, W. L., Magruder-Habib, K., Trued, S., & Broome, H. L. (1992). Alcohol abuse in elderly emergency department patients. *Journal of the American Geriatrics Society, 40,* 1236–1240.

Agbayewa, M. O. (1996). Occurrence and effects of personality disorders in depression: Are they the same in the old and young? *Canadian Journal of Psychiatry, 41*(4), 223–226.

Agronin, M. E. (2004). Sexual disorders. In D. G. Blazer, D. C. Steffens, & E. W. Busse (Eds.), *Textbook of geriatric psychiatry* (3rd ed.). Arlington, VA: American Psychiatric Publishing.

Agronin, M. E., & Maletta, G. (2000). Personality disorders in late life: Understanding and overcoming the gap in research. *American Journal of Geriatric Psychiatry, 8*(1), 4–18.

Aisen, P. S., Schafer, K. A., Grundman, M., Pfeiffer, E., Sano, M., Davis, K. L., et al. (2003). Effects of rofecoxib or naproxen vs. placebo on Alzheimer disease progression: A randomized controlled trial. *Journal of the American Medical Association, 289,* 2819–2826.

Akiskal, H. S., & McKinney, W. T. (1973). Depressive disorders: Toward a unified hypothesis. *Science, 5,* 20–29.

Albert, M. S. (1988). Assessment of cognitive function. In M. S. Albert & M. B. Moss (Eds.), *Geriatric neuropsychology* (pp. 57–81). New York: Guilford Press.

Albert, M. S., Wolfe, J., & Lafleche, G. (1990). Differences in abstraction ability with age. *Psychology and Aging, 5,* 94–100.

Alexopoulos, G. S. (1994). Biological correlates of late-life depression. In L. S. Schneider, C. F. Reynolds, B. D. Lebowitz, & A. J. Friedhoff (Eds.), *Diagnosis and treatment of depression in late life* (pp. 99–116). Washington, DC: American Psychiatric Press.

Alexopoulos, G. S., Kiosses, D. N, Choi, S. J., Murphy, C. F., & Lim, K. O. (2002). Frontal white matter microstructure and treatment response of late-life depression: A preliminary study. *American Journal of Psychiatry, 159*(11), 1929–1932.

Alexopoulos, G. S., Meyers, B. S., Young, R. C., Kakuma, T., Feder, M., Einhorn, A., et al. (1996). Recovery in geriatric depression. *Archives of General Psychiatry, 53*(4), 305–312.

Alexopoulos, G. S., Meyers, B. S., Young, R. C., Kalayam, B., Kakuma, T., Gabrielle, M., et al. (2000). Executive dysfunction and long-term outcomes of geriatric depression. *Archives of General Psychiatry, 57*(3), 285–290.

Alexopoulos, G. S., Meyers, B. S., Young, R. C., Mattis, S., & Kakuma, T. (1993). The course of geriatric depression with "reversible dementia": A controlled study. *American Journal of Psychiatry, 150,* 1693–1699.

Alexopoulos, G. S., Young, R. C., Abrams, R. C., Meyers, B., & Shamoian, C. A. (1989). Chronicity and relapse in geriatric depression. *Biological Psychiatry, 26,* 551–564.

Alexopoulos, G. S., Young, R. C., & Shindledecker, R. D. (1992). Brain computed tomography findings in geriatric depression and primary degenerative dementia. *Biological Psychiatry, 31,* 591–599.

Alwin, D. F., & Wray, L. A. (2005). A life-span developmental perspective on social status and health. *Journal of Gerontology: Social Sciences, 60,* 7–14.

Alzheimer's Disease Education and Referral Center. (2002). Frontotemporal dementia: Growing interest in a rare dementia. *Connections, 9*(4), 1–3.

American Bar Association & American Psychological Association. (2005). *Assessment of older adults with diminished capacity: A handbook for lawyers.* Washington, DC: Authors.

American Psychiatric Association. (1980). *Diagnostic and statistical manual of mental disorders* (3rd ed.). Washington, DC: Author.

American Psychiatric Association. (1994). *Diagnostic and statistical manual of mental disorders* (4th ed.). Washington, DC: Author.

American Psychiatric Association. (2001). *The practice of ECT: Recommendations for treatment, training, and privileging.* Washington, DC: Author.

American Psychological Association. (2002). Ethical principles of psychologists and code of conduct. *American Psychologist, 57*(12), 1060–1073. Retrieved October 2005 from www.apa.org/ethics/

American Psychological Association. (2004). Guidelines for psychological practice with older adults. *American Psychologist, 59*(4), 236–260.

Ames, A., & Molinari, V. (1994). Prevalence of personality disorders in community-living elderly. *Journal of Geriatric Psychiatry and Neurology, 7*(3), 189–194.

Ancill, R. J., Embury, G. D., MacEwan, G. W., & Kennedy, J. S. (1987). Lorazepam in the elderly: A retrospective study of the side-effects in 20 patients. *Journal of Psychopharmacology, 2*, 126–127.

Andrade, L., Caraveo-Anduga, J. J., Berglund, P., Biji, R. V., DeGraff, R., Volebergh, W., et al. (2003). The epidemiology of major depressive episodes: Results from the International Consortium of Psychiatric Epidemiology (ICPE) Surveys. *International Journal of Methods in Psychiatric Research, 12*(1), 3–21.

Aneshensel, C. S., Pearlin, L. I., Levy-Storms, L., & Schuler, R. H. (2000). The transition from home to nursing home mortality among people with dementia. *Journal of Gerontology: Social Sciences, 55B*(3), S152–S162.

Aneshensel, C. S., Pearlin, L. I., Mullan, J. T., Zarit, S. H., & Whitlatch, C. J. (1995). *Profiles in caregiving: The unexpected career.* New York: Academic Press.

Anthony, J. C., & Aboraya, A. (1992). The epidemiology of selected mental disorders in later life. In J. E. Birren, R. B. Sloane, & G. D. Cohen (Eds.), *Handbook of mental health and aging* (2nd ed., pp. 27–72). San Diego, CA: Academic Press.

Anthony, J. C., LeResche, L., Niaz, U., Von Korff, M. R., & Folstein, M. F. (1982). Limits of the Mini-Mental State as a screening test for dementia and delirium among hospital patients. *Psychological Medicine, 12*, 397–408.

Anthony-Bergstone, C. R., Zarit, S. H., & Gatz, M. (1988). Symptoms of psychological distress among caregivers of dementia patients. *Psychology and Aging, 3*, 245–248.

Arean, P. A., & Cook, B. L. (2002). Psychotherapy and combined psychotherapy/pharmacotherapy for late-life depression. *Biological Psychiatry, 52*(3), 293–303

Areosa Sastre, A., Sherriff, F., & McShane, R. (2005). Memantine for dementia. *CochraneDatabase of Systematic Reviews, 3*, CD003154. Retrieved August 2005 from www.interscience.wiley.com/cochrane/clsysrev/articlesCD003154/frame.html

Atkinson, R. M. (1990). Aging and alcohol use disorders: Diagnostic issues in the elderly. *International Psychogeriatrics, 2*, 55–72.

Atkinson, R. M., Ganzini, L., & Bernstein, M. J. (1992). Alcohol and substance-use disorders in the elderly. In J. E. Birren, R. B. Sloane, & G. D. Cohen (Eds.), *Handbook of mental health and aging* (2nd ed., pp. 516–556). San Diego, CA: Academic Press.

Atkinson, R. M., & Kofoed, L. L. (1982). Alcohol and drug abuse in old age: A clinical perspective. *Substance and Alcohol Actions/Misuse, 3*, 353–368.

Atkinson, R. M., Tolson, R. L., & Turner, J. A. (1990). Late versus early onset problem drinking in older men. *Alcoholism: Clinical and Experimental Research, 14*, 574–579.

Atkinson, R. M., Turner, J. A., Kofoed, L. L., & Tolson, R. L. (1985). Early versus late onset alcoholism in older persons: Preliminary findings. *Alcoholism: Clinical and Experimental Research, 9*, 513–515.

Bacellar, H., Muñoz, A., Miller, E. N., Cohen, B. A., Besley, D., Selnes, O. A., et al. (1994). Temporal trends in the incidence of HIV-1–related neurologic diseases: Multicenter AIDS Cohort Study, 1985–1992. *Neurology, 44*, 1892–1900.

Bäckman, L., Small, B. J., & Wahlin, Å. (2001). Aging and memory: Cognitive and biological perspectives. In J. E. Birren & K. W. Schaie (Eds.), *Handbook of the psychology of aging* (5th ed., pp. 349–366). San Diego, CA: Academic Press.

Baddeley, A. (1992). Working memory. *Science, 255,* 556–559.

Baldwin, R. C., & Jolley, D. J. (1986). The prognosis of depression in old age. *British Journal of Psychiatry, 149,* 574–583.

Ball, K., Berch, D. B., Helmers, K. F., Jobe, J., Leveck, M. D., Marsiske, M., et al. (2002). Effects of cognitive training interventions with older adults: A randomized controlled trial. *Journal of the American Medical Association, 288*(18), 2271–2281.

Ball, K., & Owsley, C. (2003). Driving competence: It's not a matter of age. *Journal of the American Geriatrics Society, 51,* 1499–1501.

Ballard, C., & Cream, J. (2005). Drugs used to relieve behavioral symptoms in people with dementia or an unacceptable chemical cosh? Argument. *International Psychogeriatrics, 17*(1), 12–22.

Ballard, C., Grace, J., McKeith, I., & Holmes, C. (1998). Neuroleptic sensitivity in dementia with Lewy bodies and Alzheimer's disease. *Lancet, 351,* 1032–1033.

Baltes, M. M. (1994). Aging well and institutional living: A paradox? In R. P. Abeles, H. C. Gift, & M. G. Ory (Eds.), *Aging and quality of life* (pp. 185–201). New York: Springer.

Baltes, M. M., Kindermann, T., Reisenzein, R., & Schmid, U. (1987). Further observational data on the behavioral and social world of institutions for the aged. *Psychology and Aging, 2,* 390–403.

Baltes, P. B. (1987). Theoretical propositions of life-span developmental psychology: On the dynamics between growth and decline. *Developmental Psychology, 23,* 611–626.

Baltes, P. B. (1997). On the incomplete architecture of human ontogeny: Selection, optimization, and compensation as foundation of developmental theory. *American Psychologist, 52,* 366–380.

Baltes, P. B., & Kliegl, R. (1992). Further testing of limits of cognitive plasticity: Negative age differences in a mnemonic skill are robust. *Developmental Psychology, 28,* 121–125.

Baltes, P. B., & Smith, J. (1990). Toward a psychology of wisdom and its ontogenesis. In R. J. Sternberg (Ed.), *Wisdom: Its nature, origins, and development* (pp. 87–120). New York: Cambridge University Press.

Barak, Y., Knobler, C. Y., & Aizenberg, D. (2004). Suicide attempts amongst elderly schizophrenia patients: A 10-year case-control study. *Schizophrenia Research, 71*(1), 77–81.

Barclay, L. L., Zemcov, A., Blass, J. P., & Sansone, J. (1985). Survival in Alzheimer's disease and vascular dementias. *Neurology, 35,* 834–840.

Barker, W. W., Luis, C. A., Kashuba, A., Luis, M., Harwood, D. G., Lowenstein, D., et al. (2002). Relative frequencies of Alzheimer's disease, Lewy body, vascular and frontotemporal dementia, and hippocampal sclerosis in the State of Florida Brain Bank. *Alzheimer's Disease and Associated Disorders, 16*(4), 203–212.

Barrett, L. I. (1997). Reagan's long goodbye. *Time, 149*(12), 82.

Beck, A. T. (1976). *Cognitive therapy and the emotional disorders.* New York: International Universities Press.

Beck, A. T., Emery, G., & Greenberg, R. C. (1985). *Anxiety disorders and phobias: A cognitive perspective.* New York: Basic Books.

Beck, A. T., Freeman, A., & Associates. (1990). *Cognitive therapy of personality disorders*. New York: Guilford Press.

Beck, A. T., Rush, A. J., Shaw, B. F., & Emery, G. (1979). *Cognitive therapy of depression*. New York: Guilford Press.

Beck, J. (1995). *Cognitive therapy: Basics and beyond*. New York: Guilford Press.

Beck, J. G., & Averill, P. M. (2004). Older adults: Epidemiology. In R. G. Heimberg, C. L. Turk, & D. S. Mennin (Eds.), *Generalized anxiety disorder: Advances in research and practice* (pp. 409–433). New York: Guilford Press.

Becker, J. T., Lopez, O. L., Dew, M. A., & Aizenstein, H. J. (2004). Prevalence of cognitive disorders differs as a function of age in HIV virus infection. *AIDS, 18*, 11–18.

Belanger, L., Morin, C. M., Langlois, F., & Ladouceur, R. (2004). Insomnia and generalized anxiety disorder: Effects of cognitive behavior therapy for GAD on insomnia symptoms. *Journal of Anxiety Disorders, 18*(4), 561–571.

Berg, S. (1996). Aging, behavior, and terminal decline. In J. E. Birren & K. W. Schaie (Eds.), *Handbook of the psychology of aging* (4th ed., pp. 323–336). San Diego, CA: Academic Press.

Beutler, L. E., Scogin, F., Kirkish, P., Schretlen, D., Corbishley, A., Hamblin, D., et al. (1987). Group cognitive therapy and alprazolam in the treatment of depression in older adults. *Journal of Consulting and Clinical Psychology, 55*, 550–556.

Beyer, J. L. (2004). Anxiety and panic disorders. In D. G. Blazer, D. C. Steffens, & E. W. Busse (Eds.), *Textbook of geriatric psychiatry* (3rd ed., pp. 282–294). Arlington, VA: American Psychiatric Publishing.

Bigler, E. D., Rosa, L., Schultz, F., Hall, S., & Harris, J. (1989). Rey Auditory Verbal Learning and Rey–Osterrieth Complex Figure Design performance in Alzheimer's disease and closed head injury. *Journal of Clinical Psychology, 45*, 277–280.

Bille-Brahe, U. (1993). The role of sex and age in suicidal behavior. *Acta Psychiatrica Scandinavica, 371*, 21–27.

Bird, T., Knopman, D., VanSwieten, J., Rosso, S., Feldman, H., Tanabe, H., et al. (2003). Epidemiology and genetics of frontotemporal dementia/Pick's disease. *Annals of Neurology, 54*, S29–S31.

Bird, T. D., Nochlin, D., Poorkaj, P., Cherrier, M., Kaye, J., Payami, H., et al. (1999). A clinical pathological comparison of three families with frontotemporal dementia and identical mutations in the tau gene (P301L). *Brain, 122*, 741–756.

Birks, J., & Flicker, L. (2003). Selegiline for Alzheimer's disease. *Cochrane Database of Systematic Reviews, 1*, CD000442. Retrieved March 2006 from www.mrw.interscience.wiley.com/cochrane/clsysrev/articles/CD001190/frame.html

Birks, J., Grimley Evans, E. J., Iakovidou, V., & Tsolaki, M. (2000). Rivastigmine for Alzheimer's disease. *Cochrane Database of Systematic Reviews, 2*, CD001191. Retrieved August 2005 from www.cochrane.org/reviews/en/ab001191. html

Birks, J. S., & Harvey, R. (2002). Donepezil for dementia due to Alzheimer's disease. *Cochrane Database of Systematic Reviews, 3*, CD001190. Retrieved March 2006 from www.mrw.interscience.wiley.com/cochrane/clsysrev/articles/CD001190/frame.htm

Bissette, G. (2004). Chemical messengers. In D. G. Blazer, D. C. Steffens, & E. W. Busse (Eds.), *Texbook of geriatric psychiatry* (3rd ed, pp. 83–108). Arlington, VA: American Psychiatric Publishing.

Blau, E., & Ober, B. A. (1988). The effect of depression on verbal memory in older adults. *Journal of Clinical and Experimental Neuropsychology, 10*, 81.

Blazer, D. (1994). Epidemiology of late-life depression. In L. S. Schneider, C. F. Reynolds, B. D. Lebowitz, & A. J. Friedhoff (Eds.), *Diagnosis and treatment of depression in late life* (pp. 9–20). Washington, DC: American Psychiatric Press.

Blazer, D. (2004). Alcohol and drug problems. In D. G. Blazer, D. C. Steffens, & E. W. Busse (Eds.), *Textbook of geriatric psychiatry* (3rd ed., pp. 351–368). Arlington, VA: American Psychiatric Publishing.

Blazer, D., George, L. K., & Hughes, D. (1991). The epidemiology of anxiety disorders: An age comparison. In C. Salzman & B. Lebowitz (Eds.), *Anxiety in the elderly* (pp. 17–30). New York: Springer.

Blazer, D. G. (2002). Self-efficacy and depression in late life: A primary prevention proposal. *Aging and Mental Health, 6*(4), 315–324.

Blessed, G., Tomlinson, B. E., & Roth, M. (1968). The association between quantitative measures of dementia and of senile change in the cerebral grey matter of elderly subjects. *British Journal of Psychiatry, 114,* 797–811.

Bliwise, D. L. (1994). Dementia. In M. Kryger, T. Roth, & W. Dement (Eds.), *Principles and practice of sleep medicine* (2nd ed., pp. 790–800). Philadelphia: Saunders.

Blumenthal, J. A., Babyak, M. A., Moore, K. A., Craighead, W. E., Herman, S., Khatri, P., et al. (1999). Effects of exercise training on older patients with major depression. *Archives of Internal Medicine, 159*(19), 2349–2356.

Bohnen, N., Warner, M., Kokmen, E., Beard, M., & Kurland, L. (1994). Alzheimer's disease and cumulative exposure to anesthesia: A case-control study. *Journal of the American Geriatrics Society, 42,* 198–201.

Bondi, M. W., Monsch, A. U., Galasko, D., Butters, N., Salmon, D. P., & Delis, D. C. (1994). Preclinical cognitive markers of dementia of the Alzheimer type. *Neuropsychology, 8,* 374–384.

Bonner, D., & Howard, R. (1995). Treatment-resistant depression in the elderly. *International Psychogeriatrics, 7,* 83–94.

Bootzin, R. R., Engle-Friedman, M., & Hazelwood, L. (1983). Insomnia. In P. M. Lewinsohn & L. Teri (Eds.), *Clinical geropsychology: New directions in assessment and treatment* (pp. 81–115). Elmsford, NY: Pergamon Press.

Borkovec, T., Roemer, L., & Kinyon, J. (1995). Disclosure and worry: Opposite sides of the emotional processing coin. In J. Pennebaker (Ed.), *Emotion, disclosure, and health* (pp. 47–70). Washington, DC: American Psychological Association.

Botwinick, J., & Storandt, M. (1974). *Memory, related functions and age.* Springfield, IL: Thomas.

Branconnier, R. J., Cole, J. O., Ghazvinian, S., Spera, K. F., Oxenkrug, G. F., & Bass, J. L. (1983). Clinical pharmacology of bupropion and imipramine in elderly depressives. *Journal of Clinical Psychiatry, 55*(5, Pt. 2), 130–133.

Brown, G. W., Bifulco, A., & Harris, T. O. (1987). Life events, vulnerability and onset of depression: Some refinements. *British Journal of Psychiatry, 150,* 30–42.

Brown, R., Sweeney, J., Loutsch, E., Kocsis, J., & Frances, A. (1984). Involutional melancholia revisited. *American Journal of Psychiatry, 141,* 24–28.

Brown, R. G., & Marsden, C. D. (1984). How common is dementia in Parkinson's disease? *Lancet, 2,* 1262–1265.

Buettner, L., & Fitzsimmons, S. (2002). *Dementia practice guidelines for treating disturbing behaviors.* Alexandria, VA: American Therapeutic Recreation Association.

Burgio, K. L., & Burgio, L. D. (1991). The problem of urinary incontinence. In P. A. Wisocki (Ed.), *Handbook of clinical behavior therapy with the elderly client* (pp. 317–336). New York: Plenum Press.

Burgio, L. D. (1996). Interventions for the behavioral complications of Alzheimer's disease: Behavioral approaches. *International Psychogeriatrics, 8,* 45–52.

Burgio, L. D., Engel, B. T., Hawkins, A., McCormick, K., Scheve, A. S., & Jones, L. T. (1990). A staff management system for maintaining improvements in incontinence with elderly nursing home residents. *Journal of Applied Behavior Analysis, 23,* 111–118.

Burgio, L. D., Schilley, K., Hardin, J. M., Hsu, C., & Yancey, J. (1996). Environmental "White Noise": An intervention for verbally agitated nursing home residents. *Journal of Gerontology: Psychological Sciences, 51B,* P364–P373.

Burke, K. C., Burke, J. D., Jr., Regier, D. A., & Rae, D. S. (1990). Age at onset of selected mental disorders in five community populations. *Archives of General Psychiatry, 47,* 511–518.

Burns, B. J., Wagner, H. R., Taube, J. E., Magaziner, J., Permutt, T., & Landerman, L. R. (1993). Mental health service use by the elderly in nursing homes. *American Journal of Public Health, 83,* 331–337.

Buschke, H., & Fuld, P. A. (1974). Evaluating storage, retention and retrieval in disordered memory and learning. *Neurology, 11,* 1019–1025.

Busse, A., Bischkopf, J., Riedel-Heller, S. G., & Angermeyer, M. C. (2003). Subclassifications for mild cognitive impairment: Prevalence and predictive validity. *Psychology of Medicine, 33*(6), 1029–1038.

Butters, M. A., Salmon, D. P., & Butters, N. (1994). Neuropsychological assessment of dementia. In M. Storandt & G. R. VandenBos (Eds.), *Neuropsychological assessment of dementia and depression in older adults: A clinician's guide* (pp. 33–60). Washington, DC: American Psychological Association.

Butters, N., Salmon, D. P., Cullum, C. M., Cairns, P., Troster, A. I., Jacobs, D., et al. (1988). Differentiation of amnesic and demented patients with the Wechsler Memory Scale—Revised. *Clinical Neuropsychologist, 2,* 133–144.

Caine, E. D. (1981). Pseudodementia: Current concepts and future directions. *Archives of General Psychiatry, 38,* 1359–1364.

Caine, E. D., Lyness, J. M., King, D. A., & Connors, L. (1994). Clinical and etiological heterogeneity of mood disorders in elderly patients. In L. S. Schneider, C. F. Reynolds, B. D. Lebowitz, & A. J. Friedhoff (Eds.), *Diagnosis and treatment of depression in late life* (pp. 21–54). Washington, DC: American Psychiatric Press.

Calero, M. D., & Navarro, E. (2004). Relationship between plasticity, mild cognitive impairment and cognitive decline. *Archives of Clinical Neuropsychology, 19*(5), 653–660.

Calkins, M. P. (2001). The physical and social environment of the person with Alzheimer's disease. *Aging and Mental Health, 5*(1), S74–S78.

Camp, C. J., Foss, J. W., O'Hanlon, A. M., & Stevens, A. B. (1996). Memory interventions for persons with dementia. *Applied Cognitive Psychology, 10,* 193–210.

Camp, C. J., Foss, J. W., Stevens, A. B., Reichard, C. C., McKitrick, L. A., & O'Hanlon, A. M. (1993). Memory training in normal and demented elderly populations: The E-I-E-I-O model. *Experimental Aging Research, 19,* 277–290.

Camp, C. J., & Schaller, J. R. (1989). Epilogue: Spaced-retrieval memory training in an adult day-care center. *Educational Gerontology, 15,* 641–648.

Camp, C. J., & Stevens, A. B. (1990). Spaced-retrieval: A memory intervention for dementia of the Alzheimer's type. *Clinical Gerontologist, 10,* 58–61.

Canadian Study of Health and Aging Working Group. (1994). Canadian Study of Health and Aging: Study methods and prevalence of dementia. *Canadian Medical Association Journal, 150,* 899–913.

Caplan, G. (1970). *The theory and practice of mental health consultation.* New York: Basic Books.

Carlen, P. L., McAndrews, M. P., Weiss, R. T., Doniger, M., Hill, J. M., Menzano, B., et al. (1994). Alcohol-related dementia in the institutionalized elderly. *Alcoholism: Clinical Experimental Research, 18,* 1330–1334.

Carney, S. S., Rich, C. L., Burke, P. A., & Fowler, R. C. (1994). Suicide over 60: The San Diego study. *Journal of the American Geriatrics Society, 42,* 174–180.

Carstensen, L. L. (1992). Social and emotional patterns in adulthood: Support for socioemotional selectivity theory. *Psychology and Aging, 7,* 331–338.

Carstensen, L. L., & Fisher, J. E. (1991). Treatment applications for psychological and behavioral problems of the elderly in nursing homes. In P. A. Wisocki (Ed.), *Handbook of clinical behavior therapy with the elderly client* (pp. 337–362). New York: Plenum Press.

Carstensen, L. L., Isaacowitz, D. M., & Charles, S. T. (1999). Taking time seriously: A theory of socioemotional selectivity. *American Psychologist, 54*(3), 165–181.

Carstensen, L. L., Pasupathi, M., Mayr, U., & Nesselroade, J. R. (2000). Emotional experience in everyday life across the adult life span. *Journal of Personality and Social Psychology, 79,* 1–12.

Cassel, C. K., Rudberg, M. A., & Olshansky, S. J. (1992). The price of success: Health care in an aging society. *Health Affairs, 11,* 87–99.

Cattan, R. A., Barry, P. P., Mead, G., Reefe, W. E., Gay, A., & Silverman, M. (1990). Electroconvulsive therapy in octogenarians. *Journal of the American Geriatrics Society, 38,* 753–758.

Cercy, S. P., & Bylsma, F. W. (1997). Lewy bodies and progressive dementia: A critical review and meta-analysis. *Journal of the International Neuropsychological Society, 3,* 179–194.

Chambless, D. L., Sanderson, W. C., Shoham, V., Johnson, S. B., Pope, K. S., Crits-Christoph, P., et al. (1996). An update on empirically validated therapies. *Clinical Psychologist, 49,* 5–18.

Charles, S. T., Mather, M., & Carstensen, L. L. (2003). Aging and emotional memory: The forgettable nature of negative images for older adults. *Journal of Experimental Psychology: General, 132*(2), 310–324.

Charles, S. T., Reynolds, C. A., & Gatz, M. (2001). Age related differences and change in positive and negative affect over 23 years. *Journal of Personality and Social Psychology, 80,* 136–151.

Chodosh, J., Reuben, D. B., Albert, M. S., & Seeman, T. E. (2002). Predicting cognitive impairment in high-functioning community-dwelling older persons: MacArthur Studies of Successful Aging. *Journal of Geriatric Society, 50*(6), 1051–1060.

Chui, H. C., Victoroff, J. L., Margolin, D., Jagust, W., Shankle, R., & Katzman, R. (1992). Criteria for the diagnosis of ischemic vascular dementia proposed by the State of California Alzheimer's Disease Diagnostic and Treatment Centers. *Neurology, 42,* 473–480.

Ciompi, L. (1987). Review of follow-up studies on long-term evolution and aging in schizophrenia. In N. E. Miller & G. D. Cohen (Eds.), *Schizophrenia and aging: Schizophrenia, paranoia, and schizophreniform disorders in later life* (pp. 37–51). New York: Guilford Press.

Clare, L. (2002). We'll fight it as long as we can: Coping with the onset of Alzheimer's disease. *Aging and Mental Health, 6,* 139–148.

Clare, L., Wilson, B. A., Carter, G., & Hodges, J. R. (2003). Cognitive rehabilitation as a component of early intervention in Alzheimer's disease: A single case study. *Aging and Mental Health, 7*(1), 5–6.

Clarfield, A. M. (2003). The decreasing prevalence of reversible dementias: An updated meta-analysis. *Archives of Internal Medicine, 163*(18), 2219–2229.

Clarkin, J. F., Spielman, L. A., & Klausner, E. (1999). Conceptual overview of personality disorders in the elderly. In E. Rosowsky, R. C. Abrams, & R. A. Zweig (Eds.), *Personality disorders in older adults: Emerging issues in diagnosis and treatment* (pp. 3–15). Mahwah, NJ: Erlbaum.

Clausen, J. A. (1986). A 15- to 20-year follow-up of married adult psychiatric patients. In L. Erlenmeyer-Kimling & N. E. Miller (Eds.), *Life-span research on the prediction of psychopathology* (pp. 175–194). Hillsdale, NJ: Erlbaum.

Cohen, B. J., Nestadt, G., Samuels, J. F., Romanoski, A. J., McHugh, P. R., & Rabins, P. V. (1994). Personality disorders in later life: A community study. *British Journal of Psychiatry, 165,* 493–499.

Cohen, C. I. (1990). Outcome of schizophrenia into later life: An overview. *Gerontologist, 30,* 790–797.

Cohen, G. D. (1992). The future of mental health and aging. In J. E. Birren, R. B. Sloane, G. D. Cohen, N. R. Hooyman, B. D. Lebowitz, M. Wykle, & D. E. Deutchman (Eds.), *Handbook of mental health and aging* (2nd ed., pp. 894–912). New York: Academic Press.

Cole, S. A., Woodard, J. L., Juncos, J. L., Kogos, J. L., Youngstrom, E. A., & Watts, R. L. (1996). Depression and disability in Parkinson's disease. *Journal of Neuropsychiatry and Clinical Neurosciences, 8,* 20–25.

Collins, M. W., & Abeles, N. (1996). Subjective memory complaints and depression in the able elderly. *Clinical Gerontologist, 16,* 29–54.

Conwell, Y. (1994). Suicide in elderly patients. In L. S. Schneider, C. F. Reynolds, B. D. Lebowitz, & A. J. Friedhoff (Eds.), *Diagnosis and treatment of depression in late life* (pp. 397–418). Washington, DC: American Psychiatric Press.

Conwell, Y., & Brent, D. (1995). Suicide and aging: I. Patterns of psychiatric diagnosis. *International Psychogeriatrics, 7,* 149–164.

Conwell, Y., Olsen, K., Caine, E. D., & Flannery, C. (1991). Suicide in later life: Psychological autopsy findings. *International Psychogeriatrics, 3,* 59–66.

Cooper, A. F., Garside, R. F., & Kay, D. W. K. (1976). A comparison of deaf and nondeaf patients with paranoid and affective psychoses. *British Journal of Psychiatry, 129,* 532–538.

Cooper, A. F., & Porter, R. (1976). Visual acuity and ocular pathology in the paranoid and affective psychoses of later life. *Journal of Psychosomatic Research, 20,* 107–114.

Copeland, J. R., Dewey, M. E., Scott, A., Gilmore, C., Larkin, B. A., Cleave, N., et al. (1998). Schizophrenia and delusional disorder in older age: Community prevalence, incidence, comorbidity, and outcome. *Schizophrenia Bulletin, 24*(1), 153–161.

Copeland, M. P., Daly, E., Hines, V., Mastromauro, C., Zaitchick, D., Gunther, J., et al. (2003). Psychiatric symptomatology and prodromal Alzheimer's disease. *Alzheimer Disease and Associated Disorders, 17*(1), 1–8.

Corder, E., Saunders, A., Strittmatter, W., Schmechel, D., Gaskell, P., Small, G., et al. (1993). Gene dose of apolipoprotein E type 4 allele and the risk of Alzheimer's disease in late onset families. *Science, 261,* 921–923.

Cordoliani-Mackowiak, M.-A., Hénon, H., Pruvo, J.-P., Pasquier, F., & Leys, D. (2003). Poststroke dementia: Influence of hippocampal atrophy. *Archives of Neurology, 60,* 585–590.

Corsellis, J. A. N., Bruton, C. J., & Freeman-Browne, D. (1973). The aftermath of boxing. *Psychological Medicine, 3,* 270–303.

Costa, P. T., Jr., & McCrae, R. R. (1988). From catalog to classification: Murray's needs and the five-factor model. *Journal of Personality and Social Psychology, 55,* 258–265.

Costa, P. T., Jr., & McCrae, R. R. (1989). Personality continuity and the changes of adult life. In M. Storandt & G. R. VandenBos (Eds.), *The adult years: Continuity and change* (pp. 45–77). Washington, DC: American Psychological Association.

Craik, F. I. M. (1994). Memory changes in normal aging. *Current Directions in Psychological Science, 3,* 155–158.

Crum, R. M., Anthony, J. C., Bassett, S. S., & Folstein, M. (1993). Population-based norms for the Mini-Mental State Examination by age and educational level. *Journal of the American Medical Association, 269,* 2386–2391.

Cummings, J. L. (1985). Organic delusions: Phenomenology, anatomical correlations, and review. *British Journal of Psychiatry, 146,* 184–197.

Cummings, J. L., & Benson, D. F. (1992). *Dementia: A clinical approach* (2nd ed.). Stoneham, MA: Butterworth–Heinemann.

Cummings, J. L., & Le Couteur, D. G. (2003). Benzodiazepines and risk of hip fractures in older people: A review of the evidence. *CNS Drugs, 17*(11), 825–837.

Cummings, J. L., & Mega, M. S. (2003). *Neuropsychiatry and behavioral neuroscience.* New York: Oxford University Press.

Cummings, J. L., Miller, B., Hill, M. A., & Neshkes, R. (1987). Neuropsychiatric aspects of multi-infarct dementia and dementia of the Alzheimer type. *Archives of Neurology, 44,* 389–393.

Cunningham, W. R., & Owens, W. A., Jr. (1983). The Iowa State Study of the Adult Development of Intellectual Abilities. In K. W. Schaie (Ed.), *Longitudinal studies of adult psychological development* (pp. 20–39). New York: Guilford Press.

Curtis, J. R., Geller, G., Stokes, E. J., Levine, D. M., & Moore, R. D. (1989). Characteristics, diagnosis, and treatment of alcoholism in elderly patients. *Journal of the American Geriatrics Society, 37,* 310–316.

Davey, G. (1994). Pathological worry as exacerbated problem solving. In G. C. L. Davey & F. Tallis (Eds.), *Worrying: Perspectives on theory, assessment, and treatment* (pp. 35–59). Chichester, UK: Wiley.

Davison, A. M., Walker, G. S., Oli, H., & Lewins, A. M. (1982). Water supply aluminum concentration, dialysis dementia, and effect of reverse-osmosis water treatment. *Lancet, 2,* 785–787.

DeArmond, S. J., & Prusiner, S. B. (1995). Prion protein transgenes and the neuropathology in prion diseases. *Brain Pathology, 5,* 77–89.

DeHart, S. S., & Hoffmann, N. G. (1997). Screening and diagnosis: Alcohol use disorders in older adults. In A. M. Gurnack (Ed.), *Older adults' misuse of alcohol, medicines, and other drugs* (pp. 25–53). New York: Springer.

de la Monte, S. M., & Wands, J. R. (2005). Review of insulin and insulin-like growth factor expression, signaling, and malfunction in central nervous system: Relevance to Alzheimer's disease. *Journal of Alzheimer's Disease, 7*(1), 45–61.

De Leo, D., & Diekstra, R. F. (1990). *Depression and suicide in late life.* Toronto, Ontario, Canada: Hogrefe & Huber.

D'Elia, L. F., Boone, K. B., & Mitrushina, M. (1995). *Handbook of normative data for neuropsychological assessment.* New York: Oxford University Press.

Delis, D. C., Kramer, J. H., Kaplan, E., & Ober, B. A. (1987). *The California Verbal Learning Test.* New York: Psychological Corporation.

Delis, D. C., Massman, P. J., Butters, N., Salmon, D. P., Kramer, J. H., & Cermak, L. (1991). Profiles of demented and amnesic patients on the California Verbal Learning Test: Implications for the assessment of memory disorders. *Psychological Assessment: A Journal of Clinical and Consulting Psychology, 3,* 19–26.

Dennis, H. (2002). The retirement planning specialty. *Generations, 26,* 55–60.

Dennis, M. S., & Lindesay, J. (1995). Suicide in the elderly: The United Kingdom perspective. *International Psychogeriatrics, 7,* 263–274.

DeRubeis, R. J., Gelfand, L. A., Tang, T. Z., & Simons, A. D. (1999). Medications versus cognitive behavior therapy for severely depressed outpatients: Meta-analysis of four randomized comparisons. *American Journal of Psychiatry, 156*(7), 1007–1013.

Devanand, D. P., Adorno, E., Cheng, J., Burt, T., Belton, G. H., Roose, S. P., et al. (2004). Late onset dysthymic disorder and major depression differ from early onset dysthymic disorder and major depression in elderly outpatients. *Journal of Affective Disorders, 78*(3), 259–267.

Diamond, M. C., Johnson, R. E., Protti, A. M., Ott, C., & Kajisa, L. (1985). Plasticity in the 904-day-old male rat cerebral cortex. *Experimental Neurology, 87,* 309–317.

Ditter, S. M., & Mirra, S. S. (1987). Neuropathologic and clinical features of Parkinson's disease in Alzheimer's disease patients. *Neurology, 37,* 754–760.

Ditto, P. H. (2006). What would Terri want? On the psychological challenges of surrogate decision making. *Death Studies, 30*(2), 135–148.

Dobbs, A. R., Heller, R. B., & Schopflocher, D. (1998). A comparative approach to identify unsafe older drivers. *Accident Analysis and Prevention, 30*(3), 363–370.

Doubleday, E. K., Snowden, J. S., Varma, A. R., & Neary, D. (2002). Qualitative performance characteristics differentiate dementia with Lewy bodies and Alzheimer's disease. *Journal of Neurology, Neurosurgery, and Psychiatry, 72,* 602–607.

Dowling, G. A. (1996). Specific interventions: Behavioral intervention strategies for sleep-activity disruption. *International Psychogeriatrics, 8,* 77–86.

Drebing, C. E., Van Gorp, W. G., Stuck, A. E., Mitrushina, M., & Beck, J. (1994). Early detection of cognitive decline in higher cognitively functioning older adults: Sensitivity and specificity of a neuropsychological screening battery. *Neuropsychology, 8,* 31–43.

Dresser, R. S. (1992). Autonomy revisited: The limits of anticipatory choices. In R. H. Binstock, S. G. Post, & P. J. Whitehouse (Eds.), *Dementia and aging: Ethics, values and policy choices* (pp. 71–85). Baltimore: Johns Hopkins University Press.

Duff, K., Patton, D., Schoenberg, M. R., Mold, J., Scott, J. G., & Adams, R. L. (2003).

Age- and education-corrected independent normative data for the RBANS in a community dwelling elderly sample. *Clinical Neuropsychology, 17*(3), 351–366.

Edland, S. D., Rocca, W. A., Petersen, R. C., Cha, R. H., & Kokmen, E. (2002). Dementia and Alzheimer's disease incidence rates do not vary by sex in Rochester, Minn. *Archives of Neurology, 59,* 1589–1593.

Egbert, A. M. (1993). Clinical clues to active alcoholism in the older patient. *Geriatrics, 48*(7), 63–69.

Ekerdt, D., & Dennis, H. (Eds.). (2002). Retirement: New chapters in American life. *Generations, 26.*

Elder, G. H., Jr. (1998). The life course and human development. In W. Damon & R. M. Lerner (Eds.), *Handbook of child psychology: Vol. 1. Theoretical models of human development* (pp. 939–991). New York: Wiley.

Elder, G. H., Jr., Shanahan, M. J., & Clipp, E. C. (1994). When war comes to men's lives: Life-course patterns in family, work, and health. *Psychology and Aging, 9,* 5–16.

Elkin, J., Shea, M. T., Watkins, J. T., Imber, S. D., Sotsky, S. M., Collins, J. R., et al. (1989). National Institute of Mental Health Treatment of Depression Collaborative Research Program: General effectiveness of treatment. *Archives of General Psychiatry, 46,* 971–983.

Engelhart, M. J., Geerlings, M. I., Ruitenberg, A., van Swieten, J. C. Hofman, A., Witteman, J. C., et al. (2002). Dietary intake of antioxidants and risk of Alzheimer disease. *Journal of the American Medical Association, 287*(24), 3223–3229.

Engels, G. I., Duijsens, I. J., Haringsma, R., & van Putten, C. M. (2003). Personality disorders in the elderly compared to four younger age groups: A cross-sectional study of community residents and mental health patients. *Journal of Personality Disorders, 17*(5), 447–459.

Engle-Friedman, M., Bootzin, R. R., Hazlewood, L., & Tsao, C. (1992). An evaluation of behavioral treatments for insomnia in the older adult. *Journal of Clinical Psychology, 48,* 77–90.

Erikson, E. H. (1950). *Childhood and society.* New York: Norton.

Erikson, E. H., Erikson, J. M., & Kivnick, H. Q. (1986). *Vital involvement in old age.* New York: Norton.

Erlangsen, A., Jeune, B., Bille-Brahe, U., & Vaupel, J. W. (2004). Loss of partner and suicide risks among oldest old: A population-based register study. *Age and Ageing, 33*(4), 378–383.

Erlangsen, A., Mortensen, P. B., Vach, W., & Jeune, B. (2005). Psychiatric hospitalisation and suicide among the very old in Denmark: Population-based register study. *British Journal of Psychiatry, 187,* 43–48.

Erlangsen, A., Vach, W., & Jeune, B. (2005). The effect of hospitalization with medical illnesses on the suicide risk in the oldest old: A population-based register study. *Journal of the American Geriatric Society, 53*(5), 771–776.

Evans, D. A., Funkenstein, H., Albert, M. S., Scherr, P. A., Cook, N. R., Chown, M. J., et al. (1989). Prevalence of Alzheimer's disease in a community population of older persons. *Journal of the American Medical Association, 262,* 2551–2556.

Evans, L. K. (1987). Sundown syndrome in institutionalized elderly. *Journal of the American Geriatrics Society, 35,* 101–108.

Farberow, N. L., Gallagher-Thompson, D., Gilewski, M., & Thompson, L. (1992). The role of social supports in the bereavement process of surviving spouses of suicide and natural deaths. *Suicide and Life-Threatening Behavior, 22,* 107–124.

Farrell, K. R., & Ganzini, L. (1995). Misdiagnosing delirium as depression in medically ill elderly patients. *Archives of Internal Medicine, 155,* 2459–2464.

Femia, E. E., Braungart, E. R., Zarit, S. H., & Stephens, M. A. P. (2004, August). *Adult day care use: Impact on clients' mood and behavior.* Poster presented at the annual meeting of the American Psychological Association, Honolulu, HI.

Femia, E. E., Zarit, S. H., & Johansson, B. (1997). Predicting change in activities of daily living: A longitudinal study of the oldest old. *Journal of Gerontology: Psychological Sciences, 52B,* P292–P304.

Ferman, T. J., Lucas, J. A., Ivnik, R. J., Smith, G. E., Willis, F. B., Petersen, R. C., et al. (2005). Mayo's Older African American Normative Studies: Auditory Verbal Learning Test norms for African American elders. *Clinical Neuropsychology, 19*(2), 214–228.

Ferman, T. J., Smith, G. E., Boeve, B. F., Ivnik, R. J., Petersen, R. C., Knopman, D., et al. (2004). DLB fluctuations: Specific features that reliably differentiate DLB from AD and normal aging. *Neurology, 62,* 181–187.

Ferrier, I. N., & McKeith, I. G. (1991). Neuroanatomical and neurochemical changes in affective disorders in old age. *International Journal of Geriatric Psychiatry, 6,* 445–451.

Ferrucci, L., Cecchi, F., Guralnik, J. M., Giampaoli, S., Lo Noce, C., Salani, B., et al. (1996). Does the clock drawing test predict cognitive decline in older persons independent of the Mini-Mental State Examination? *Journal of the American Geriatric Society, 44,* 1326–1331.

Fick, D. M., Agostini, J. V., & Inouye, S. K. (2002). Delirium superimposed on dementia: A systematic review. *Journal of the American Geriatric Society, 50*(10), 1723–1732.

Filipp, S. H. (1996). Motivation and emotion. In J. E. Birren & K. W. Schaie (Eds.), *Handbook of the psychology of aging* (4th ed., pp. 218–235). San Diego, CA: Academic Press.

Fingerman, K. L. (2000). "We had a nice little chat": Age and generational differences in mothers' and daughters' descriptions of enjoyable visits. *Journals of Gerontology: Psychological Sciences, 55B*(2), P95–P106.

Finkel, S. I., & Rosman, M. (1995). Six elderly suicides in a 1-year period in a rural midwestern community. *International Psychogeriatrics, 7,* 221–230.

Finlayson, R. D. (1997). Misuse of prescription drugs. In A. M. Gurnack (Ed.), *Older adults' misuse of alcohol, medicines, and other drugs* (pp. 158–184). New York: Springer.

Finlayson, R. D., & Davis, L. J. (1994). Prescription drug dependence in the elderly population: Demographic and clinical features of 100 inpatients. *Mayo Clinic Proceedings, 69,* 1137–1145.

Fishel, M. A., Watson, G. S., Montine, T. J., Wang, Q., Green, P. S., Kulstad, J. J., et al. (2005). Hyperinsulinemia provokes synchronous increases in central inflammation and beta-amyloid in normal adults. *Archives of Neurology, 62,* 1539–1544.

Fisher, N. M., Pendergast, D. R., & Calkins, E. (1991). Muscle rehabilitation in impaired elderly nursing home residents. *Archives of Physical Medicine and Rehabilitation, 72,* 181–185.

Fisher, P. L., & Durham, R. C. (1999). Recovery rates in generalized anxiety disorder following psychological therapy: An analysis of clinically significant change in the STAI-T across outcome studies since 1990. *Psychological Medicine, 29*(6), 1425–1434.

Fitten, L. J., Ortiz, F., & Ponton, M. (2001). Frequency of Alzheimer's disease and other dementias in a community outreach sample of Hispanics. *Journal of the American Geriatrics Society, 49*(10), 1393–1394.

Fitzpatrick, A. L., Kuller, L. H., Ives, D. G., Lopez, O. L., Jagust, W., Breitner, J. C., et al. (2004). Incidence and prevalence of dementia in the Cardiovascular Health Study. *Journal of the American Geriatrics Society, 52,* 195–204.

Flicker, C. (1988). Neuropsychological evaluation of treatment effects in the elderly: A critique of tests in current use. *Psychopharmacology Bulletin, 24,* 535–556.

Flicker, C., Ferris, S. H., Crook, T., Bartus, R. T., & Reisberg, B. (1986). Cognitive decline in advanced age: Future directions for psychometric differentiation of normal and pathological age changes in cognitive function. *Developmental Neuropsychology, 2,* 309–322.

Flicker, C., Ferris, S. H., & Reisberg, B. (1993). A longitudinal study of cognitive function in elderly persons with subjective memory complaints. *Journal of the American Geriatrics Society, 41,* 1029–1032.

Floyd, M., & Scogin, F. (1996). Effects of memory training on the subjective memory functioning and mental health of older adults: A meta-analysis. *Psychology and Aging, 12,* 150–161.

Folstein, M. F., Anthony, J. C., Parhad, I., Duffy, B., & Gruenberg, E. M. (1985). The meaning of cognitive impairment in the elderly. *Journal of the American Geriatrics Society, 33,* 228–235.

Folstein, M. F., Bassett, S. S., Romanoski, A. J., & Nestadt, G. (1991). The epidemiology of delirium in the community: The Eastern Baltimore Mental Health Survey. *International Psychogeriatrics, 3,* 169–176.

Folstein, M. F., Folstein, S. E., & McHugh, P. R. (1975). "Mini-Mental State": A practical method for grading the cognitive state of patients for the clinician. *Journal of Psychiatric Research, 12,* 189–198.

Frank, E. (1994). Long-term prevention of recurrences in elderly patients. In L. S. Schneider, C. F. Reynolds, B. D. Lebowitz, & A. J. Friedhoff (Eds.), *Diagnosis and treatment of depression in late life* (pp. 317–329). Washington, DC: American Psychiatric Press.

Frank, E., Kupfer, D. J., Perel, J. M., Cornes, C., Jarrett, D. B., Mallinger, A. G., et al. (1990). Three-year outcomes for maintenance therapies in recurrent depression. *Archives of General Psychiatry, 47,* 1093–1099.

Freedman, M. (2002). Civic windfall? Realizing the promise in an aging America. *Generations, 26,* 86–89.

Friedman, R., & Tappen, R. M. (1991). The effect of planned walking on communication in Alzheimer's disease. *Journal of the American Geriatrics Society, 39,* 650–654.

Friend, K. B., & Grattan, L. (1998). Use of the North American Adult Reading Test to estimate premorbid intellectual function in patients with multiple sclerosis. *Journal of Clinical and Experimental Neuropsychology, 20,* 846–851.

Fries, J. F. (1983). The compression of morbidity. *Milbank Memorial Fund Quarterly, 61,* 397–419.

Fritsch, T., McClendon, M. J., Smyth, K. A., & Ogrocki, P. K. (2002). Effects of educational attainment and occupational status on cognitive and functional decline in persons with Alzheimer-type dementia. *International Psychogeriatrics, 14*(4), 347–363.

Froehlich, T. E., Bogardus, S. T., Jr., & Inouye, S. K. (2001). Dementia and race: Are there differences between African Americans and Caucasians? *Journal of the American Geriatrics Society, 49*(4), 477–484.

Fuld, P. A. (1978). Psychological testing in the differential diagnosis of the dementias. In R. Katzman, R. D. Terry, & K. L. Bick (Eds.), *Alzheimer's disease, senile dementia and related disorders* (pp. 185–193). New York: Raven Press.

Funkenstein, H. H. (1988). Cerebrovascular disorders. In M. S. Albert & M. B. Moss (Eds.), *Geriatric neuropsychology* (pp. 179–210). New York: Guilford Press.

Gallagher, D., Rose, J., Rivera, P., Lovett, S., & Thompson, L. W. (1989). Prevalence of depression in family caregivers. *Gerontologist, 29,* 449–456.

Gallagher, D., Thompson, L. W., Baffa, G., Piatt, C., Ringering, L., & Stone, V. (1981). *Depression in the elderly: A behavioral treatment manual.* Unpublished manuscript, Andrus Gerontology Center, University of Southern California, Los Angeles.

Gallagher-Thompson, D., & Thompson, L. W. (1995). Psychotherapy with older adults in theory and practice. In B. Bonger & L. Beutler (Eds.), *Comprehensive textbook of psychotherapy* (pp. 357–379). New York: Oxford University Press.

Gallagher-Thompson, D., & Thompson, L. W. (1996). Applying cognitive-behavioral therapy to the common psychological problems of later life. In S. H. Zarit & B. G. Knight (Eds.), *A guide to psychotherapy and aging* (pp. 61–82). Washington, DC: American Psychological Association.

Gatz, M. (1994). Application of assessment to therapy and intervention with older adults. In M. Storandt & G. R. VandenBos (Eds.), *Neuropsychological assessment of dementia and depression in older adults: A clinician's guide* (pp. 155–176). Washington, DC: American Psychological Association.

Gatz, M., Fiske, A., Fox, L. S., Kaskie, B., Kasl-Godley, J. E., McCallum, T. J., et al. (1998). Empirically validated psychological treatments for older adults. *Journal of Mental Health and Aging, 4*(1), 9–46.

Gatz, M., Fiske, A., Reynolds, C. A., Wetherell, J. L., Johansson, B., Pedersen, N. L. (2003). Sex differences in genetic risk for dementia. *Behavioral Genetics, 33*(2), 95–105.

Gatz, M., & Hurwicz, M. L. (1990). Are old people more depressed? Cross-sectional data on Center for Epidemiological Studies depression scale factors. *Psychology and Aging, 5,* 284–290.

Gatz, M., Lowe, B., Berg, S., Mortimer, J., & Pedersen, N. (1994). Dementia: Not just a search for the gene. *Gerontologist, 34,* 251–255.

Gatz, M., Pedersen, N. L., Berg, S., Johansson, B., Johansson, K., Mortimer, J. A., et al. (1997). Heritability for Alzheimer's disease: The study of dementia in Swedish twins. *Journals of Gerontology: Medical Sciences, 52A,* M117–M125.

Gatz, M., Pedersen, N. L., Plomin, R., Nesselroade, J. R., & McClearn, G. E. (1992). Importance of shared genes and shared environments for symptoms of depression in older adults. *Journal of Abnormal Psychology, 101,* 701–708.

Gatz, M., Svedberg, P., Pedersen, N. L., Mortimer, J. A., Berg, S., & Johannsson, B. (2001). Education and the risk of Alzheimer's disease: Findings from the study of dementia in Swedish twins. *Journal of Gerontology, 56*(5), 292–300.

Gatz, M., & Warren, C. (1989, November). *Pathways to electroconvulsive therapy: Depressed elders and distressed families.* Paper presented at the annual meeting of the Gerontological Society of America, Minneapolis, MI.

Gaugler, J. E. (Ed.). (2005). *Promoting family involvement in long-term care settings: A guide to programs that work.* Baltimore: Health Professions Press.

Gearing, M., Mirra, S. S., Hedreen, J. C., Sumi, S. M., Hansen, L. A., & Heyman, A. (1995). The Consortium to Establish a Registry for Alzheimer's Disease (CERAD): Part 10. Neuropathology confirmation of the clinical diagnosis of Alzheimer's disease. *Neurology, 45*(3), 461–466.

Genensky, S., Zarit, S. H., & Amaral, P. (1992). Visual care and rehabilitation of the elderly patient. In A. A. Rosenblum, Jr., & M. W. Morgan (Eds.), *Vision and aging: General and clinical perspectives* (2nd ed., pp. 424–444). New York: Professional Press.

German, P. S., Shapiro, S., & Kramer, M. (1986). Nursing home study of the Eastern Baltimore Epidemiological Catchment Area Study. In M. S. Harper & B. D. Lebowitz (Eds.), *Mental illness in nursing homes: Agenda for research* (pp. 27–40). Rockville, MD: National Institute of Mental Health.

Gildengers, A. G., Butters, M. A., Seligman, K., McShea, M., Miller, M. D., Mulsant, B. H., et al. (2004). Cognitive functioning in late-life bipolar disorder. *American Journal of Psychiatry, 161*(4), 736–738.

Girolamo, G., & Reich, J. H. (1993). *Personality disorders.* Geneva: World Health Organization.

Gislason, T. B., Sjogren, M., Larsson, L., & Skoog, I. (2003). The prevalence of frontal variant frontotemporal dementia and the frontal lobe syndrome in a population-based sample of 85-year-olds. *Journal of Neurology and Neurosurgery, 74*(7), 867–871.

Glasscote, R. M., Gudemen, J. E., & Miles, D. G. (1977). *Creative mental health services for the elderly.* Washington, DC: American Psychiatric Association

Golden, R. N., Gaynes, B. N., Ekstrom, R. D., Hamer, R. M., Jacobsen, F. M., Suppes, T., et al. (2005). The efficacy of light therapy in the treatment of mood disorders: A review and meta-analysis of the evidence. *American Journal of Psychiatry, 162*(4), 656–662.

Goldsilver, P. M., & Gruneir, M. R. (2001). Early stage dementia group: An innovative model of support for individuals in the early stages of dementia. *American Journal of Alzheimer's Disease, 16*, 109–114.

Gontkovsky, S. T., Mold, J. W., & Beatty, W. W. (2002). Age and educational influences on RBANS index scores in a nondemented geriatric sample. *Clinical Neuropsychology, 16*(3), 258–263.

Goodwin, F. K., & Bunney, W. E., Jr. (1973). Psychobiological aspects of stress and affective illness. In J. P. Scott & E. C. Senay (Eds.), *Separation and depression: Clinical and research aspects* (pp. 91–112). Washington, DC: American Association for the Advancement of Science.

Gorelick, P. B., Erkinjuntti, T., Hofman, A., Rocca, W. A., Skoog, I., & Winblad, B. (1999). Prevention of vascular dementia. *Alzheimers Disease and Associated Disorders, 13*(3), S131–S132.

Grant, B. F., Hasin, D. S., Stinson, F. S., Dawson, D. A., Chou, S. P., Ruan, W. J., et al.. (2004). Prevalence, correlates, and disability of personality disorders in the

United States: Results from the national epidemiologic survey on alcohol and related conditions. *Journal of Clinical Psychiatry, 65*(7), 948–958.

Grant, R. W., & Casey, D. A. (1995). Adapting cognitive behavioral therapy for the frail elderly. *International Psychogeriatrics, 7,* 561–571.

Graves, A. B., White, E., Koepsell, T., Reifler, B., Van Belle, G., & Larson, E. (1990). The association between aluminum-coating products and Alzheimer's disease. *Journal of Clinical Epidemiology, 43,* 35–44.

Graves, R. E., Bezeau, S. C., Fogarty, J., & Blair, R. (2004). Boston Naming Test short forms: A comparison of previous forms with new item response theory based forms. *Journal of Clinical and Experimental Neuropsychology, 26*(7), 891–902.

Green, G. R., Linsk, N. L., & Pinkson, E. M. (1986). Modification of verbal behavior of the mentally impaired elderly by their spouses. *Journal of Applied Behavior Analysis, 19,* 329–336.

Green, R. C., Cupples, L. A., Kurz, A., Auerbach, S., Go, R., Sadovnick, D., et al. (2003). Depression as a risk factor for Alzheimer disease: The MIRAGE Study. *Archives of Neurology, 60*(5), 753–759.

Gregoire, J., & Van der Linden, M. (1997). Effects of age on forward and backward digit span. *Aging, Neuropsychology, and Cognition, 4,* 140–149.

Griffin, S. L., Mindt, M. R., Rankin, E. J., Ritchie, A. J., & Scott, J. G. (2002). Estimating premorbid intelligence: Comparison of traditional and contemporary methods across the intelligence continuum. *Archives of Clinical Neuropsychology, 17*(5), 497–507.

Griffith, H. R., Belue, K., Sicola, A., Krzywanski, S., Zamrini, E., Harrell, L., et al. (2003). Impaired financial abilities in mild cognitive impairment: A direct assessment approach. *Neurology, 60*(12), 449–457.

Grisso, T. (1994). Clinical assessments for legal competence of older adults. In M. Storandt & G. R. VandenBos (Eds.), *Neuropsychological assessment of dementia and depression in older adults: A clinician's guide* (pp. 119–140). Washington, DC: American Psychological Association.

Grisso, T. (2003). *Evaluating competencies: Forensic assessments and instruments* (2nd ed.). New York: Plenum Press.

Gross, J. J., Carstensen, L. L., Pasupathi, M., Tsai, J., Skorpen, C. G., & Hsu, A. Y. C. (1997). Emotion and aging: Experience, expression, and control. *Psychology and Aging, 12,* 590–599.

Gruber-Baldini, A. L., Boustani, M., Sloane, P. D., & Zimmerman, S. (2004). Behavioral symptoms in residential care/assisted living facilities: Prevalence, risk factors, and medication management. *Journal of the American Geriatrics Society, 52*(10), 1771–1773.

Gruber-Baldini, A. L., Schaie, K. W., & Willis, S. L. (1995). Similarity in married couples: A longitudinal study of mental abilities and flexibility–rigidity. *Journal of Personality and Social Psychology: Personality Processes and Individual Differences, 69,* 191–203.

Gurian, B., & Miner, J. H. (1991). Clinical presentation of anxiety in the elderly. In C. Salzman & B. Lebowitz (Eds.), *Anxiety in the elderly* (pp. 31–46). New York: Springer.

Gurland, B., Wilder, D., Cross, P., Lantigua, R., Teresi, J., Barrett, V., et al. (1995). Relative rates of dementia by multiple case definitions, over two prevalence periods, in three sociocultural groups. *American Journal of Geriatric Psychiatry, 3,* 6–20.

Gurland, B. J., Copeland, J., Kuriansky, J., Kelleher, M. J., Sharpe, L., & Dean, L. (1983). *The mind and mood of aging.* New York: Haworth Press.

Gurland, B. J., & Cross, P. S. (1982). Epidemiology of psychopathology in old age. *Psychiatric Clinics of North America, 5,* 11–26.

Gustafson, L., Brun, A., & Passant, U. (1992). Frontal lobe degeneration of non-Alzheimer type. *Baillieres Clinical Neurology, 1,* 559–582.

Haan, M. N., Shemanski, L., Jagust, W. J., Manolio, T. A., & Kuller, L. (1999). The role of APO e4 in modulating effects of other risk factors for cognitive decline in elderly persons. *Journal of the American Medical Association, 282*(1), 40–46

Haan, N., Millsap, R., & Hartka, E. (1986). As time goes by: Change and stability in personality over fifty years. *Psychology and Aging, 1,* 220–232.

Hachinski, V. C., Iliff, L. D., Zilhka, E., DuBoulay, G. H., McAllister, V. L., Marshall, J., et al. (1975). Cerebral blood flow in dementia. *Archives of Neurology, 32*(9), 632–637.

Haley, J. (1976). *Problem-solving therapy.* San Francisco: Jossey-Bass.

Haley, W. E. (1983). A family-behavioral approach to the treatment of the cognitively impaired elderly. *Gerontologist, 23,* 18–20.

Halpain, M. C., Harris, M. J., McClure, F. S., & Jeste, D. V. (1999). Training in geriatric mental health: Needs and strategies. *Psychiatric Services, 50*(9), 1205–1208.

Hamilton, J. M., Salmon, D. P., Galasko, D., Delis, D. C., Hansen, L. A., Masliah, E., et al. (2004). A comparison of episodic memory deficits in neuropathologically-confirmed dementia with Lewy bodies and Alzheimer's disease. *Journal of International Neuropsychology and Sociology, 10*(5), 689–697.

Harding, C. M., Brooks, G. W., Ashikaga, T., Strauss, J. S., & Breier, A. (1987). The Vermont Longitudinal Study of Persons with Severe Mental Illness: I. Methodology, study sample and overall status 32 years later. *American Journal of Psychiatry, 144,* 18–26.

Hardy, J. (1993). Genetic mistakes point the way for Alzheimer's disease. *Journal of National Institutes of Health Research, 5,* 46–49.

Harris, M. E., Ivnik, R. J., & Smith, G. E. (2002). Mayo's older Americans normative studies: Expanded AVLT Recognition Trial norms for ages 57–98. *Journal of Clinical and Experimental Neuropsychology, 24*(2), 214–220.

Harvey, R. J., & Rossor, M. N. (1995). Does early-onset Alzheimer disease constitute a distinct subtype? The contribution of molecular genetics. *Alzheimer Disease and Associated Disorders, 9*(Suppl. 1), S7–13.

Harwood, D., Hawton, K., Hope, T., & Jacoby, R. (2001). Psychiatric disorder and personality factors associated with suicide in older people: A descriptive and case-control study. *International Journal of Geriatric Psychiatry, 16*(2), 155–165.

Hassing, L. B., Johansson, B., Nilsson, S. E., Berg, S., Pedersen, N. L., Gatz, M., et al. (2002). Diabetes mellitus is a risk factor for vascular dementia, but not for Alzheimer's disease: A population-based study of the oldest old. *International Psychogeriatrics, 14*(3), 239–248.

Hayden, C. M., & Camp, C. J. (1995). Spaced-retrieval: A memory intervention for dementia in Parkinson's disease. *Clinical Gerontologist, 16,* 80–82.

Haynie, D. A., Berg, S., Johansson, B., Gatz, M., & Zarit, S. H. (2001). Symptoms of depression in the oldest old: A longitudinal study. *Journal of Gerontology: Psychological Sciences, 56B*, P111–P118.

Heikkinen, M. E., & Lönnqvist, J. K. (1995). Recent life events in elderly suicide: A nationwide study in Finland. *International Psychogeriatrics, 7*, 287–300.

Heikkinen, R. L., & Kauppinen, M. (2004). Depressive symptoms in late life: A 10-year follow-up. *Archives of Gerontology and Geriatrics, 38*(3), 239–250.

Hejl, A., Høgh, P., & Waldemar, G. (2002). Potentially reversible conditions in 1,000 consecutive memory clinic patients. *Journal of Neurology, Neurosurgery, and Psychiatry, 73*, 390–394.

Helson, R., & Moane, G. (1987). Personality change in women from college to midlife. *Journal of Personality and Social Psychology, 53*, 176–186.

Henon, H., Durieu, I., Guerouaou, D., Lebert, F., Pasquier, F., & Leys, D. (2001). Poststroke dementia: Incidence and relationship to prestroke cognitive decline. *Neurology, 57*(7), 1216–1222.

Herr, J. J., & Weakland, J. H. (1979). *Counseling elders and their families*. New York: Springer.

Hetzel, L., & Smith, A. (2001). *The 65 years and over population: 2000—Census 2000 Brief*. Washington, DC: U.S. Census Bureau.

Heuzenroeder, L., Donnelly, M., Haby, M. M., Mihalopoulos, C. Rossell, R., Carter, R., et al. (2004). Cost-effectiveness of psychological and pharmacological interventions for generalized anxiety disorder and panic disorder. *Australian and New Zealand Journal of Psychiatry, 38*(8), 602–612.

Heyman, A., Fillenbaum, G., Prosnitz, B., Raiford, K., Burchett, B., & Clark, C. (1991). Estimated prevalence of dementia among elderly black and white community residents. *Archives of Neurology, 48*(6), 594–598.

Heyman, A., Fillenbaum, G. G., Gearing, M., Mirra, S. S., Welsh-Bohmer, D. A., Peterson, B., et al. (1999). Consortium to Establish a Registry for Alzheimer's Disease: Part 19. Comparison of Lewy body variant of Alzheimer's disease with pure Alzheimer's disease. *Neurology, 52*(9), 1839–1844.

Heyman, A., Peterson, B., Fillenbaum, G., & Pieper, C. (1996). Consortium to Establish a Registry for Alzheimer's Disease: Part 14. Demographic and clinical predictors of survival in patients with Alzheimer's disease. *Neurology, 46*(3), 656–660.

Hijman, R., Hulshoff Pol, H. E., Sitskoorn, M. M., & Kahn, R. S. (2003). Global intellectual impairment does not accelerate with age in patients with schizophrenia: A cross-sectional analysis. *Schizophrenia Bulletin, 29*(3), 509–517.

Hill, R. D., Sheikh, J. I., & Yesavage, J. A. (1988). Pretraining enhances mnemonic training in elderly adults. *Experimental Aging Research, 14*, 207–211.

Hinchliffe, A. C., Hyman, I. L., Blizard, B., & Livingston, G. (1995). Behavioural complications of dementia: Can they be treated? *International Journal of Geriatric Psychiatry, 10*, 839–847.

Hinrichsen, G. A. (1992). Recovery and relapse from major depressive disorder in the elderly. *American Journal of Psychiatry, 149*, 1575–1579.

Hinrichsen, G. A., & Hernandez, N. A. (1993). Factors associated with recovery from and relapse into major depressive disorder in the elderly. *American Journal of Psychiatry, 150*, 1820–1825.

Hinrichsen, G. A., & Zweig, R. A. (1994). Family issues in late-life depression. *Journal of Long Term Home Health Care, 13*, 4–15.

Hirschfeld, R. M., Dunner, D. L., Keitner, G., Klein, D. N., Koran, L. M., Kornstein, S. G., et al. (2002). Does psychosocial functioning improve independent of depressive symptoms? A comparison of nefazodone, psychotherapy, and their combination. *Biological Psychiatry, 51*(2), 123–133.

Hobbs, F. B., & Damon, B. L. (1996). 65+ in the United States. *Current population reports: Special studies* (No. P23-190). Washington, DC: U.S. Census Bureau.

Hodges, J. R., Patterson, K., Ward, R. Garrard, P., Bak, T., Perry, R., et al. (1999). The differentiation of semantic dementia and frontal lobe dementia (temporal and frontal variants of frontotemporal dementia) from early Alzheimer's disease: A comparative neuropsychological study. *Neuropsychology, 13*(1), 31–40.

Hofer, S. M., Christensen, H., Mackinnon, A. J., Korten, A. E., Jorm, A. F., Henderson, A. D., et al. (2002). Change in cognitive functioning associated with ApoE genotype in a community sample of older adults. *Psychology and Aging, 17*(2), 194–208.

Hofland, B. F. (1995). Resident autonomy in long-term care: Paradoxes and challenges. In L. M. Gamroth, J. Semradek, & E. M. Tornquist (Eds.), *Enhancing autonomy in long-term care: Concepts and strategies* (pp. 15–33). New York: Springer.

Hogan, D. B., Maxwell, C. J., Fung, T. S., & Ebly, E. M. (2003). Prevalence and potential consequences of benzodiazepine use in senior citizens: Results from the Canadian Study of Health and Aging. *Canadian Journal of Clinical Pharmacology, 10*(2), 72–77.

Holland, J. C., & Tross, S. (1985). The psychosocial and neuropsychiatric sequelae of the acquired immunodeficiency syndrome and related disorders. *Annals of Internal Medicine, 103,* 760–764.

Holmes, D., Splaine, M., Teresi, J., Ory, M., Barret, V., Monaco, C., et al. (1994). What makes special care special?: Concept mapping as a definitional tool. *Alzheimer's Disease and Associated Disorders, 8,* S41–S59.

Homack, S., Lee, D., & Riccio, C. A. (2005). Test review: Delis–Kaplan Executive Function System. *Journal of Clinical and Experimental Neuropsychology, 27*(5), 599–609.

Horowitz, A., Reinhardt, J. P., & Kennedy, G. (2005). Major and subthreshold depression among older adults seeking vision rehabilitation services. *American Journal of Geriatric Psychiatry, 13,* 180–187.

Howard, R., Rabins, P. V., Seeman, M. V., Jeste, D. V., and the International Late-Onset Schizophrenia Group. (2000). Late-onset schizophrenia and very-late-onset schizophrenia-like psychosis: An international consensus. *American Journal of Psychiatry, 157*(2), 172–178.

Huber, G. (1997). The heterogeneous course of schizophrenia. *Schizophrenia Research, 28*(2–3), 177–185.

Huber, T. J., Borsutzky, M., Schneider, U., & Emrich, H. M. (2004). Psychotic disorders and gonadal function: Evidence supporting the oestrogen hypothesis. *Acta Psychiatrica Scandinavica, 109*(4), 269–274.

Hughes, C. P., Berg, L., Danziger, W. L., Coben, L. A., & Martin, R. L. (1982). A new clinical scale for the staging of dementia. *British Journal of Psychiatry, 140,* 566–572.

Hultsch, D. (1971). Adult age differences in free classification and free recall. *Developmental Psychology, 4,* 338–342.

Hunt, L., Morris, J. C., Edwards, D., & Wilson, B. S. (1993). Driving performance in persons with mild senile dementia of the Alzheimer type. *Journal of the American Geriatrics Society, 41,* 747–753.

Hussian, R. A. (1986). Severe behavioral problems. In L. Teri & P. M. Lewinsohn (Eds.), *Geropsychological assessment and treatment* (pp. 121–143). New York: Springer.

Hussian, R. A., & Davis, R. L. (1985). *Responsive care: Behavioral interventions with elderly persons.* Champaign, IL: Research Press.

Hustey, F. M., & Meldon, S. W. (2002). The prevalence and documentation of impaired mental status in elderly emergency department patients. *Annals of Emergency Medicine, 39*(3), 338–341.

Hypericum Depression Trial Study Group. (2002). Effect of *hypericum perforatum* (St. John's wort) in major depressive disorder: A randomized controlled trial. *Journal of the American Medical Association, 287*(14), 1807–1814.

Iliffe, S., & Manthorpe, J. (2004). The hazards of early recognition of dementia: A risk assessment. *Aging and Mental Health, 8*(2), 99–105.

Imamura, T., Takatsuki, Y., Fujimori, M., Hirono, N., Ikejiri, Y. Shimomura, T., et al. (1988). Age at onset and language disturbances in Alzheimer's disease. *Neuropsychologia, 36*(9), 945–949.

Inouye, S. K. (1994). The dilemma of delirium: Clinical and research controversies regarding diagnosis and evaluation of delirium in hospitalized elderly medical patients. *American Journal of Medicine, 97*(3), 278–288.

Inouye, S. K., Bogardus, S. T., Jr., Charpentier, P. A., Leo-Summers, L., Acampora, D., Holford, T. R., et al. (1999). A multicomponent intervention to prevent delirium in hospitalized older patients. *New England Journal of Medicine, 340*(9), 669–676.

Inouye, S. K., & Charpentier, P. A. (1996). Precipitating factors for delirium in hospitalized elderly persons: Predictive model and interrelationship with baseline vulnerability. *Journal of the American Medical Association, 275,* 852–857.

Inouye, S. K., vanDyck, C. H., Alessi, C. A., Balkin, S., Siegal, A. P., & Horwitz, R. I. (1990). Clarifying confusion: The confusion assessment method. *Annals of Internal Medicine, 113,* 941–948.

in t'Veld, B. A., Ruitenberg, A., Hofman, A., Launer, L. J., van Duijn, C. M., Stijnen, T., et al. (2001). Nonsteroidal antiinflamatory drugs and the risk of Alzheimer's disease. *New England Journal of Medicine, 345,* 1515–1521.

Ivnik, R. J., Malec, J. F., Smith, G. E., Tangalos, E. G., Peterson, R. C., Kokmen, E., et al. (1992a). Mayo's older Americans normative studies: Updated AVLT norms for ages 56–97. *Clinical Neuropsycholgist, 6,* 83–104.

Ivnik, R. J., Malec, J. F., Smith, G. E., Tangalos, E. G., Petersen, R. C., Kokmen, E., et al. (1992b). Mayo's older Americans normative studies: WAIS-R norms for ages 56–97. *Clinical Neuropsychologist, 6,* 1–30.

Ivnik, R. J., Smith, G. E., Cerhan, J. H., Boeve, B. F., Tangalos, E. G., & Petersen, R. C. (2001). Understanding the diagnostic capabilities of cognitive tests. *Clinical Neuropsychology, 15*(1), 114–124.

Ivnik, R. J., Smith, G. E., Malec, J. F., Kokmen, E., & Tangalos, E. G. (1994). Mayo cognitive factor scales: Distinguishing normal and clinical samples by profile variability. *Neuropsychology, 8,* 203–209.

Jackson, S. W. (1969). Galen on mental disorders. *Journal of the History of the Behavioral Sciences, 5,* 365.

Jacobs, D., Sano, M., Marder, K., Bell, K., Bylsma, F., Lafleche, G., et al. (1994). Age at onset of Alzheimer's disease: Relation to pattern of cognitive dysfunction and rate of decline. *Neurology, 44*(7), 1215–1220.

Jacobs, D., Troster, A. I., Butters, N., Salmon, D. P., & Cermak, L. S. (1990). Intrusion errors on the Visual Reproduction test of the Wechsler Memory Scale and the Wechsler Memory Scale—Revised: An analysis of demented and amnesic patients. *Clinical Neuropsychology, 4,* 177–191.

Jacobson, S. A., Pies, R. W., & Greenblatt, D. J. (2002). *Handbook of geriatric psychopharmacology.* Washington, DC: American Psychiatric Publishing.

Jang, K. L., Livesley, W. J., Taylor, S., Stein, M. B., & Moon, E. C. (2004). Heritability of individual depressive symptoms. *Journal of Affective Disorders, 80*(2–3), 125–133.

Jansson, M., Gatz, M., Berg, S., Johansson, B., Malmberg, B., McClearn, G. E., et al. (2004). Gender differences in heritability of depressive symptoms in the elderly. *Psychology of Medicine, 34*(3), 471–479.

Jeste, D. V., Wetherell, J. L., & Dolder, C. R. (2004). Schizophrenia and paranoid disorders. In D. G. Blazer, D. C. Steffens, & E. W. Busse (Eds.), *Textbook of geriatric psychiatry* (3rd ed., pp. 269–282). Arlington, VA: American Psychiatric Publishing.

Jinks, M. J., & Raschko, R. R. (1990). A profile of alcohol and prescription drug abuse in a high-risk community-based elderly population. *DICP: Annals of Pharmacology, 24*(10), 971–975.

Johansson, B. (1988–1989). *The MIR—Memory-in-Reality Test.* Stockholm, Sweden: Psykologiförlaget AB.

Johansson, B., Allen-Burge, R., & Zarit, S. H. (1997). Self-reports on memory functioning in a longitudinal study of the oldest old: Relation to current, prospective, and retrospective performance. *Journal of Gerontology: Psychological Sciences, 52B,* P139–P146.

Johansson, B., & Zarit, S. H. (1991). Dementia and cognitive impairment in the oldest old: A comparison of two rating methods. *International Psychogeriatrics, 3,* 29–38.

Johansson, B., & Zarit, S. H. (1995). Prevalence and incidence of dementia in the oldest old: A study of a population based sample of 84–90-year-olds in Sweden. *International Journal of Geriatric Psychiatry, 10,* 359–366.

Johansson, B., & Zarit, S. H. (1997). Early cognitive markers of the incidence of dementia and mortality: A longitudinal population-based study of the oldest old. *International Journal of Geriatric Psychiatry, 12,* 53–59.

Johansson, B., Zarit, S. H., & Berg, S. (1992). Changes in cognitive functioning of the oldest old. *Journals of Gerontology: Psychological Sciences, 47,* P75–P80.

Johnson, C. L., & Barer, B. M. (1997). *Life beyond 85 years: The aura of survivorship.* New York: Springer.

Jones, C. J., & Meredith, W. (1996). Patterns of personality change across the life span. *Psychology and Aging, 11*(1), 57–65.

Jones, C. J., & Meredith, W. (2000). Developmental paths of psychological health from early adolescence to later adulthood. *Psychology and Aging, 15,* 351–360.

Jongsma, A. E., Jr. (Ed.). (2004). *The complete anxiety treatment and homework planner.* Hoboken, NJ: Wiley.

Jorm, A. F., Rodgers, B., & Christensen, H. (2004). Use of medications to enhance memory in a large community sample of 60–64-year-olds. *International Psychogeriatrics 16*(2), 209–217.

Judd, L. L., Kessler, R. C., Paulus, M. P., Zeller, P. V., Wittchen, H. U., & Kunovac, J. L. (1998). Comorbidity as a fundamental feature of generalized anxiety disorders: Results from the National Comorbidity Study (NCS). *Acta Psychiatrica Scandinavica, 393*(Suppl.), 6–11.

Jung, C. G. (1933). *Modern man in search of a soul.* New York: Harcourt Brace Jovanovich.

Jungwirth, S., Fischer, P., Weissgram, S., Kirchmeyr, W., Bauer, P., & Tragl, K. H. (2004). Subjective memory complaints and objective memory impairment in the Vienna–Transdanube aging community. *Journal of the American Geriatrics Society, 52*(2), 263–268.

Juni, P., Nartely, L., Reichenbach, S., Sterchi, R., Dieppe, P. A., & Egger, M. (2004). Risk of cardiovascular events and rofecoxib: Cumulative meta-analysis. *Lancet, 364,* 2021–2029.

Kagan, J. (1996). Three pleasing ideas. *American Psychologist, 51,* 901–908.

Kahn, R., & Fink, M. (1959). Personality factors in behavioral response to electroshock therapy. *Journal of Neuropsychiatry, 1,* 45–49.

Kahn, R. L. (1975). The mental health system and the future aged. *Gerontologist, 15*(1, Pt. 2), 24–31.

Kahn, R. L., Goldfarb, A. I., Pollack, M., & Peck, A. (1960). Brief objective measures for the determination of mental status in the aged. *American Journal of Psychiatry, 117,* 326–328.

Kahn, R. L., & Miller, N. E. (1978). Assessment of altered brain function in the aged. In M. Storandt, I. C. Siegler, & M. F. Elias (Eds.), *The clinical psychology of aging* (pp. 43–69). New York: Plenum Press.

Kahn, R. L., Pollack, M., & Goldfarb, A. I. (1961). Factors related to individual differences in mental status of institutionalized aged. In P. Hoch & J. Zubin (Eds.), *Psychopathology of aging* (pp. 104–113). New York: Grune & Stratton.

Kahn, R. L., Zarit, S. H., Hilbert, N. M., & Niederehe, G. A. (1975). Memory complaint and impairment in the aged: The effect of depression and altered brain function. *Archives of General Psychiatry, 32,* 1569–1573.

Kamboh, M., Sanghera, D., Ferrell, R., & DeKosky, S. (1995). APO e4–associated Alzheimer's disease risk is modified by alpha 1–antichymotrypsin polymorphism. *Nature Genetics, 10,* 486–488.

Kaplan, E., Goodglass, H., & Weintraub, S. (1983). *Boston Naming Test.* Philadelphia: Lea & Febiger.

Kapp, M. B. (1996). Alternatives to guardianship: Enhanced autonomy for diminished capacity. In M. Smyer, K. W. Schaie, & M. B. Kapp (Eds.), *Older adults' decision-making and the law* (pp. 182–201). New York: Springer.

Kaszniak, A. W. (1986). The neuropsychology of dementia. In I. Grant & K. M. Adams (Eds.), *Neuropsychological assessment of neuropsychiatric disorders* (pp. 172–220). New York: Oxford University Press.

Kaszniak, A. W. (1987). Neuropsychological consultation to geriatricians: Issues in the assessment of memory complaints. *Clinical Neuropsychologist, 1,* 35–46.

Kaszniak, A. W. (1990). Psychological assessment of the aging individual. In J. E. Birren & K. W. Schaie (Eds.), *Handbook of the psychology of aging* (3rd ed., pp. 427–445). New York: Academic Press.

Kaszniak, A. W. (1996). Techniques and instruments for assessment of the elderly. In S. H. Zarit & B. G. Knight (Eds.), *A guide to psychotherapy and aging* (pp. 163–219). Washington, DC: American Psychological Association.

Kaszniak, A. W., & DiTraglia Christenson, G. (1994). Differential diagnosis of dementia and depression. In M. Storandt & G. R. VandenBos (Eds.), *Neuropsychological assessment of dementia and depression in older adults: A clinician's guide* (pp. 81–118). Washington, DC: American Psychological Association.

Kaszniak, A. W., Keyl, P., & Albert, M. (1991). Dementia and the older driver. *Human Factors, 33,* 527–537.

Katz, I. R., Parmalee, P., & Brubaker, K. (1991). Toxic and metabolic encephalopathies in long-term care patients. *International Psychogeriatrics, 3,* 337–348.

Katzelnick, D. J., Simon, G. E., Pearson, S. D., Manning, W. G., Heistad, C. P., Henk, H. J., et al. (2000). Randomized trial of a depression management program in high utilizers of mental care. *Archives of Family Medicine, 9,* 345–351.

Kay, D. W. K. (1995). The epidemiology of age-related neurological disease and dementia. *Reviews of Clinical Gerontology, 5,* 39–56.

Kay, D. W. K., Cooper, A. F., Garside, R. F., & Roth, M. (1976). The differentiation of paranoid from affective psychoses by patients' premorbid characteristics. *British Journal of Psychiatry, 129,* 207–215.

Kay, D. W. K., Henderson, A. S., Scott, R., Wilson, J., Rickwood, D., & Grayson, D. A. (1985). Dementia and depression among the elderly living in the Hobart community: The effect of the diagnostic criteria on the prevalence rates. *Psychological Medicine, 15,* 771–788.

Kempen, G. I. J. M., van Sonderen, E., & Ormel, J. (1999). The impact of psychological attributes on changes in disability among low-functioning older persons. *Journals of Gerontology: Psychological Sciences, 54,* P23–P29.

Kemper, P., & Murtaugh, C. M. (1991). Lifetime use of nursing home care. *New England Journal of Medicine, 324,* 595–629.

Kessler, R. C., Berglund, P., Demler, O., Jin, R., Koretz, D., Merikangas, K. R., et al. (2003). The epidemiology of major depressive disorder. *Journal of the American Medical Association, 289*(23), 3095–3105.

Kessler, R. C., Nelson, C. B., McGonagle, K. A., Liu, J., Swartz, M., & Blazer, D. G. (1996, June). Comorbidity of DSM-III-R major depressive disorder in the general population: Results from the U.S. National Comorbidity Survey. *British Journal of Psychiatry, 30*(Suppl.), 17–30.

Kessler, R. C., Stang, P. E., Wittchen, H. U., Ustun, T. B., Roy-Burne, P. P., & Walters, E. E. (1998). Lifetime panic-depression comorbidity in the National Comorbidity Survey. *Archives of General Psychiatry, 55*(9), 801–808.

Kessler, R. C., Walters, E. E., & Wittchen, H. (2004). Epidemiology. In R. G. Heimberg, C. L. Turk, & D. S. Mennin (Eds.), *Generalized anxiety disorder: Advances in research and practice* (pp. 29–50). New York: Guilford Press.

Kiecolt-Glaser, J. K., Dura, J. R., Speicher, C. E., Trask, O. J., & Glaser, R. (1991). Spousal caregivers of dementia victims: Longitudinal changes in immunity and health. *Psychosomatic Medicine, 53,* 345–362.

Kiely, D. K., Bergmann, M. A., Jones, R. N., Murphy, K. M., Orav, E. J., &

Marcantonio, E. R. (2004). Characteristics associated with delirium persistence among newly admitted post-acute facility patients. *Journals of Gerontology: Series A. Biological Science and Medical Science, 59*(4), 344–349.

Kiloh, L. G. (1961). Pseudo-dementia. *Acta Psychiatrica Scandinavica, 37*, 336–351.

Kim, J., Jeong, I., Chun, J. H., & Lee, S. (2003). The prevalence of dementia in a metropolitan city of South Korea. *International Journal of Geriatric Psychiatry, 18*(7), 617–622.

Kingdon, D. G., & Turkington, D. (2005). *Cognitive therapy of schizophrenia.* New York: Guilford Press.

Kinsella, K., & Velkoff, V. Z. (2001). *An aging world: 2001.* Washington, DC: U.S. Census Bureau.

Kirby, M., & Lawlor, B. A. (1995). Biologic markers and neurochemical correlates of agitation and psychosis in dementia. *Journal of Geriatric Psychiatry and Neurology, 8*(Suppl. 1), S2–S7.

Kitwood, T. (1997). *Dementia reconsidered: The person comes first.* Bristol, PA: Open University Press.

Klatka, L. A., Louis, E. D., & Schiffer, R. B. (1996). Psychiatric features in diffuse Lewy body disease: A clinicopathologic study using Alzheimer's disease and Parkinson's disease comparison groups. *Neurology, 47*, 1148–1152.

Klerman, G. L., Weissman, M. M., Rounsaville, B. J., & Chevron, E. (1984). *Interpersonal psychotherapy of depression.* New York: Basic Books.

Kliegl, R., Smith, J., & Baltes, P. B. (1989). Testing the limits and the study of adult age differences in cognitive plasticity of a mnemonic skill. *Developmental Psychology, 25*, 247–256.

Knapp, M. J., Knopman, D., Solomon, P., Pendlebury, W., Davis, C., & Gracon, S. A. (1994). 30–week randomized controlled trial of high-dose tacrine in patients with Alzheimer's disease. *Journal of the American Medical Association, 271*, 985–991.

Knight, B. (1992). *Older adults in psychotherapy: Case histories.* Newbury Park, CA: Sage.

Knight, B. (1996). *Psychotherapy with older adults* (2nd ed.). Beverly Hills, CA: Sage.

Knopman, D. S., Parisi, J. E., Boeve, B. F., Cha, R. H., Apaydin, H., Salviati, A., et al. (2003). Vascular dementia in a population-based autopsy study. *Archives of Neurology, 60*(4), 569–575.

Kocsis, J. H., Zisook, S., Davidson, J., Shelton, R., Yonkers, K., Hellerstein, D. J., et al. (1997). Double-blind comparison of sertraline, imipramine, and placebo in the treatment of dysthymia: Psychosocial outcomes. *American Journal of Psychiatry, 154*, 390–395.

Koenig, H. G., & Blazer, D. G. (1992). Mood disorders and suicide. In J. E. Birren, R. B. Sloane, G. D. Cohen, N. R. Hooyman, B. D. Lebowitz, M. Wykle, & D. E. Deutchman (Eds.), *Handbook of mental health and aging* (2nd ed., pp. 380–400). New York: Academic Press.

Koenig, H. G., & Blazer, D. G. (2004). Mood disorders. In D. G. Blazer, D. C. Steffens, & E. W. Busse (Eds.), *Textbook of geriatric psychiatry* (3rd ed., pp. 241–268). Arlington, VA: American Psychiatric Publishing.

Kokmen, E., Beard, C. M., Offord, K. P., & Kurland, L. T. (1989). Prevalence of medically diagnosed dementia in a defined United States population: Rochester, Minnesota, January 1, 1975. *Neurology, 39*, 773–776.

Kosaka, K., Tsuchiya, K., & Yoshimura, M. (1988). Lewy body disease with and without dementia: A clinicopathological study of 35 cases. *Clinical Neuropathology,* *7,* 299–305.

Kramer, A. F., Fabiani, M., & Colcombe, S. J. (2006). Contributions of cognitive neuroscience to the understanding of behavior and aging. In J. E. Birren & K. W. Schaie (Eds.), *Handbook of the psychology of aging* (6th ed., pp. 57–84). Boston: Academic Press.

Kryger, M., Monjan, A., Bliwise, D., & Ancoli-Israel, S. (2004). Sleep, health, and aging: Bridging the gap between science and clinical practice. *Geriatrics, 59*(1), 29–30.

Kuhn, D. R. (1998). Caring for relatives with early-stage Alzheimer's disease: An exploratory study. *American Journal of Alzheimer's Disease, 13,* 189–196.

Kuller, L. H., Lopez, O. L., Newman, A., Beauchamp, N. J., Burke, G., Dulberg, C., et al. (2003). Risk factors for dementia in the cardiovascular health cognition study. *Neuroepidemiology, 22,* 13–22.

Labouvie-Vief, G., Hakim-Larson, J., DeVoe, M., & Schoeberlein, S. (1989). Emotions and self-regulation: A life span view. *Human Development, 32,* 279–299.

Lachman, J. L., & Lachman, R. (1980). Age and actualization of knowledge. In L. W. Poon, J. L. Fozard, L. S. Cermak, D. Arenberg, & L. W. Thompson (Eds.), *New directions in memory and aging* (pp. 313–343). Hillsdale, NJ: Erlbaum.

Langer, E. J., & Rodin, J. (1976). The effects of choice and enhanced personal responsibility for the aged: A field experiment in an institutional setting. *Journal of Personality and Social Psychology, 34,* 191–198.

Lansbury, P. T., Jr., Costa, P. R., Griffiths, J. M., Simon, E. J., Auger, M., Halverson, K. J., et al. (1995). Structural model for the beta-amyloid fibril based on interstrand alignment of an antiparallel-sheet comprising a C-terminal peptide. *Nature Structural Biology, 2,* 990–998.

Larrieu, S., Letenneur, L., Orgogozo, J. M., Fabrigoule, C., Amieva, H., Le Carret, N., et al. (2002). Incidence and outcome of mild cognitive impairment in a population-based prospective cohort. *Neurology, 59,* 1594–1599.

Laurila, J. V., Pitkala, K. H., Strandberg, T. E., & Tilvis, R. S. (2002). Confusion assessment method in the diagnostics of delirium among aged hospital patients: Would it serve better in screening than as a diagnostic instrument? *International Journal of Geriatric Psychiatry, 17,* 1112–1119.

Laurila, J. V., Pitkala, K. H., Strandberg, T. E., & Tilvis, R. S. (2004). Detection and documentation of dementia and delirium in acute geriatric wards. *Annals of General Hospital Psychiatry, 26*(1), 31–35.

Lawton, M. P. (1986). *Environment and aging.* Albany, NY: Center for the Study of Aging.

Lawton, M. P., & Brody, E. (1969). Assessment of older people: Self-maintaining and instrumental activities of daily living. *Gerontologist, 9,* 179–186.

Lawton, M. P., Kleban, M. H., Rajagopal, D., & Dean, J. (1992). Dimensions of affective experience in three age groups. *Psychology and Aging, 7,* 171–184.

Lawton, M. P., & Nahemow, L. (1973). Ecology and the aging process. In C. Eisdorfer & M. P. Lawton (Eds.), *The psychology of adult development and aging* (pp. 619–674). Washington, DC: American Psychological Association.

Lee, R., & Haaga, J. (2002). Government spending in an older America. *Population Reference Bureau: Reports on America, 3,* 1.

Lee, V. M., Balin, B. J., Otvos, L., Jr., & Trojanowski, J. Q. (1991). A68: A major subunit of paired helical filaments and derivatized forms of normal tau. *Science, 251,* 675–678.

Lee, V. M., Giasson, B. I., & Trojanowski, J. Q. (2004). More than just two peas in a pod: Common amyloidogenic properties of tau and alpha-synuclein in neurodegenerative diseases. *Trends in Neurosciences, 27*(3), 129–134.

Lehtovirta, M., Soininen, H., Helisalmi, S., Mannermaa, A., Helkala, E. L., Hartikainen, P., et al. (1996). Clinical and neuropsychological characteristics in familial and sporadic Alzheimer's disease: Relation to apolipoprotein e polymorphism. *Neurology, 46*(2), 413–419.

Lenze, E. J., Mulsant, B. H., Mohlman, J., Shear, M. K., Dew, M. A., Schulz, R., et al. (2005). Generalized anxiety disorder in late life: Lifetime course and comorbidity with major depressive disorder. *American Journal of Geriatric Psychiatry, 13*(1), 77–80.

Lenze, E. J., Pollock, B. G., Shear, M. K., Mulsant, B. H., Bharucha, A., & Reynolds, C. F. (2003). Treatment considerations for anxiety in the elderly. *CNS Spectrums, 8*(12), 6–13.

Leuchter, A. F. (1994). Brain structural and functional correlates of late-life depression. In L. S. Schneider, C. F. Reynolds, B. D. Lebowitz, & A. J. Friedhoff (Eds.), *Diagnosis and treatment of depression in late life* (pp. 117–130). Washington, DC: American Psychiatric Press.

Levinson, D. J. (1986). A conception of adult development. *American Psychologist, 41,* 3–13.

Levkoff, S., Cleary, P., Liptzin, B., & Evans, D. A. (1991). Epidemiology of delirium: An overview of research issues and findings. *International Psychogeriatrics, 3,* 149–167.

Levkoff, S., Liptzin, B., Cleary, P., Reilly, C. H., & Evans, D. (1991). Review of research instruments and techniques used to detect delirium. *International Psychogeriatrics, 3,* 253–271.

Lewinsohn, P. M. (1975). The behavioral study and treatment of depression. In M. Hersen, R. M. Eisler, & P. M. Miller (Eds.), *Progress in behavior modification* (pp. 19–64). New York: Academic Press.

Lewinsohn, P. M., Antonuccio, D. O., Steinmetz, J. L., & Teri, L. (1984). *The coping and depression course: A psychoeducational intervention for unipolar depression.* Eugene, OR: Castalia.

Lewinsohn, P. M., Biglan, A., & Zeiss, A. M. (1976). Behavioral treatment of depression. In P. O. Davidson (Ed.), *The behavioral management of anxiety, depression and pain* (pp. 91–146). New York: Brunner/Mazel.

Lewinsohn, P. M., & Libet, L. (1972). Pleasant events, activity schedules and depression. *Journal of Abnormal Psychology, 79,* 291–295.

Lewinsohn, P. M., & MacPhillamy, D. (1974). The relationship between age and engagement in pleasant activities. *Journal of Gerontology, 29,* 290–294.

Lewinsohn, P. M., Muñoz, R. F., Youngren, M. A., & Zeiss, A. M. (1992). *Control your depression* (Rev. ed.). New York: Simon & Schuster.

Lewinsohn, P. M., Rohde, P., Fischer, S. A., & Seeley, J. R. (1991). Age and depression: Unique and shared effects. *Psychology and Aging, 6,* 247–260.

Lezak, M. D. (1995). *Neuropsychological assessment* (3rd ed.). New York: Oxford University Press.

Lezak, M. D., Howieson, D. B., & Loring, D. W. (2004). *Neuropsychological assessment* (4th ed.). New York: Oxford University Press.

Libon, D. J., Bogdanoff, B., Bonavita, J., Skalina, S., Cloud, B. S., Resh, R., et al. (1997). Dementia associated with periventricular and deep white matter alterations: A subtype of subcortical dementia. *Archives of Neuropsychology, 12*(3), 239–250.

Lichtenberg, P. A., Smith, M., Frazer, D., Molinari, V., Rosowsky, E., Corse, R., et al. (1998). Standards for psychological services in long-term care facilities. *Gerontologist, 38*(1), 122–127.

Lindesay, J., Briggs, K., & Murphy, E. (1989). The Guy's/Age Concern Survey: Prevalence rates of cognitive impairment, depression and anxiety in an urban elderly community. *British Journal of Psychiatry, 155,* 317–329.

Lindesay, J., Rockwood, K., & Rolfson, D. (2002). The epidemiology of delirium. In J. Lindesay, K. Rockwood, & A. Macdonald (Eds.), *Delirium in old age* (pp. 27–50). New York: Oxford University Press.

Linehan, M. M. (1993). *Cognitive-behavioral treatment of borderline personality disorder.* New York: Guilford Press.

Lipowski, Z. J. (1990). *Delirium: Acute confusional states.* New York: Oxford University Press.

Liu, H., Lin, K., Teng, E., Wang, S., Fuh, J., Guo, N., et al. (1995). Prevalence and subtypes of dementia in Taiwan: A community survey of 5,297 individuals. *Journal of the American Geriatrics Society, 43,* 144–149.

Liu, U., Stern, Y., Chun, M. R., Jacobs, D. M., Yau, P., & Goldman, J. E. (1977). Pathological correlates of extrapyramidal signs in Alzheimer's disease. *Annals of Neurology, 41,* 368–374.

Livingston, G., Hawkins, A., Graham, N., Blizard, B., & Mann, A. (1990). The Gospel Oak Study: Prevalence rates of dementia, depression and activity limitation among elderly residents in inner London. *Psychological Medicine, 20,* 137–146.

Loeb, P. (1983). *Validity of the Community Competence Scale with the elderly.* Unpublished doctoral dissertation, St. Louis University, MO.

Loevinger, J. (1976). *Ego development: Conception and theory.* San Francisco: Jossey-Bass.

Logsdon, R. G., & Teri, L. (1995). Depression in Alzheimer's disease patients: Caregivers as surrogate reporters. *Journal of American Geriatrics Society, 43,* 150–155.

Lohr, J. B., Jeste, D. V., Harris, M. J., & Salzman, C. (1992). Treatment of disordered behavior. In C. Salzman (Ed.), *Clinical geriatric psychopharmacology* (pp. 79–114). Baltimore: Williams & Wilkins.

Looman, W. J., Noelker, L. S., Schur, D., Whitlatch, C. J., & Ejaz, F. K. (2002). Impact of family members on nurse assistants: What helps, what hurts. *American Journal of Alzheimers Disease and other Dementia, 17*(6), 350–356.

Lopez, O. L., Becker, J. T., Kaufer, D. I., Hamilton, R. L., Sweet, R. A., Klunk, W., et al. (2002). Research evaluation and prospective diagnosis of dementia with Lewy bodies. *Archives of Neurology, 59,* 43–46.

Lopez, O. L., Jagust, W. J., DeKosky, S. T., Becker, J. T., Fitzpatrick, A., Dulberg, C., et al. (2003). Prevalence and classification of mild cognitive impairment in the Cardiovascular Health Study Cognition Study: Part 1. *Archive of Neurology, 60*(10), 1385–1389.

Lopez, O. L., Jagust, W. J., Dulberg, C., Becker, J. T., DeKosky, S. T., Fitzpatrick, A., et al. (2003). Risk factors for mild cognitive impairment in the cardiovascular Health Study Cognition Study: Part 2. *Archives of Neurology, 60*(10), 1394–1399.

Lopez, O. L., Litvan, I., Catt, K. E., Stowe, R., Klunk, W., Kaufer, D. I., et al. (1999). Accuracy of four clinical diagnostic criteria for the diagnosis of neurodegenerative dementias. *Neurology, 53*(6), 1292–1299.

Louza, M. R., Marques, A. P., Elkis, H., Bassitt, D., Diegoli, M., & Gattaz, W. F. (2004). Conjugated estrogens as adjuvant therapy in the treatment of acute schizophrenia: A double-blind study. *Schizophrenia Research, 66*(2–3), 97–100.

Lowenstein, D. A., Acevedo, A., Czaja, S. J., & Duara, R. (2004). Cognitive rehabilitation of mildly impaired Alzheimer disease patients on cholinesterase inhibitors. *American Journal of Geriatric Psychiatry,12*(4), 395–402.

Lowenstein, D. A., Amigo, E., Duara, R., Guterman, A., Hurwitz, D., Berkowitz, N., et al. (1989). A new scale for the assessment of functional status in Alzheimer's disease and related disorders. *Journal of Gerontology, 44,* 114–121.

Lowenstein, D. A., Duara, R., Rubert, M. P., Arguelles, T., Lapinski, K. J., & Eisdorfer, C. (1995). Deterioration of functional capacities in Alzheimer's disease after a 1-year period. *International Psychogeriatrics, 7*(4), 495–503.

Loy, C., & Schneider, L. (2004). Galantamine for Alzheimer's disease. *Cochrane Database of Systematic Reviews, 4,* CD001747. Retrieved May 21, 2005, from www.cochrane.org/reviews/en/ab001747.html

Lucas, J. A., Ivnik, R. J., Smith, G. E., Bohac, D. L., Tangalos, E. G., Kokmen, E., et al. (1998). Normative data for the Mattis Dementia Rating Scale. *Journal of Clinical and Experimental Neuropsychology, 20*(4), 536–547.

Lucas, J. A., Ivnik, R. J., Smith, G. E., Ferman, T. J., Willis, F. B., Petersen, R. C., et al. (2005a). A brief report on WAIS-R normative data collection in Mayo's Older African Americans Normative Studies. *Clinical Neuropsychology, 19*(2), 184–188.

Lucas, J. A., Ivnik, R. J., Smith, G. E., Ferman, T. J., Willis, F. B., Petersen, R. C., et al. (2005b). Mayo's Older African Americans Normative Studies: Norms for Boston Naming Test, Controlled Oral Word Association, Category Fluency, Animal Naming, Token Test, WRAT-3 Reading, Trail Making Test, Stroop Test, and Judgment of Line Orientation. *Clinical Neuropsychology, 19*(2), 243–269.

Lucas, J. A., Ivnik, R. J., Smith, G. E., Ferman, T. J., Willis, F. B., Petersen, R. C., et al. (2005c). Mayo's Older African Americans Normative Studies: WMS-R norms for African American elders. *Clinical Neuropsychology, 19*(2), 189–213.

Luchsinger, J. A., Tang, M. X., Shea, S., & Mayeux, R. (2003). Antioxidant vitamin intake and risk of Alzheimer disease. *Archives of Neurology, 60*(2), 203–208.

Lund, D. A., Hill, R. D., Caserta, M. S., & Wright, S. D. (1995). Video Respite: An innovative resource for family, professional caregivers, and persons with dementia. *Gerontologist, 35,* 683–687.

Lustig, C., & Buckner, R. L. (2004). Preserved neural correlates of priming in old age dementia. *Neuron, 42,* 865–875.

Lyness, J. M. (2002). The cerebrovascular model of depression in late life. *CNS Spectrums, 7*(10), 712–715.

Lyness, J. M., King, D. A., Conwell, Y., Cox, C., & Caine, E. (2000). Cerebrovascular risk factors and 1-year depression outcome in older primary care patients. *American Journal of Psychiatry, 157*(9), 1499–1501.

Lyness, J. M., King, D. A., Cox, C., Yoediono, Z., & Caine, E. D. (1999). The importance of subsyndromal depression in older primary care patients: Prevalence and associated functional disability. *Journal of the American Geriatrics Society, 47*(6), 647–652.

Madhusoodanan, S., & Bogunovic, O. J. (2004). Safety of benzodiazepines in the geriatric population. *Expert Opinions on Drug Safety, 3*(5), 485–493.

Mahurin, R. K., DeBettignies, B. H., & Pirozzolo, F. J. (1991). Structured Assessment of Independent Living Skills: Preliminary report of a performance measure of functional abilities in dementia. *Journals of Gerontology: Psychological Sciences, 46*, P58–P66.

Maletta, G. (1990). The concept of "reversible" dementia: How nonreliable terminology may impair effective treatment. *Journal of the American Geriatrics Society, 38*, 136–140.

Malmberg, B. (1999). Swedish group homes for people with dementia. *Generations, 23*(3), 82–87.

Malmberg, B., & Zarit, S. H. (1993). Group homes for dementia patients: An innovative model in Sweden. *Gerontologist, 31*, 682–686.

MaloneBeach, E. E., & Zarit, S. H. (1995). Dimensions of social support and social conflict as predictors of caregiver depression. *International Psychogeriatrics, 7*, 25–38.

MaloneBeach, E. E., Zarit, S. H., & Spore, D. L. (1992). Caregivers' perceptions of case management and community-based services: Barriers to service use. *Journal of Applied Gerontology, 11*, 146–159.

Malouf, R., & Birks, J. (2004). Donepezil for vascular cognitive impairment. *Cochrane Database of Systematic Reviews, 1*, CD004395. Retrieved April 30, 2005, from www.cochrane.org/reviews/en/ab004395.html

Mangion, D. M., Platt, J. S., & Syam, V. (1992). Alcohol and acute medical admission of elderly people. *Age and Ageing, 21*, 362–367.

Mann, D. A. (1997). Frontal lobe dementia. In C. Holmes & R. Howard (Eds.), *Advances in old age psychiatry: Chromosomes to community care* (pp. 64–78). Bristol, PA: Wrightson Biomedical.

Marcantonio, E. (2002). The management of delirium. In J. Lindesay, K. Rockwood, & A. Macdonald (Eds.), *Delirium in old age* (pp. 123–152). New York: Oxford University Press.

Marcantonio, E. R., Simon, S. E., Bergmann, M. A., Jones, R. N., Murphy, K. M., & Morris, J. N. (2003). Delirium symptoms in post-acute care: Prevalent, persistent, and associated with poor functional recovery. *Journal of the American Geriatrics Society, 51*(1), 4–9.

Marcopulos, B., & McLain, C. (2003). Are our norms "normal"? A 4-year follow-up study of a biracial sample of rural elders with low education. *Clinical Neuropsychology, 17*(1), 19–33.

Marsiske, M., & Willis, S. L. (1995). Dimensionality of everyday problem solving in older adults. *Psychology and Aging, 10*, 269–283.

Martiny, K., Lunde, M., Unden, M., Dam, H., & Bech, P. (2005). Adjunctive bright light in nonseasonal major depression: Results from patient-reported symptom and well-being scales. *Acta Psychiatrica Scandinavica, 111*(6), 453–459.

Maslow, K. (1994). Current knowledge about special care units: Findings of a study by the U.S. Office of Technology Assessment. *Alzheimer's Disease and Associated Disorders, 8*, S14–S40.

Mason, E., Clare, L., & Pistrang, N. (2005). Processes and experiences of mutual support in professionally led support groups for people with early-stage dementia. *Dementia, 4*(1), 87–112.

Massman, P. J., Delis, D. C., Butters, N., Dupont, R. M., & Gillin, J. C. (1992). The subcortical dysfunction hypothesis of memory deficits in depression: Neuropsychological validation in subgroup patients. *Journal of Clinical and Experimental Neuropsychology, 14*, 687–706.

Massoud, F., Devi, G., Stern, Y., Lawton, A., Goldman, J. E., Liu, Y., et al. (1999). A clinicopathological comparison of community-based and clinic-based cohorts of patients with dementia. *Archives of Neurology, 56*(11), 1368–1373.

Mast, B. T., MacNeill, S. E., & Lichtenberg, P. A. (2002). A MIMIC model approach for neuropsychological research: The case of vascular dementia. *Aging, Neuropsychology, and Cognition, 9*, 21–37.

Mast, B. T., Neufeld, S., MacNeill, S. E., & Lichtenberg, P. A. (2004). Longitudinal support for the relationship between vascular risk factors and late-life depressive symptoms. *American Journal of Geriatric Psychiatry, 12*(1), 93–101.

Masterman, D., & Swanberg, M. (2003). Neurologic aspects of dementia with Lewy bodies and Parkinson's disease with dementia. In P. A. Lichtenberg, D. L. Murman, & A. M. Mellow (Eds.), *Handbook of dementia* (pp. 49–82). Hoboken, NJ: Wiley.

Masur, D. M., Fuld, P. A., Blau, A. D., Thal, L. J., Levin, H. S., & Aronson, M. K. (1989). Distinguishing normal and demented elderly with the selective reminding test. *Journal of Clinical and Experimental Neuropsychology, 11*, 615–630.

Matarazzo, J. D. (1972). *Wechsler's measurement and appraisal of adult intelligence* (5th ed.). Baltimore: Williams & Wilkins.

Mattis, S. (1976). Mental status examination for organic mental syndrome in the elderly patient. In L. Bellack & T. B. Karasu (Eds.), *Geriatric psychiatry* (pp. 77–121). New York: Grune & Stratton.

Mattis, S. (1989). *Dementia Rating Scale*. Odessa, FL: Psychological Assessment Resources.

Maxwell, C. J., Hicks, M. S., Hogan, D. B., Basran, J., & Ebly, E. M. (2005). Supplemental use of antioxidant vitamins and subsequent risk of cognitive decline and dementia. *Dementia and Geriatric Cognitive Disorders, 20*(1), 45–51.

Mayeux, R. (2003). Apolipoprotein E, Alzheimer disease, and African Americans. *Archives of Neurology, 60*, 161–163.

McArthur, J. C., Hoover, D. R., Bacellar, H., Miller, E. N., Cohen, B. A., Becker, J. T., et al. (1993). Dementia in AIDS patients: Incidence and risk factors: Multicenter AIDS cohort study. *Neurology, 43*, 2245–2252.

McArthur, J. C., Sacktor, N., & Selnes, O. (1999). Human immunodeficiency virus–associated dementia. *Seminars in Neurology, 19*(2), 129–150.

McCrae, R. R., & Costa, P. T., Jr. (1990). *Personality in adulthood*. New York: Guilford Press.

McCurry, S. M., Gibbons, L. E., Logsdon, R. G., Vitiello, M. V., & Teri, L. (2005). Nighttime insomnia treatment and education for Alzheimer's disease: A randomized, controlled trial. *Journal of the American Geriatrics Society, 53*(5), 793–802.

McGwin, G., Jr., Sims, R. V., Pulley, L., & Roseman, J. M. (2000). Relations among chronic medical conditions, medications, and automobile crashes in the elderly: A population-based case-control study. *American Journal of Epidemiology, 152*(5), 424–431.

McIntosh, J. L., Santos, J. F., Hubbard, R. W., & Overholser, J. C. (1994). *Elder suicide: Research, theory and treatment.* Washington, DC: American Psychological Association.

McKeith, I., Mintzer, J., Aarsland, D., Burn, D., Chiu, H., Cohen-Mansfield, J., et al. (2004). Dementia with Lewy bodies. *Lancet: Neurology, 3,* 19–28.

McKeith, I. G. (1997). Dementia with Lewy bodies. In C. Holmes & R. Howard (Eds.), *Advances in old age psychiatry: Chromosomes to community care* (pp. 52–63). Bristol, PA: Wrightson Biomedical.

McKeith, I. G., Dickson, D. W., Lowe, J., Emre, M., O'Brien, J. T., Feldman, H., et al. (2005). Diagnosis and management of dementia with Lewy bodies: Third report of the DLB consortium. *Neurology, 65,* 1863–1872.

McKeith, I. G., Galasko, D., Koska, K., Perry, E. K., Dickinson, D. W., Hansen, L. A., et al. (1996). Consensus guidelines for the clinical and pathologic diagnosis of dementia with Lewy bodies (DLB): Report of the Consortium on DLB International Workshop. *Neurology, 47*(5), 1113–1124.

McKenzie, J. E., Roberts, G. W., & Royston, M. C. (1996). Comparative investigation of neurofibrillary damage in the temporal lobe in Alzheimer's disease, Down's syndrome and dementia pugilistica. *Neurodegeneration, 5,* 259–264.

McKhann, G. M., Albert, M. S., Grossman, M., Miller, B., Dickson, D., & Trojanowski, J. Q. (2001). Clinical and pathological diagnosis of frontotemporal dementia. *Archives of Neurology, 58,* 1803–1809.

McNicoll, L., Pisani, M. A., Zhang, Y., Ely, E. W., Siegel, M. D., & Inouye, S. K. (2003). Delirium in the intensive care unit: Occurrence and clinical course in older patients. *Journal of the American Geriatrics Society, 51*(5), 591–598.

McNulty, J. A., & Caird, W. (1966). Memory loss with age: Retrieval or storage? *Psychological Reports, 19,* 229–230.

Meeks, S., Carstensen, L. L., Stafford, P. B., Brenner, L. L., Weathers, F., Welch, R., et al. (1990). Mental health needs of the chronically mentally ill elderly. *Psychology and Aging, 5,* 163–171.

Mendez, M. F., & Cummings, J. L. (2003). *Dementia: A clinical approach* (3rd ed.). Philadelphia: Butterworth-Heinemann.

Mendez, M. F., Mastri, A. R., Sung, J. H., & Frey, W. H., II. (1992). Clinically diagnosed Alzheimer disease: Neuropathologic findings in 650 cases. *Alzheimer's Disease and Associated Disorders, 6*(1), 35–43.

Mendez, M. F., & Perryman, K. M. (2002). Neuropsychiatric features of frontotemporal dementia: Evaluation of consensus criteria and review. *Journal of Neuropsychiatry and Clinical Neuroscience, 14*(4), 424–429.

Meyer, B. J. F., Young, C. J., & Bartlett, B. J. (1989). *Memory improved: Reading and memory enhancement across the life span through strategic text structures.* Hillsdale, NJ: Erlbaum.

Meyers, B. S., & Greenberg, R. (1986). Late-life delusional depression. *Journal of Affective Disorders, 11,* 133–137.

Miller, B. (1990). Gender differences in spouse caregiver strain: Socialization and role expectation. *Journal of Marriage and the Family, 52,* 311–321.

Miller, L. J. (2004). The role of cholesterol and statins in Alzheimer's disease. *Annals of Pharmacotherapy, 38*(1), 91–98.

Miller, M. D., & Silberman, R. I. (1996). Using interpersonal psychotherapy with depressed elders. In S. H. Zarit & B. G. Knight (Eds.), *A guide to psychotherapy and aging* (pp. 83–100). New York: American Psychological Association.

Milstein, A., Pollack, A., Kleinman, G., & Barak, Y. (2002). Confusion/delirium following cataract surgery: An incidence study of 1-year duration. *International Psychogeriatrics, 14*(3), 301–306.

Mishara, B. L., & Kastenbaum, R. (1980). *Alcohol and old age.* New York: Grune & Stratton.

Mittelman, M. A., Epstein, C., & Peirzchalla, A. (2002). *Counseling the Alzheimer's caregiver: A resource for health care professionals.* Chicago: American Medical Association.

Mittelman, M. S., Ferris, S. H., Shulman, E., Steinberg, G., Ambinder, A., Mackell, J., et al. (1995). A comprehensive support program: Effect on depression in spouse-caregivers of AD patients. *Gerontologist, 35,* 792–802.

Mittelman, M. S., Ferris, S. H., Shulman, E., Steinberg, G., & Levin, B. (1996). A family intervention to delay nursing home placement of patients with Alzheimer disease: A randomized controlled trial. *Journal of the American Medical Association, 276*(21), 1725–1731.

Mittelman, M. S., Roth, D. L., Coon, D. W., & Haley, W. E. (2004). Sustained benefit of supportive intervention for depressive symptoms in caregivers of patients with Alzheimer's disease. *American Journal of Psychiatry, 161*(5), 850–856.

Mohlman, J. (2004). Psychosocial treatment of late-life generalized anxiety disorder: Current status and future directions. *Clinical and Psychological Review, 24*(2), 149–169.

Mohlman, J., Gorenstein, E. E., Kleber, M., deJesus, M., Gorman, J. M., & Papp, L. A. (2003). Standard and enhanced cognitive-behavior therapy for late-life generalized anxiety disorder: Two pilot investigations. *American Journal of Geriatric Psychiatry, 11*(1), 24–32.

Moniz-Cook, E., Agar, S., Gibson, G., Win, T., & Wang, M. (1998). A preliminary study of the effects of early intervention with people with dementia and their families in a memory clinic. *Aging and Mental Health, 2,* 199–211.

Moody, H. R. (1992). A critical view of ethical dilemmas in dementia. In R. H. Binstock, S. G. Post, & P. J. Whitehouse (Eds.), *Dementia and aging: Ethics, values and policy choices* (pp. 86–100). Baltimore: Johns Hopkins University Press.

Moore, K. A., Danks, J. H., Ditto, P. H., Druley, J. A., Townsend, A., & Smucker, W. D. (1994). Elderly outpatients' understanding of a physician-initiated advance directive discussion. *Archives of Family Medicine, 3,* 1057–1063.

Moos, R. H., Brennan, P. L., Schutte, K. K., & Moos, B. S. (2005). Older adults' health and changes in late-life drinking patterns. *Aging and Mental Health, 9*(1), 49–59.

Morgan, D. G. (1992). Neurochemical changes with aging: Predisposition towards age-related mental disorders. In J. E. Birren, R. B. Sloan, & G. D. Cohen (Eds.), *Handbook of mental health and aging* (2nd ed., pp. 175–200). San Diego, CA: Academic Press.

Morgan, L. A., Eckert, J. K., & Lyon, S. M. (1995). *Small board-and-care homes: Residential care in transition.* Baltimore: Johns Hopkins University Press.

Morin, C. M., Colecchi, C., Stone, J., Sood, R., & Brink, D. (1999). Behavioral and pharmacological therapies for late-life insomnia: A randomized controlled trial. *Journal of the American Medical Association, 28*(11), 991–999.

Morris, J. C., Heyman, A., Mohs, R. C., Hughes, J. P., Van Belle, G., Fillenbaum, G. G., et al. (1989). The Consortium to Establish a Registry for Alzheimer's Disease (CERAD). *Neurology, 39,* 1159–1165.

Morris, J. C., McKeel, D. W., Jr., Storandt, M., Rubin, E. H., Price, J. L, Grant, E. A., et al. (1991). Very mild Alzheimer's disease: Informant-based clinical, psychometric, and pathologic distinction from normal aging. *Neurology, 41,* 469–478.

Morris, J. C., Storandt, M., Miller, J. P., McKeel, D. W., Price, J. L., Rubin, E. H., et al. (2001). Mild cognitive impairment represents early-stage Alzheimer disease. *Archives of Neurology, 58,* 397–405.

Morris, M. C., Evans, D. A., Bienias, J. L., Tangney, C. C., Bennett, D. A., Aggarwal, N., et al. (2003). Dietary fats and the risk of incident of Alzheimer disease. *Archives of Neurology, 60,* 194–200.

Morris, M. C., Evans, D. A., Bienias, J. L., Tangney, C. C., Bennett, D. A., Wilson, R. S., et al. (2003). Consumption of fish and n-3 fatty acids and risk of incident Alzheimer disease. *Archives of Neurology, 60*(7), 923–924.

Morrison, J. (1997). *When psychological problems mask medical disorders: A guide for psychotherapists.* New York: Guilford Press.

Moscicki, E. K. (1995). Epidemiology of suicide. *International Psychogeriatrics, 7,* 137–148.

Mossey, J. M., Knott, K. A., Higgins, M., & Talerico, K. (1996). Effectiveness of a psychosocial intervention, interpersonal counseling, for subdysthymic depression in medically ill elderly. *Journal of Gerontology, 51A*(4), M172–M178.

Mowry, B. J., & Burvill, P. W. (1988). A study of mild dementia in the community using a wide range of diagnostic criteria. *British Journal of Psychiatry, 153,* 328–334.

Mroczek, D. K., & Almeida, D. M. (2004). The effect of daily stress, personality, and age on daily negative affect. *Journal of Personality, 72*(2), 355–378.

Mroczek, D. K., & Kolarz, C. M. (1998). The effect of age on positive and negative affect: A developmental perspective on happiness. *Journal of Personality and Social Psychology, 75,* 1333–1349.

Mroczek, D. K., & Spiro, A., III (2003). Modeling intraindividual change in personality traits: Findings from the normative aging study. *Journals of Gerontology: Psychological Sciences, 58,* P153–P165.

Mukamal, K. J., Kuller, L. H., Fitzpatrick, A. L., Longstreth, W. T., Jr., Mittleman, M. A., & Siscovick, D. S. (2003). Prospective study of alcohol consumption and risk of dementia in older adults. *Journal of the American Medical Association, 289*(11), 1405–1413.

Mulsant, B. H., & Pollock, B. G. (2004). Psychopharmacology. In D. G. Blazer, D. C. Steffens, & E. W. Busse (Eds.), *Textbook of geriatric psychiatry* (3rd ed., pp. 387–412). Arlington, VA: American Psychiatric Publishing.

Murden, R. A., McRae, T. D, Kaner, S., & Bucknam, M. E. (1991). Mini-Mental State Exam scores vary with education in blacks and whites. *Journal of the American Geriatrics Society, 39,* 149–155.

Murman, D. L. (2003). Neurologic aspect of prion diseases and frontotemporal dementias. In P. A. Lichtenberg, D. L. Murman, & A. M. Mellow (Eds.), *Handbook of dementia* (pp. 83–114). Hoboken, NJ: Wiley.

Murphy, E. (1994). The course and outcome of depression in late life. In L. S. Schneider, C. F. Reynolds, B. D. Lebowitz, & A. J. Friedhoff (Eds.), *Diagnosis and treatment of depression in late life* (pp. 81–98). Washington, DC: American Psychiatric Press.

Myers, A. J., & Goate, A. M. (2001). The genetics of late-onset Alzheimer's disease. *Current Opinion in Neurology, 14*(4), 433–440.

Myers, R. S., Ball, K. K., Kalina, T. D., Roth, D. L., & Goode, K. T. (2000). Relation of useful field of view and other screening tests to on-road driving performance. *Perception and Motor Skills, 91*(1), 279–290.

Nasar, S. (1998). *A beautiful mind: A biography of John Forbes Nash, Jr.* New York: Simon & Schuster.

National Institute of Aging Task Force. (1980). Senility reconsidered. *Journal of the American Medical Association, 244,* 259–263.

National Institute of Neurological Disorders and Stroke, National Institutes of Health. (2006). *The dementias: Hope through research.* Retrieved from www.ninds.nih. gov/disorders/alzheimersdisease/detail_alzheimersdisease.htm#58683045

National Institute of Neurological Disorders and Stroke, National Institutes of Health. (2006). *NINDS frontotemporal dementia information page.* Bethesda, MD: Author. Retrieved April 26, 2006, at www.ninds.nih.gov/disorders/picks/ picks.htm#What_is

National Institute on Alcohol Abuse and Alcoholism. (2005). *Harmful interactions: Mixing alcohol with medications.* Retrieved from http://pubs.niaaa.nih.gov/publications/Medicine/medicine.htm

National Institutes of Health. (1987). Differential diagnosis of dementing diseases. *Consensus Development Conference Statement, 6,* 6–9.

National Institutes of Health Consensus Development Program. (2004). *National Institutes of Health State-of-the-Science Conference statement on improving end-of-life care.* Retrieved June 20, 2005, from www.consensus.nih.gov/2004/2004-EndOfLifeCareSOS024html.htm

Neary, D. (1990). Dementia of frontal lobe type. *Journal of the American Geriatrics Society, 38,* 71–72.

Neary, D., Snowden, J. S., Gustafson, L., Passant, U., Stuss, D., Black, S., et al. (1998). Frontotemporal lobar degeneration: A consensus on clinical diagnostic criteria. *Neurology, 51*(6), 1546–1554.

Neikrug, S. M. (2003). Worrying about a frightening old age. *Aging and Mental Health, 7*(5), 326–333.

Nelson, H. E. (1976). A modified card sorting test sensitive to frontal lobe defects. *Cortex, 12,* 313–324.

Neugarten, B. L. (1974). Age groups in American society and the rise of the young-old. *Annals of the American Academy of Political and Social Science, 415,* 187–198.

Neugarten, B. L., Moore, J. W., & Lowe, J. C. (1968). Age norms, age constraints, and adult socialization. In B. L. Neugarten (Ed.), *Middle age and aging: A reader in social psychology* (pp. 22–28). Chicago: University of Chicago Press.

Newman, A. B., Fitzpatrick, A. L., Lopez, O., Jackson, S., Lyketsos, C., Jagust, W., et al. (2005). Dementia and Alzheimer's disease incidence in relationship to cardiovascular disease in the cardiovascular health study cohort. *Journal of the American Geriatrics Society, 53*(7), 1257–1258.

Newman, M. F., Kirchner, J. L., Phillips-Bute, B., Gaver, V., Grocott, H., Jones, R. H., et al. (2001). Longitudinal assessment of neurocognitive function after coronary-artery bypass surgery. *New England Journal of Medicine, 344*(6), 395–402.

Newmann, J. P., Engel, R. J., & Jensen, J. E. (1991). Changes in depressive-symptom experiences among older women. *Psychology and Aging, 6*, 212–222.

Niederehe, G., & Yoder, C. (1989). Metamemory perceptions in depressions of young and older adults. *Journal of Nervous and Mental Disease, 177*, 4–14.

Nordhus, I. H., & Pallesen, S. (2003). Psychological treatment of late-life anxiety: An empirical review. *Journal of Consulting and Clinical Psychology, 71*(4), 643–651.

Norris, M. P., MacNeill, S. E., & Haines, M. E. (2003). Psychological and neuropsychological aspects of vascular and mixed dementia. In P. A. Lichtenberg, D. L. Murman, & A. M. Mellow (Eds.), *Handbook of dementia* (pp. 173–196). Hoboken, NJ: Wiley.

Nuland, S. B. (1993). *How we die: Reflections on life's final chapter.* New York: Knopf.

Nuti, A., Ceravolo, R., Piccinni, A., Dell'Agnello, G., Bellini, G., Gambaccini, G., et al. (2004). Psychiatric comorbidity in a population of Parkinson's disease patients. *European Journal of Neurology, 11*(5), 315–320.

Ober, B. A., Dronkers, N. F., Koss, E., Delis, D. C., & Friedland, R. P. (1986). Retrieval from semantic memory in Alzheimer-type dementia. *Journal of Clinical and Experimental Neuropsychology, 8*, 75–92.

O'Brien, J. T., Erkinjuntti, T., Reisberg, B., Roman, G., Sawada, T., Pantoni, L., et al. (2003). Vascular cognitive impairment. *Lancet Neurology, 2*(2), 89–98.

O'Connell, H., Chin, A., Cunningham, C., & Lawlor, B. (2003). Alcohol use disorders in elderly people: Redefining an age-old problem in old age. *British Medical Journal, 327*, 664–667.

O'Connor, M. K., Knapp, R., Husain, M., Rummans, T. A., Petrides, G., Smith, G., et al. (2001). The influence of age on the response of major depression to electroconvulsive therapy: A C.O.R.E. report. *American Journal of Geriatric Psychiatry, 9*(4), 382–390.

Odenheimer, G. L., Beaudet, M., Jette, A. M., Albert, M. S., Grande, L., & Minaker, K. L. (1994). Performance-based driving evaluation of the elderly driver: Safety, reliability, and validity. *Journal of Gerontology, 49*, M153–M159.

Orne, M. T., & Wender, P. H. (1968). Anticipatory socialization for psychotherapy. *American Journal of Psychiatry, 124*, 1201–1212.

Orrell, M., Spector, A., Thorgrimsen, L., & Woods, B. (2005). A pilot study examining the effectiveness of Maintenance Cognitive Stimulation Therapy (MCST) for people with dementia. *International Journal of Geriatric Psychiatry, 20*(5), 446–451.

Ortiz, D., & Shea, T. B. (2004). Apple juice prevents oxidative stress induced by amyloid-beta in culture. *Journal of Alzheimer's Disease, 6*(1), 27–30.

Osterrieth, P. A. (1944). Le test de copie d'une figure complexe. *Archives de Psychologie, 30*, 206–356.

Ott, A., Breteler, M. M., van Harskamp, F., Claus, J. J., van der Cammen, T. J., Grobbee, D. E., et al. (1995). Prevalence of Alzheimer's disease and vascular dementia: Association with education. The Rotterdam study. *British Medical Journal, 310*, 970–973.

Owsley, C., Ball, K., McGwin, G., Jr., Sloane, M. E., Roenker, D. L., White, M. F., et al. (1998). Visual processing impairment and risk of motor vehicle crash among older adults. *Journal of the American Medical Association, 279*(14), 1083–1088.

Pantoni, L., Leys, D., Fazekas, F., Longstreth, W. T., Jr., Inzitari, D., Wallin, A., et al. (1999). Role of white matter lesions in cognitive impairment of vascular origin. *Alzheimer's Disease and Associated Disorders, 13*(3), S49–S54.

Parkinson, S. R., & Perey, A. (1980). Aging, digit span, and the stimulus suffix effect. *Journal of Gerontology, 35,* 736–742.

Parks, R. W., Zec, R. F., & Wilson, R. S. (Eds.). (1993). *Neuropsychology of Alzheimer's disease and other dementias.* New York: Oxford University Press.

Parmalee, P. A., Katz, I. R., & Lawton, M. P. (1992). Incidence of depression in long-term care settings. *Journal of Gerontology, 47,* M189–M196.

Parmelee, P. A., & Lawton, M. P. (1990). The design of special environments for the aged. In J. E. Birren & K. W. Schaie (Eds.), *Handbook of the psychology of aging* (3rd ed., pp. 464–488). San Diego, CA: Academic Press.

Patient Self-Determination Act. Sections 4206 and 4751 of OBRA, 1990, Public Law 101-508.

Paykel, E. S. (1974). Recent life events and clinical depression. In E. K. E. Gunderson & R. H. Rahe (Eds.), *Life stress and illness* (pp. 134–163). Springfield, IL: Thomas.

Paykel, E. S. (1982). Life events and early environment. In E. S. Paykel (Ed.), *Handbook of affective disorders* (pp. 146–161). New York: Guilford Press.

Payne, J. L., Sheppard, J. M., Steinberg, M., Warren, A., Baker, A., Steele, C., et al. (2002). Incidence, prevalence, and outcomes of depression in residents of a long-term care facility with dementia. *International Journal of Geriatric Psychiatry, 17*(3) 247–253.

Pearlin, L. I., Mullan, J. T., Semple, S. J., & Skaff, M. M. (1990). Caregiving and the stress process: An overview of concepts and their measures. *Gerontologist, 30*(5), 583–594.

Pearman, A., & Storandt, M. (2004). Predictors of subjective memory in older adults. *Journals of Gerontology: Psychological Sciences, 59*(1): P4–6.

Peisah, C., Sachdev, P., & Brodaty, H. (1993). Vascular dementia. *International Review of Psychiatry, 5,* 381–395.

Penninx, B. W., Rejeski, W. J., Pandya, J., Miller, M. E., DiBari, M., Applegate, W. B., et al. (2002). Exercise and depressive symptoms: A comparison of aerobic and resistance exercise effects on emotional and physical function in older persons with high and low depressive symptomatology. *Journals of Gerontology: Psychological Sciences, 57B*(2), P124–P132.

Perlmutter, M. (1978). What is memory aging the aging of? *Developmental Psychology, 14,* 330–345.

Petersen, R. C., Smith, G. E., Waring, S. C., Ivnik, R. J., Tangalos, E. G., & Kokmen, E. (1999). Mild cognitive impairment: Clinical characterization and outcome. *Archives of Neurology, 56*(3), 303–308.

Petersen, R. C., Thomas, R. G., Grundman, M., Bennett, D., Doody, R., Ferris, S., et al. (2005). Vitamin E and donepezil for the treatment of mild cognitive impairment. *New England Journal of Medicine, 352*(23), 2439–2441.

Pfeiffer, E. (1975). A short portable mental status questionnaire for the assessment of organic brain deficit in elderly patients. *Journal of the American Geriatrics Society, 23,* 433–439.

Piguet, O., Ridley, L., Grayson, D. A., Bennett, H. P., Creasey, H., Lye, T. C., et al. (2003). Are MRI white matter lesions clinically significant in the "old-old"? Evidence from the Sidney Older Persons Study. *Dementia and Geriatric Cognitive Disorders, 15,* 143–150.

Pinkston, E. M., & Linsk, N. L. (1984). Behavioral family intervention with the impaired elderly. *Gerontologist, 24,* 576–583.

Pirozzolo, F. J., Hansch, E. C., Mortimer, J. A., Webster, D. D., & Kuskowski, M. A. (1982). Dementia in Parkinson disease: A neuropsychological analysis. *Brain and Cognition, 1,* 71–83.

Pisani, M. A., McNicoll, L., & Inouye, S. K. (2003). Cognitive impairment in the intensive care unit. *Clinics in Chest Medicine, 24*(4), 727–737.

Plomin, R., Pedersen, N. L., McClearn, G. E., Nesselroade, J. R., & Bergeman, C. S. (1988). EAS temperaments during the last half of the life span: Twins reared apart and twins reared together. *Psychology and Aging, 3,* 43–50.

Pollan, S. M., & Levine, M. (2004). *Second acts: Creating the life you really want: Building the career you truly desire.* New York: HarperCollins.

Pompei, P., Foreman, M., Rudberg, M. A., Inouye, S. K., Braund, V., & Casel, C. K. (1994). Delirium in hospitalized older persons: Outcomes and predictors. *Journal of the American Geriatrics Society, 42,* 809–815.

Popkin, S. J., Gallagher, D., Thompson, L. W., & Moore, M. (1982). Memory complaint and performance in normal and depressed older adults. *Experimental Aging Research, 8,* 141–145.

Post, F. (1966). *Persistent persecutory states in the elderly.* New York: Pergamon Press.

Post, F. (1973). Paranoid disorders in the elderly. *Postgraduate Medicine, 53,* 52–56.

Post, F. (1980). Paranoid, schizophrenia-like and schizophrenic states in the aged. In J. E. Birren & R. B. Sloane (Eds.), *Handbook of mental health and aging* (pp. 591–615). Englewood Cliffs, NJ: Prentice-Hall.

Post, S. G., Whitehouse, P. J., Binstock, R. H., Bird, T. D., Eckert, S. K., Farrer, L. A., et al. (1997). The clinical introduction of genetic testing for Alzheimer disease: An ethical perspective. *Journal of the American Medical Association, 277,* 832–836.

Preston, J. D., O'Neal, J. H., & Talaga, M. C. (2002). *Handbook of clinical psychopharmacology for therapists* (3rd ed.). Oakland, CA: New Harbinger.

Preston, T., & Kelly, M. (2006). A medical ethics assessment of the case of Terri Schiavo. *Death Studies, 30*(2), 121–133.

Qiu, C., von Strauss, E., Fasborn, J., Winblad, B., & Fratiglioni, L. (2003). Low blood pressure and risk of dementia in the Kungsholmen Project. *Archives of Neurology, 60,* 223–228.

Quayhagen, M. P., & Quayhagen, M. (1989). Differential effects of family-based strategies on Alzheimer's disease. *Gerontologist, 29,* 150–155.

Rabins, P., McHugh, P. R., Pauker, S., & Thomas, J. (1987). The clinical features of late onset schizophrenia. In N. E. Miller & G. D. Cohen (Eds.), *Schizophrenia and aging: Schizophrenia, paranoia, and schizophreniform disorders in later life* (pp. 235–238). New York: Guilford Press.

Rabins, P. V. (1992). Schizophrenia and psychotic states. In J. E. Birren, R. B. Sloane, G. D. Cohen, N. R. Hooyman, B. D. Lebowitz, M. Wykle, & D. E. Deutchman

(Eds.), *Handbook of mental health and aging* (2nd ed., pp. 464–475). New York: Academic Press.

Rabins, P. V., Lyketsos, C. G., & Steele, C. D. (1999). *Practical dementia care.* New York: Oxford University Press.

Rabins, P. V., Merchant, A., & Nestadt, G. (1984). Criteria for diagnosing reversible dementia caused by depression. *British Journal of Psychiatry, 144,* 488–492.

Radloff, L. S. (1977). The CES-D Scale: A self-report depression scale for research in the general population. *Applied Psychological Measurement, 1,* 385–401.

Randolph, C., Tierney, M. C., Mohr, E., & Chase, T. N. (1998). The Repeatable Battery for the Assessment of Neuropsychological Status (RBANS): Preliminary clinical validity. *Journal of Clinical and Experimental Neuropsychology, 20*(3), 310–319.

Rank, M. R., & Hirschl, T. A. (1999). Estimating the proportion of Americans ever experiencing poverty during their elderly years. *Journals of Gerontology: Social Sciences, 54,* S184–S193.

Raskind, M. A., Carta, A., & Bravi, D. (1995). Is early-onset Alzheimer disease a distinct subgroup within the Alzheimer disease population? *Alzheimer's Disease and Associated Disorders, 9*(Suppl. 1), S2–S6.

Ratnavalli, E., Brayne, C., Dawson, K., & Hodges, J. R. (2002). The prevalence of frontotemporal dementia. *Neurology, 58,* 1615–1621.

Reger, M. A., Welsh, R. K., Watson, G. S., Cholerton, B., Baker, L. D., & Craft, S. (2004). The relationship between neuropsychological functioning and driving ability in dementia: A meta-analysis. *Neuropsychology, 18*(1), 85–93.

Regestein, Q. R. (1992). Treatment of insomnia in the elderly. In C. Salzman (Ed.), *Clinical geriatric psychopharmacology* (2nd ed., pp. 236–254). Baltimore: Williams & Wilkins.

Regier, D. A., Boyd, J. H., Burke, J. D., Jr., Rae, D. S., Myers, J. K., Kraemer, M., et al. (1988). One-month prevalence of mental disorders in the United States. *Archives of General Psychiatry, 45,* 977–986.

Reifler, B. V., Larson, E., & Hanley, R. (1982). Coexistence of cognitive impairment and depression in geriatric outpatients. *American Journal of Psychiatry, 139,* 623–626.

Reifler, B. V., Larson, E., Teri, L., & Poulsen, M. (1986). Dementia of the Alzheimer's type and depression. *Journal of the American Geriatrics Society, 34,* 855–859.

Reifler, B. V., Teri, L., Raskind, M., Veith, R., Barnes, R., White, E., et al. (1989). Double-blind trial of imipramine in Alzheimer's disease patients with and without depression. *American Journal of Psychiatry, 146,* 45–49.

Reisberg, B., Doody, R., Stöffler, A., Schmitt, F., Ferris, S., Möbius, J., et al. (2003). Memantine in moderate-to-severe Alzheimer's disease. *New England Journal of Medicine, 348,* 1333–1341.

Reisberg, B., Ferris, S. H., de Leon, M. J., & Crook, T. (1982). The Global Deterioration Scale for the assessment of primary degenerative dementia. *American Journal of Psychiatry, 139,* 1136–1139.

Reitan, R. M. (1958). Validity of the Trail Making Test as an indication of organic brain damage. *Perceptual and Motor Skills, 8,* 271–276.

Reynolds, C. F., III, Frank, E., Perel, J. M., Imber, S. D., Cornes, C., Miller, M. D., et al. (1999). Nortriptyline and interpersonal psychotherapy as maintenance therapies for recurrent major depression: A randomized controlled trial in patients older than 59 years. *Journal of the American Medical Association, 281,* 39–45.

Reynolds, C. F., III, Frank, E., Perel, J. M., Imber, S. D., Cornes, C., Morycz, R. K., et al. (1992). Combined pharmacotherapy and psychotherapy in the acute and continuation treatment of elderly patients with recurrent major depression: A preliminary report. *American Journal of Psychiatry, 149*(12), 1687–1692.

Rhoden, N. K. (1988). Litigating life and death. *Harvard Law Review, 102,* 375–446.

Rilling, L. M., Lucas, J. A., Ivnik, R. J., Smith, G. E., Willis, F. B., Ferman, T. J., et al. (2005). Mayo's older African American normative studies: Norms for the Mattis Dementia Rating Scale. *Clinical Neuropsychology, 19*(2), 229–242.

Ritchie, K., Artero, S., Beluche, I., Ancelin, M. L., Mann, A., Dupuy, A. M., et al. (2004). Prevalence of DSM-IV psychiatric disorder in the French elderly populations. *British Journal of Psychiatry, 184,* 147–152.

Ritchie, K., Artero, S., & Touchon, J. (2001). Classification criteria for mild cognitive impairment: A population-based validation study. *Neurologia, 56,* 37–42.

Roach, G. W., Kanchuger, M., Mangano, C. M., Newman, M., Nussmeier, N., Wolman, R., et al. (1996). Adverse cerebral outcomes after coronary bypass surgery: Multicenter Study of Perioperative Ischemia Research Group and the Ischemia Research and Education Foundation Investigators. *New England Journal of Medicine, 335,* 1857–1863

Robertsson, B. (2002). The instrumentation of delirium. In J. Lindesay, K. Rockwood, & A. Macdonald (Eds.), *Delirium in old age* (pp. 9–26). New York: Oxford University Press.

Robinson, L. A., Berman, J. S., & Neimeyer, R. A. (1990). Psychotherapy for the treatment of depression: A comprehensive review of controlled outcome research. *Psychological Bulletin, 108,* 30–49.

Robison, J., Curry, L., Gruman, C., Covington, T., Gaztambide, S., & Blank, K. (2003). Depression in later-life Puerto Rican primary care patients: The role of illness, stress, social integration, and religiosity. *International Psychogeriatrics, 15*(3), 239–251.

Rockwood, K., Goodman, J., Flynn, M., & Stolee, P. (1996). Cross-validation of the delirium rating scale in older patients. *Journal of the American Geriatrics Society, 44,* 839–842.

Rogers, C. R. (1951). *Client-centered therapy: Its current practice, implications, and theory.* Boston: Houghton Mifflin.

Román, G. C. (2003). Neurologic aspects of vascular dementia: Basic concepts, diagnosis, and management. In P. A. Lichtenberg, D. L. Murman, & A. M. Mellow (Eds.), *Handbook of dementia* (pp. 149–172). Hoboken, NJ: Wiley.

Román, G. C., Tatemichi, T. K., Erkinjuntti, T., Cummings, J. L., Masedeu, J. C., Garcia, J. H., et al. (1993). Vascular dementia: Diagnostic criteria for research studies: Report of the NINDS-AIREN International Workshop. *Neurology, 43,* 250–260.

Rosen, H. J., Hartikainen, K. M., Jagust, W., Kramer, J. H., Reed, B. R., Cummings, J. L., et al. (2002). Utility of clinical criteria in differentiating frontotemporal lobar degeneration (FTLD) from AD. *Neurology, 58,* 1608–1615.

Rosenthal, C., & Dawson, P. (1991). Wives of institutionalized elderly men: The first stage of the transition to quasi-widowhood. *Journal of Aging and Health, 3,* 315–334.

Ross, C. A., Peyser, C. E., Shapiro, I., & Folstein, M. F. (1991). Delirium: Phenotypic and etiologic subtypes. *International Psychogeriatrics, 3,* 135–145.

Roth, M. (1955). The natural history of mental disorder in old age. *Journal of Mental Science, 101,* 281–289.

Roth, M. (1987). Late paraphrenia: Phenomenology and etiological factors and their bearing upon problems of the schizophrenic family of disorders. In N. E. Miller & G. D. Cohen (Eds.), *Schizophrenia and aging: Schizophrenia, paranoia, and schizophreniform disorders in later life* (pp. 217–234). New York: Guilford Press.

Roth, M. (1991). Clinical perspectives. *International Psychogeriatrics, 3,* 309–317.

Roth, M., & Myers, D. H. (1975). The diagnosis of dementia. *British Journal of Psychiatry, 9,* 87–99.

Rovner, B. W., Kafonek, S., Filipp, L., Lucas, M. J., & Folstein, M. F. (1986). Prevalence of mental illness in a community nursing home. *American Journal of Psychiatry, 143,* 1446–1449.

Rowe, J. W., & Kahn, R. L. (1987). Human aging: Usual and successful. *Science, 237,* 143–149.

Rowe, J. W., & Kahn, R. L. (1997). Successful aging. *Gerontologist, 37*(4), 433–440.

Roy-Byrne, P. P., Craske, M. G., Stein, M. B., Sullivan, G., Bystritsky, A., Katon, W., et al. (2005). A randomized effectiveness trial of cognitive-behavioral therapy and medication for primary care panic disorder. *Archives of General Psychiatry, 62*(3), 290–298.

Rubin, K. H., Bukowski, W., & Parker, J. (1998). Peer interactions, relationships, and groups. In W. Damon & N. Eisenberg (Eds.), *Handbook of child psychology: Vol. 4. Child psychology in practice* (5th ed., pp. 619–700). New York: Wiley.

Rusin, M. J., & Lawson, K. J. (2001). Behavioral interventions and families: A medical rehabilitation perspective. *Journal of Clinical Geropsychology, 7*(4), 255–269.

Ryan, J. J., Paolo, A. M., & Brungardt, T. M. (1990). Standardization of the Wechsler Adult Intelligence Scale—Revised for persons 75 years and older. *Psychological Assessment: A Journal of Consulting and Clinical Psychology, 2,* 404–411.

Rybarczyk, B., Lopez, M., Benson, R., Alsten, C., & Stepanski, E. (2002). Efficacy of two behavioral treatment programs for comorbid geriatric insomnia. *Psychology and Aging, 17,* 288–298.

Ryff, C. D. (1989). Happiness is everything, or is it?: Explorations on the meaning of psychological well-being. *Journal of Personality and Social Psychology, 57,* 1069–1081.

Sabatino, C. P. (1996). Competency: Refining our legal fictions. In M. A. Smyer, K. W. Schaie, & M. B. Kapp (Eds.), *Older adults' decision-making and the law* (pp. 1–28). New York: Springer.

Sackeim, H. A. (1992). The cognitive effects of electroconvulsive therapy. In W. H. Moos, E. R. Gamzu, & L. J. Thal (Eds.), *Cognitive disorders: Pathophysiology and treatment* (pp. 183–228). New York: Dekker.

Sackeim, H. A. (1994). Use of electroconvulsive therapy in late-life depression. In L. S. Schneider, C. F. Reynolds, B. D. Lebowitz, & A. J. Friedhoff (Eds.), *Diagnosis and treatment of depression in late life* (pp. 259–278). Washington, DC: American Psychiatric Press.

Sackeim, H. A., Haskett, R. F., Mulsant, B. H., Thase, M. E., Mann, J. J., Pettinati, H. M., et al. (2001). Continuation pharmacotherapy in the prevention of relapse following electroconvulsive therapy: A randomized controlled trial. *Journal of the American Medical Association, 285*(10), 1299–1307.

Sadavoy, J., & Fogel, B. (1992). Personality disorders in old age. In J. E. Birren, R. B. Sloane, G. D. Cohen, N. R. Hooyman, B. D. Lebowitz, M. Wykle, & D. E. Deutchman (Eds.), *Handbook of mental health and aging* (2nd ed., pp. 433–463). New York: Academic Press.

Sakauye, K. M., Camp, C. J., & Ford, P. A. (1993). Effects of buspirone on agitation associated with dementia. *American Journal of Geriatric Psychiatry, 1,* 82–84.

Salmon, D. P., Thal, L. J., Butters, N., & Heindel, W. C. (1990). Longitudinal evaluation of dementia of the Alzheimer type: A comparison of 3 standardized mental status examinations. *Neurology, 40,* 1225–1230.

Salokangas, R. K., Honkonen, T., & Saarinen, S. (2003). Women have later onset than men in schizophrenia—but only in its paranoid form: Results of the DSP project. *European Psychiatry, 18*(6), 274–281.

Salthouse, T. A. (1984). Effects of age and skill in typing. *Journal of Experimental Psychology: General, 113,* 345–371.

Salthouse, T. A. (1990). Cognitive competence and expertise in aging. In J. E. Birren & K. W. Schaie (Eds.), *Handbook of the psychology of aging* (3rd ed., pp. 310–391). New York: Academic Press.

Salthouse, T. A. (1994a). The aging of working memory. *Neuropsychology, 8,* 535–543.

Salthouse, T. A. (1994b). The nature of the influence of speed on adult age differences in cognition. *Developmental Psychology, 30,* 240–259.

Salthouse, T. A., & Babcock, R. L. (1991). Decomposing adult age differences in working memory. *Developmental Psychology, 27,* 763–776.

Salzman, C. (1992). Treatment of anxiety. In C. Salzman (Ed.), *Clinical geriatric psychopharmacology* (2nd ed., pp. 189–212). Baltimore: Williams & Wilkins.

Salzman, C. (1993). Pharmacologic treatment of depression in the elderly. *Journal of Clinical Psychiatry, 54*(2, Suppl.), 23–27.

Salzman, C. S. (1994). Pharmacological treatment of depression in elderly patients. In L. S. Schneider, C. F. Reynolds, B. D. Lebowitz, & A. J. Friedhoff (Eds.), *Diagnosis and treatment of depression in late life* (pp. 181–206). Washington, DC: American Psychiatric Press.

Samuels, J. F., Nestadt, G., Romanoski, A. J., Folstein, M. F., & McHugh, P. R. (1994). DSM-III personality disorders in the community. *American Journal of Psychiatry, 151,* 1055–1062.

Sandberg, O., Gustafson, Y., Brannstrom, B., & Buch, G. (1999). Clinical profile of delirium in older patients. *Journal of the American Geriatrics Society, 47,* 1300–1306.

Santos, F. S., Velasco, I. T., & Fráguas, R., Jr. (2004). Risk factors for delirium in the elderly after coronary artery bypass graft surgery. *International Psychogeriatrics, 16*(2), 175–193.

Schaie, K. W. (1967). Age changes and age differences. *Gerontologist, 7,* 128–132.

Schaie, K. W. (1983). The Seattle Longitudinal Study: A twenty-one-year exploration of psychometric intelligence in adulthood. In K. W. Schaie (Ed.), *Longitudinal studies of adult psychological development* (pp. 64–135). New York: Guilford Press.

Schaie, K. W. (1985). *Manual for the Schaie–Thurstone Adult Mental Abilities Test (STAMAT).* Palo Alto, CA: Consulting Psychologists Press.

Schaie, K. W. (1995). Intellectual development in adulthood. In J. E. Birren & K. W. Schaie (Eds.), *Handbook of the psychology of aging* (4th ed., pp. 266–286). New York: Academic Press.

Schaie, K. W. (1996). *Intellectual development in adulthood: The Seattle Longitudinal Study.* Cambridge, UK: Cambridge University Press.

Schaie, K. W. (2005). *Developmental influences on adult intelligence: The Seattle longitudinal study.* New York: Oxford University Press.

Schaie, K. W., & Hertzog, C. (1986). Toward a comprehensive model of adult intellectual development: Contributions of the Seattle Longitudinal Study. In R. J. Sternberg (Ed.), *Advances in human intelligence* (Vol. 3, pp. 79–118). Hillsdale, NJ: Erlbaum.

Schaie, K. W., & Hofer, S. M. (2001). Longitudinal studies in aging research. In J. E. Birren & K. W. Schaie (Eds.), *Handbook of the psychology of aging* (5th ed., pp. 53–77). San Diego, CA: Academic Press.

Schaie, K. W., & Labouvie-Vief, G. (1974). Generational versus ontogenetic components of change in adult cognitive behavior: A fourteen-year cross-sequential study. *Developmental Psychology, 10,* 305–320.

Schaie, K. W., & Willis, S. L. (1986). Can intellectual decline in the elderly be reversed? *Developmental Psychology, 22,* 223–232.

Schaie, K. W., & Willis, S. L. (2002). *Adult development and aging* (5th ed.). Upper Saddle River, NJ: Prentice-Hall.

Schellenberg, G. D., Bird, T. D., Wijsman, E. M., Orr, H. T., Anderson, L., Nemens, E., et al. (1992). Genetic linkage evidence for a familial Alzheimer's disease locus on chromosome 14. *Science, 258,* 668–671.

Schmidt, M. L., Martin, J. A., Lee, V. M., & Trojanowski, J. Q. (1996). Convergence of Lewy bodies and neurofibrillary tangles in amygdala neurons of Alzheimer's disease and Lewy body disorders. *Acta Neuropathologica, 91,* 475–481.

Schmidt, R., Fazekas, F., Offenbacher, H., Dusek, T., Zach, E., Reinhart, B., et al. (1993). Neuropsychologic correlates of MRI white matter hyperintensities: A study of 150 normal volunteers. *Neurology, 43,* 2490–2494.

Schneider, L. S. (1996). Meta-analysis of controlled pharmacologic trials. *International Psychogeriatrics, 8,* 375–380.

Schneider, L. S., & Olin, J. T. (1995). Efficacy of acute treatment for geriatric depression. *International Psychogeriatrics, 7,* 7–26.

Schneider, L. S., Pollock, V. E., & Lyness, S. A. (1990). A meta-analysis of controlled trials of neuroleptic treatment in dementia. *Journal of the American Geriatrics Society, 38,* 553–563.

Schnelle, J. F., Newman, D. R., & Fogarty, T. (1990). Management of patient continence in long-term-care nursing facilities. *Gerontologist, 30,* 373–376.

Schnelle, J. F., Traughber, B., Sowell, V. A., Newman, D. R., Petrill, C. O., & Ory, M. (1989). Prompted voiding treatment of urinary incontinence in nursing home patients: A behavior management approach for nursing home staff. *Journal of the American Geriatrics Society, 31,* 1051–1057.

Schoeni, R. F., Freedman, V. A., & Wallace, R. B. (2001). Persistent, consistent, widespread, and robust? Another look at recent trends in old-age disability. *Journals of Gerontology: Social Sciences, 56B,* S206–S218.

Schofield, P. W., Tang, M., Marder, K., Bell, K., Dooneief, G., Chun, M., et al. (1997). Alzheimer's disease after remote head injury: An incidence study. *Journal of Neurology, Neurosurgery and Psychiatry, 62,* 119–124.

Schonfield, D., & Robertson, B. A. (1966). Memory storage and aging. *Canadian Journal of Psychology, 20,* 228–236.

Schooler, C., Mulatu, M. S., & Oates, G. (1999). The continuing effects of substantively complex work on the intellectual functioning of older workers. *Psychology and Aging, 14,* 483–506.

Schulz, R., & Beach, S. R. (1999). Caregiving as a risk factor for mortality: The Caregiver Health Effects Study. *Journal of the American Medical Association, 282,* 2215–2219.

Schulz, R., & Heckhausen, J. (1999). Aging, culture and control: Setting a new research agenda. *Journals of Gerontology: Psychological Science, 54,* P139–P145.

Schulz, R., O'Brien, A. T., Bookwala, J., & Fleissner, K. (1995). Psychiatric and physical morbidity effects of dementia caregiving: Prevalence, correlates, and causes. *Gerontologist, 35,* 771–791.

Scogin, F. (2000). *The first session with seniors: A step-by-step guide.* San Francisco: Jossey-Bass.

Scogin, F., Jamison, C., & Gochneaur, K. (1989). Comparative efficacy of cognitive and behavioral bibliotherapy for mildly and moderately depressed older adults. *Journal of Consulting and Clinical Psychology, 57,* 403–407.

Scogin, F., & McElreath, L. (1994). Efficacy of psychosocial treatments for geriatric depression: A quantitative review. *Journal of Consulting and Clinical Psychology, 62,* 69–74.

Scogin, F., Rickard, H. C., Keith, S., Wilson, J., & McElreath, L. (1992). Progressive and imaginal relaxation training for elderly persons with subjective anxiety. *Psychology and Aging, 7,* 419–424.

Segal, D. L., Hersen, M., Van Hasselt, V. B., Silberman, C. S., & Roth, L. (1996). Diagnosis and assessment of personality disorders in older adults: A critical review. *Journal of Personality Disorders, 10*(4), 384–399.

Seligman, M. (1975). *Helplessness: On depression, development and death.* San Francisco: Freeman.

Seligman, M. (1991). *Learned optimism.* New York: Knopf.

Semple, S. J. (1992). Conflict in Alzheimer's caregiving families: Its dimensions and consequences. *Gerontologist, 32,* 648–655.

Settersten, R. H. (1999). *Lives in time and place: The problems and promises of developmental science.* Amityville, NY: Baywood.

Shea, D., Streit, A., & Smyer, M. (1994). Use of specialist mental health services by nursing home residents. *Health Services Research, 29,* 169–185.

Shea, D. G. (2003). Swimming upstream: Geriatric mental health workforce. *Public Policy and Aging Report, 13*(2), 3–7.

Shelton, R. C., Keller, M. B., Gelenbert, A., Dunner, D. L., Hirschfeld, R., Thase, M. E., et al. (2001). Effectiveness of St. John's wort in major depression: A randomized controlled trial. *Journal of the American Medical Association, 285*(15), 1978–1986.

Shuchter, S. R., Downs, N., & Zisook, S. (1996). *Biologically informed psychotherapy for depression.* New York: Guilford Press.

Shumaker, S. A., Legault, C., Thal, L., Wallace, R. B., Ockene, J. K., Hendrix, S. L., et al. (2003). Estrogen plus progestin and the incidence of dementia and mild cognitive impairment in postmenopausal women. *Journal of the American Medical Association, 289*(20), 2651–2662.

Siegler, I. C. (1983). Psychological aspects of the Duke Longitudinal Studies. In K. W. Schaie (Ed.), *Longitudinal studies of adult psychological development* (pp. 136–190). New York: Guilford Press.

Siegler, I. C., George, L. K., & Okun, M. A. (1979). Cross-sequential analysis of adult personality. *Developmental Psychology, 15*, 350–351.

Sims, R. V., McGwin, G., Jr., Allman, R. M., Ball, K., & Owsley, C. (2000). Exploratory study of incident vehicle crashes among older drivers. *Journals of Gerontology: Medical Sciences, 55*(1), M22–M27.

Sink, K. M., Holden, K. F., & Yaffe, K. (2005). Pharmacological treatment of neuropsychiatric symptoms of dementia: A review of the evidence. *Journal of the American Medical Association, 293*(5), 596–608.

Skaff, M. M., & Pearlin, L. I. (1992). Caregiving: Role engulfment and the loss of self. *Gerontologist, 32*(5), 656–664.

Skene, L. (2005). The Schiavo and Korp cases: Conceptualising end-of-life decisionmaking. *Journal of Law and Medicine, 13*(2), 223–229.

Skoog, I. (1994). Risk factors for vascular dementia: A review. *Dementia, 5*, 137–144.

Skoog, I. (2003). Hypertension and cognition. *International Psychogeriatrics, 15*(1), 139–146.

Skoog, I., Berg, S., Johansson, B., Palmertz, B., & Andreasson, L.-A. (1996). The influence of white matter lesions on neuropsychological functioning in demented and nondemented 85-year-olds. *Acta Neurologica Scandinavica, 93*, 142–148.

Skoog, I., Nilsson, L., Palmertz, B., Andreasson, L. A., & Svanborg, A. (1993). A population-based study of dementia in 85-year-olds. *New England Journal of Medicine, 328*, 153–158.

Sliwinski, M., Lipton, R. B., Buschke, H., & Stewart, W. F. (1996). The effect of preclinical dementia on estimates of normal cognitive function in aging. *Journals of Gerontology: Psychological Sciences, 51B*, P217–P225.

Sloane, P. D., Davidson, S., Buckwalter, K., Lindsey, B. A., Ayers, S., Lenker, V., et al. (1997). Management of the patient with disruptive vocalization. *Gerontologist, 37*(5), 675–682.

Sloane, P. D., Hoeffer, B., Mitchell, C. M., McKenzie, D. A., Barrick, A. L., Rader, J., et al. (2004). Effect of person-centered showering and the towel bath on bathing-associated aggression, agitation, and discomfort in nursing home residents with dementia: A randomized, controlled trial. *Journal of the American Geriatrics Society, 52*(11), 1795–1804.

Sloane, P. D., & Mathew, L. J. (1991). *Dementia units in long-term care*. Baltimore: Johns Hopkins University Press.

Small, B. J., Hertzog, C., Hultsch, D. F., & Dixon, R. A. (2003). Stability and change in adult personality over 6 years: Findings from the Victoria Longitudinal Study. *Journals of Gerontology: Psychological Science, 58*, P166–P176.

Smith, A. D. (1996). Memory. In J. E. Birren & K. W. Schaie (Eds.), *Handbook of the psychology of aging* (4th ed., pp. 236–250). San Diego, CA: Academic Press.

Smith, D. (2003). *The older population in the United States: March 2002*. Washington, DC: U.S. Census Bureau.

Smith, D. M., & Atkinson, R. M. (1995). Alcoholism and dementia. *International Journal of Addictions, 30*(13–14), 1843–1869.

Smith, G. C. (2004). Predictors of the stage of residential planning among aging families of adults with severe mental illness. *Psychiatric Services, 55*(7), 804–810.

Smith, G. C., Clarke, D. M., Handrinos, D., & Dunsis, A. (1998). Consultation–liaison psychiatrists management of depression. *Psychosomatics, 39*(3), 244–252.

Smith, M. T., Perlis, M. L., Park, A., Smith, M. S., Pennington, J., Giles, D. E., et al. (2002). Comparative meta-analysis of pharmacotherapy and behavior therapy for persistent insomnia. *American Journal of Psychiatry, 159*(1), 5–11.

Smyer, M. A. (1989). Nursing homes as a setting for psychological practice. *American Psychologist, 44,* 1307–1314.

Smyer, M. A., Cohn, M. D., & Brannon, D. (1988). *Mental health consultation in nursing homes.* New York: New York University Press.

Smyer, M. A., Zarit, S. H., & Qualls, S. H. (1990). Psychological intervention with aging individuals. In J. E. Birren & K. W. Schaie (Eds.), *Handbook of the psychology of aging* (3rd ed., pp. 375–403). San Diego, CA: Academic Press.

Snowdon, D. A., Greiner, L. H., Mortimer, J. A., Riley, K. P., Greiner, P. A., & Markesbery, W. R. (1997). Brain infarction and the clinical expression of Alzheimer disease: The nun study. *Journal of the American Medical Association, 277,* 813–817.

Solomon, P. R., Hirschoff, A., Kelly, B., Relin, M., Breush, M., DeVeaux, R. D., et al. (1998). A 7 minute neurocognitive screening battery highly sensitive to Alzheimer's disease. *Archives of Neurology, 55*(3), 349–355.

Somboontanont, W., Sloane, P. D., Floyd, F. J., Holditch-Davis, D., Hogue, C. C., & Mitchel, C. M. (2004). Assaultive behavior in Alzheimer's disease: Identifying immediate antecedents during bathing. *Journal of Gerontological Nursing, 30*(9), 22–29.

Spayd, C., & Smyer, M. A. (1996). Psychological interventions in nursing homes. In S. H. Zarit & B. G. Knight (Eds.), *A guide to psychotherapy and aging: Effective clinical interventions in a life-stage context* (pp. 241–268). Washington, DC: American Psychological Association.

Spector, A., Orrell, M., Davies, S., & Woods, B. (2000). Reality orientation for dementia. *Cochrane Database Systematic Review, 17*(3), 247–253.

Spector, A., Thorgrimsen, L., Woods, B., Royan, L., Davies, S., Butterworth, M., et al. (2003). Efficacy of an evidence-based cognitive stimulation therapy programme for people with dementia: Randomised controlled trial. *British Journal of Psychiatry, 183,* 248–254.

Sperber, K., & Shao, L. (2003). Neurologic consequences of HIV infection in the era of HAART. *AIDS Patient Care STDS, 17*(10), 509–518.

Spreen, D., & Strauss, E. (1991). *A compendium of neuropsychological tests.* New York: Oxford University Press.

Squire, L. R. (1974). Remote memory as affected by aging. *Neuropsychologia, 12,* 429–435.

St. George-Hyslop, P. H., Haines, J. L., Farrer, L. A., Polinsky, R., Van Broeckhoven, C., Goate, A., et al. (1990). Genetic linkage studies suggest that Alzheimer's disease is not a single homogeneous disorder. *Nature, 347,* 194–197.

St. George-Hyslop, P. H., Tanzi, R. E., Polinsky, R. J., Haines, J. L., Nee, L., Watkins, P. C., et al. (1987). The genetic defect causing familial Alzheimer's disease maps on chromosome 21. *Science, 235,* 885–890.

Stanford, E. P., & Usita, P. M. (2002). Retirement: Who is at risk? *Generations, 26*(2), 45–48.

Stanley, M. A., & Beck, J. G. (2000). Anxiety disorders. *Clinical Psychology Review, 20*(6), 731–754.

Stanley, M. A., Diefenbach, G. J., & Hopko, D. R. (2004). Cognitive behavioral treatment for older adults with generalized anxiety disorder: A therapist manual for primary care settings. *Behavioral Modification, 28*(1), 73–117.

Stanley, M. A., Hopko, D. R., Diefenbach, G. J., Bourland, S. L., Rodriguez, H., & Wagener, P. (2003). Cognitive-behavior therapy for late-life generalized anxiety disorder in primary care: Preliminary findings. *American Journal of Geriatric Psychiatry, 11*(1), 92–96.

Staudinger, U. M. (1999). Older and wiser?: Integrating results on the relationship between age and wisdom-related performance. *International Journal of Behavioral Development, 23*, 641–664.

Staudinger, U. M., & Baltes, P. B. (1996). Interactive minds: A facilitative setting for wisdom-related performance? *Journal of Personality and Social Psychology, 71*, 746–762.

Staudinger, U. M., Lopez, D. F., & Baltes, P. B. (1997). The psychometric location of wisdom-related performance. *Personality and Social Psychology Bulletin, 23*, 1200–1214.

Staudinger, U. M., Marsiske, M., & Baltes, P. B. (1995). Resilience and reserve capacity in later adulthood: Potentials and limits of development across the life span. In D. Cicchetti & D. J. Cohen (Eds.), *Developmental psychopathology: Vol. 2. Risk, disorder, and adaptation* (pp. 801–847). New York: Wiley.

Stek, M. L., Gussekloo, J., Beekman, A. T., van Tilburg, W., & Westendorp, R. G. (2004). Prevalence, correlates and recognition of depression in the oldest old: The Leiden 85–plus study. *Journal of Affective Disorders, 78*(3), 193–200.

Stephenson, J. (1997). Researchers find evidence of a new gene for late-onset Alzheimer disease. *Journal of the American Medical Association, 277*, 775.

Stern, Y., Gurland, B., Tatemichi, T., Tang, M., Wilder, D., & Mayeux, R. (1994). Influence of education and occupation on the incidence of Alzheimer's disease. *Journal of the American Medical Association, 271*, 1004–1010.

Stokes, G. (1996). Challenging behaviour in dementia: A psychological approach. In R. T. Woods (Ed.), *Handbook of the clinical psychology of ageing* (pp. 601–628). New York: Wiley.

Stone, M., & Stone, H. (2004). *Too young to retire: 101 ways to start the rest of your life.* New York: Plume Books.

Stone, R., Cafferata, G. L., & Sangl, J. (1987). Caregivers of the frail elderly: A national profile. *Gerontologist, 27*, 616–626.

Storandt, M., Botwinick, J., Danziger, W. L., Berg, L., & Hughes, C. P. (1984). Psychometric differentiation of mild senile dementia of the Alzheimer type. *Archives of Neurology, 41*, 497–499.

Storandt, M., & Hill, R. D. (1989). Very mild senile dementia of the Alzheimer type. *Archives of Neurology, 46*, 383–386.

Strassburger, T. L., Lee, H. C., Daly, E. M., Szczepanik, J., Krasuski, J. S., Mentis, M. J., et al. (1997). Interactive effects of age and hypertension on volumes of brain structures. *Stroke, 28*, 1410–1417.

Strauss, J. S. (1987). Schizophrenia and aging: Meeting point of diagnosis and conceptual questions. In N. E. Miller & G. D. Cohen (Eds.), *Schizophrenia and aging:*

Schizophrenia, paranoia, and schizophreniform disorders in later life (pp. 3–8). New York: Guilford Press.

Sultzer, D., Levin, H. S., Mahler, M. E., High, W. M., & Cummings, J. L. (1993). A comparison of psychiatric symptoms in vascular dementia and Alzheimer's disease. *American Journal of Psychiatry, 15*, 1806–1812.

Sunderland, T., Lawlor, B. A., Martinez, R., & Molchan, S. (1991). Anxiety in the elderly: Neurobiological and clinical interface. In C. Salzman & B. Lebowitz (Eds.), *Anxiety in the elderly* (pp. 105–130). New York: Springer.

Swartz, K. L. (2005). *The Johns Hopkins white papers: Depression and anxiety.* Baltimore: Johns Hopkins Medical Institutions.

Swartz, K. L., & Margolis, S. (2004). The *Johns Hopkins white papers: Depression and anxiety.* Baltimore: Johns Hopkins Medical Institutions.

Swearer, J. M., O'Donnell, B. F., Drachman, D. A., & Woodward, B. M. (1992). Neuro-psychological features of familial Alzheimer's disease. *Annals of Neurology, 32*(5), 687–694.

Swearer, J. M., O'Donnell, B. F., Ingram, S. M., & Drachman, D. A. (1996). Rate of progression in familial Alzheimer's disease. *Journal of Geriatric Psychiatry and Neurology, 9*(1), 22–25.

Takkinen, S., Gold, C., Pedersen, N. L., Malmberg, B., Nilsson, S., & Rovine, M. (2004). Gender differences in depression: A study of older unlike-sex twins. *Aging and Mental Health, 8*(3), 187–195.

Task Force on Benzodiazepine Dependency. (1990). *Benzodiazepine dependence, toxicity and abuse.* Washington, DC: American Psychiatric Association.

Teaster, P. B., & Roberto, K. A. (2004). Sexual abuse of older adults: APS cases and outcomes. *Gerontologist, 44*(6), 788–796.

Teri, L., Gibbons, L. E., McCurry, S. M., Logsdon, R. G., Buchner, D. M., Barlow, W. E., et al. (2003). Exercise plus behavioral management in patients with Alzheimer's disease: A randomized controlled trial. *Journal of the American Medical Association, 290*(15), 2015–2022.

Teri, L., Hughes, J., & Larson, E. (1990). Cognitive deterioration in Alzheimer's disease: Behavioral and health factors. *Journal of Gerontology, 45*, 58–63.

Teri, L., & Lewinsohn, P. M. (1982). Modification of the pleasant and unpleasant events schedules for use with the elderly. *Journal of Consulting and Clinical Psychology, 50*, 444–445.

Teri, L., & Logsdon, R. G. (1991). Identifying pleasant activities for Alzheimer's disease patients: The Pleasant Events Schedule—AD. *Gerontologist, 31*, 124–127.

Teri, L., Logsdon, R. G., Peskind, E., Raskind, M., Weinerm M. F., Tractenberg, R. E., et al. (2000). Treatment of agitation in AD: A randomized, placebo-controlled clinical trial. *Neurology, 55*(9), 1271–1278.

Teri, L., Logsdon, R. G., Uomoto, J., & McCurry, S. M. (1997). Behavioral treatment of depression in dementia patients: A controlled clinical trial. *Journal of Gerontology: Psychological Sciences, 52B*(4), 159–166.

Teri, L., & Truax, P. (1994). Assessment of depression in dementia patients: Association of caregiver mood with depression ratings. *Gerontologist, 34*, 213–234.

Teri, L., & Wagner, A. (1992). Alzheimer's disease and depression. *Journal of Consulting and Clinical Psychology, 60*, 379–391.

Terry, R. D., & Katzman, R. (1983). Senile dementia of the Alzheimer's type. *Annals of Neurology, 14*, 153–176.

Thal, L. J., Thomas, R. G., Mulnard, R., Sano, M., Grundman, M., & Schneider, L. (2003). Estrogen levels do not correlate with improvement in cognition. *Archives of Neurology, 60*, 209–212.

Thomas, V. S., & Rockwood, K. J. (2001). Alcohol abuse, cognitive impairment, and mortality among older people. *Journal of the American Geriatrics Society, 49*(4), 415–420.

Thomasma, D. C. (1992). Mercy killing of elderly people with dementia: A counter-proposal. In R. H. Binstock, S. G. Post, & P. J. Whitehouse (Eds.), *Dementia and aging: Ethics, values and policy choices* (pp. 101–117). Baltimore: Johns Hopkins University Press.

Thompson, L. W., Coon, D. W., Gallagher-Thompson, D., Sommer, B. R., & Koin, D. (2001). Comparison of desipramine and cognitive/behavioral therapy in the treatment of elderly outpatients with mild-to-moderate depression. *American Journal of Geriatric Psychiatry, 9*(3), 225–240.

Thompson, L. W., Gallagher, D., Nies, G., & Epstein, D. (1983). Evaluation of the effectiveness of professionals and nonprofessionals as instructors of "coping with depression" classes for elders. *Gerontologist, 23*, 390–396.

Thompson, L. W., Kaye, J. L., Tang, P. C. Y., & Gallagher-Thompson, D. (2004). Bereavement and adjustment disorders. In D. G. Blazer, D. C. Steffens, & E. W. Busse (Eds.), *Textbook of geriatric psychiatry* (3rd ed., pp. 319–338). Arlington, VA: American Psychiatric Publishing.

Thurstone, L. L., & Thurstone, T. G. (1949). *Examiner manual for the SRA Primary Abilities Test*. Chicago: Science Research Associates.

Tiemeier, H., van Dijck, W., Hofman, A., Witteman, J. C., Stijnen, T., & Breteler, M. M. (2004). Relationship between atherosclerosis and late-life depression: The Rotterdam Study. *Archives of General Psychiatry, 61*(4), 369–376.

Tombaugh, T. N., & McIntyre, N. J. (1992). The Mini-Mental State Examination: A comprehensive review. *Journal of the American Geriatrics Society, 40*, 922–935.

Toseland, R. W., Rossiter, C. M., Peak, T., & Smith, G. C. (1990). Comparative effectiveness of individual and group interventions to support family caregivers. *Social Work, 35*, 209–217.

Treas, J. (1995). Older Americans in the 1990s and beyond. *Population Bulletin, 50*(2), 1–45.

Troll, L. E., & Skaff, M. M. (1997). Perceived continuity of self in very old age. *Psychology and Aging, 12*, 162–169.

Trzepacz, P. T., & Dew, M. A. (1995). Further analyses of the delirium rating scale. *General Hospital Psychiatry, 17*, 75–79.

Tsuang, M. T. (1986). Predictors of poor and good outcome in schizophrenia. In L. Erlenmeyer-Kimling & N. E. Miller (Eds.), *Life-span research on the prediction of psychopathology* (pp. 195–203). Hillsdale NJ: Erlbaum.

Tune, L. E. (1991). Postoperative delirium. *International Psychogeriatrics, 3*, 325–332.

Tune, L. E., & Folstein, M. F. (1986). Post-operative delirium. *Advances in Psychosomatic Medicine, 15*, 51–68.

Tuokko, H., & Frerichs, R. J. (2000). Cognitive impairment with no dementia (CIND): Longitudinal studies, the findings, and the issues. *Clinical Neuropsychology, 14*(4), 504–525.

Tuokko, H., Hadjistavropoulos, T., Miller, J. A., & Beattie, B. L. (1992). The clock test: A sensitive measure to differentiate normal elderly from those with Alzheimer disease. *Journal of the American Geriatrics Society, 40,* 579–584.

Tuokko, H., Kristjansson, E., & Miller, J. (1995). Neuropsychological detection of dementia: An overview of the neuropsychological component of the Canadian Study of Health and Aging. *Journal of Clinical and Experimental Neuropsychology, 17,* 352–373.

Tuokko, H., Tallman, K., Beattie, B. L., Cooper, P., & Weir, J. (1995). An examination of driving records in a dementia clinic. *Journals of Gerontology: Social Sciences, 50B,* S173–S181.

Tyrer, P. (1995). Are personality disorders well classified in DSM-IV? In W. J. Livesley (Ed.), *The DSM-IV personality disorders* (pp. 29–44). New York: Guilford Press.

Tyrer, P., & Seivewright, H. (1988). Studies of outcome. In P. Tyrer (Ed.), *Personality disorders: Diagnosis, management and course* (pp. 119–136). London: Wright.

Uc, E. Y., Rizzo, M., Anderson, S. W., Shi, Q., & Dawson, J. D. (2004). Driver route-following and safety errors in early Alzheimer disease. *Neurology, 63*(5), 832–837.

Uhlmann, R. F., & Larson, E. B. (1991). Effect of education on the Mini-Mental State Examination as a screening test for dementia. *Journal of the American Geriatrics Society, 39,* 876–880.

U.S. Census Bureau. (1998). *Marital status and living arrangements: March 1998.* Washington, DC: Author.

U.S. Census Bureau. (2003). *Statistical abstract of the United States.* Washington, DC: Author.

U.S. Department of Health and Human Services. (2003). *Health, United States, 2003, special excerpt: Trend tables on 65 and older population* (DHHS Publication No. 2004–0152). Hyattsville, MD: Author.

Vaillant, G. E., & Vaillant, C. O. (1990). Natural history of male psychological health: 12. A 45-year study of predictors of successful aging. *American Journal of Psychiatry, 147,* 31–37.

Van Everbroeck, B., Dobbeleir, I., De Waele, M., De Deyn, P., Martin, J. J., & Cras, P. (2004). Differential diagnosis of 201 possible Creutzfeldt–Jakob disease patients. *Journal of Neurology, 251*(3), 298–304.

Van Gorp, W. G., Satz, P., Kiersch, M. E., & Henry, R. (1986). Normative data on the Boston Naming Test for a group of normal older adults. *Journal of Clinical and Experimental Neuropsychology, 8,* 702–705.

Verbrugge, L. M. (1984). Longer life but worsening health? Trends in health and mortality of middle-aged and older persons. *Milbank Memorial Fund Quarterly/ Health and Society, 62,* 474–519.

Vinters, H. V. (2001). Aging and the human nervous system. In J. E. Birren & K. W. Schaie (Eds.), *Handbook of the psychology of aging* (5th ed., pp. 135–160). San Diego, CA: Academic Press.

Vitaliano, P. P., Persson, R., Kiyak, A., Saini, H., & Echeverria, D. (2005). Caregiving and gingival symptom reports: Psychophysiologic mediators. *Psychosomatic Medicine, 67*(6), 930–938.

Vitaliano, P. P., Zhang, J., & Scanlan, J. M. (2003). Is caregiving hazardous to one's physical health? A meta-analysis. *Psychological Bulletin, 129*(6), 946–972.

Walsh, D., Till, R. E., & Williams, M. V. (1978). Age differences in peripheral perceptual processing: A monoptic backward masking investigation. *Journal of Experimental Psychology: Human Perception and Performance, 4,* 232–243.

Wang, X., DeKosky, S. T., Ikonomovic, M. D., & Kamboh, M. I. (2002). Distribution of plasma alpha 1–antichymotrypsin levels in Alzheimer disease patients and controls and their genetic controls. *Neurobiology and Aging, 23*(3), 377–382.

Watson, L. C., Garrett, J. M., Sloane, P. D., Gruber-Baldini, A. L., & Zimmerman, S. (2003). Depression in assisted living: Results from a four-state study. *American Journal of Geriatric Psychiatry, 11*(5), 534–542.

Watson, Y. I., Arfken, C. L., & Birge, S. J. (1993). Clock competition: An objective screening test for dementia. *Journal of the American Geriatrics Society, 41,* 1235–1240.

Wechsler, D. (1958). *The measurement and appraisal of adult intelligence.* Baltimore: Williams & Wilkins.

Wechsler, D. (1981). *Manual for Wechsler Adult Intelligence Scale—Revised.* New York: Psychological Corporation.

Wechsler, D. (1987). *Wechsler Memory Scale—Revised.* San Antonio, TX: Psychological Corporation.

Wechsler, D. (1997a). *WAIS-III: Administration and scoring manual.* San Antonio, TX: Psychological Corporation.

Wechsler, D. (1997b). *Wechsler Memory Scale* (3rd ed). San Antonio, TX: Psychological Corporation.

Wechsler, D. (2001). *Wechsler Test of Adult Reading (WTAR).* San Antonio, TX: Harcourt Assessment.

Weihs, K. L., Settle, E. C., Jr., Batey, S. R., Houser, T. L., Donahue, R. M., & Ascher, J. A. (2000). Bupropion sustained release versus paroxetine for the treatment of depression in the elderly. *Journal of Clinical Psychiatry, 61*(3), 196–202.

Weinstein, E. A., & Kahn, R. L. (1955). *Denial of illness: Symbolic and physiological aspects.* Springfield, IL: Thomas.

Weissman, M. M., Leaf, P. J., Tischler, G. L., Blazer, D. G., Karno, M., Bruce, M. L., et al. (1988). Affective disorders in five United States communities. *Psychological Medicine, 18,* 141–153.

Weissman, M. M., & Myers, J. K. (1978). Affective disorders in a U.S. urban community. *Archives of General Psychiatry, 35,* 1304–1311.

Wells, C. (1979). Pseudodementia. *American Journal of Psychiatry, 136,* 895–900.

Welsh, K., Butters, N., Hughes, J., Mohs, R., & Heyman, A. (1991). Detection of abnormal memory decline in mild cases of Alzheimer's disease using CERAD neuropsychological measures. *Archives of Neurology, 48,* 278–281.

Werner, E. E. (2001). *Journeys from childhood to midlife: Risk, resilience, and recovery.* Ithaca, NY: Cornell University Pres.

Wetherell, J. L., Gatz, M., & Craske, M. G. (2003). Treatment of generalized anxiety disorder in older adults. *Journal of Consulting and Clinical Psychology, 71*(1), 31–40.

Wetherell, J. L., Gatz, M., & Pedersen, N. L. (2001). A longitudinal analysis of anxiety and depressive symptoms. *Psychology and Aging, 16*(2), 187–195.

Wetherell, J. L., Sorrell, J. T., Thorp, S. R., & Patterson, T. L. (2005). Psychological interventions for late-life anxiety: A review and early lessons from the CALM study. *Journal of Geriatric Psychiatry and Neurology, 18*(2), 72–82.

White, P. D. (1992). Essays in the aftermath of Cruzan. *Journal of Medicine and Philosophy, 17*, 563–571.

Whitlatch, C. J., Judge, K., Zarit, S. H., & Femia, E. E. (in press). A dyadic intervention for family caregivers and care receivers in early stage dementia. *Gerontologist.*

Whitlatch, C. J., & Zarit, S. H. (1988). Sexual dysfunction in an aged married couple: A case study of a behavioral intervention. *Clinical Gerontologist, 8*, 43–62.

Whitlatch, C. J., Zarit, S. H., Goodwin, P. E., & von Eye, A. (1995). Influence of the success of psychoeducational interventions on the course of family care. *Clinical Gerontologist, 16*, 17–30.

Whitlatch, C. J., Zarit, S. H., & von Eye, A. (1991). Efficacy of interventions with caregivers: A reanalysis. *Gerontologist, 31*, 9–14.

Whitmer, R. A., Gunderson, E. P., Barrett-Connor, E., Quesenberry, C. P., Jr., & Yaffe, K. (2005). Obesity in middle age and future risk of dementia: A 27-year longitudinal population-based study. *British Medical Journal, 330*(7504), 1360.

Whyte, E. M., Mulsant, B. H., Vanderbilt, J., Dodge, H. H., & Ganguli, M. (2004). Depression after stroke: A prospective epidemiological study. *Journal of the American Geriatrics Society, 52*(5), 774–778.

Widiger, T. A. (2005). A dimensional model of psychopathology. *Psychopathology, 38*(4), 211–214.

Widiger, T. A., & Sanderson C. J. (1995). Toward a dimensional model of personality disorders. In W. J. Livesley (Ed.), *The DSM-IV personality disorders* (pp. 433–458). New York: Guilford Press.

Widiger, T. A., & Simonsen, E. (2005). Alternative dimensional models of personality disorder: Finding a common ground. *Journal of Personality Disorders, 19*(2), 110–130.

Wilcox, S., Evenson, K. R., Aragaki, A., Wassertheil-Smoller, S., Mouton, C. P., & Loevinger B. L. (2003). The effects of widowhood on physical and mental health, health behaviors, and health outcomes: The women's health initiative. *Health Psychology, 22*(5), 513–522.

Willis, S. L. (1996). Assessing everyday competence in the cognitively challenged elderly. In M. Smyer, K. W. Schaie, & M. B. Kapp (Eds.), *Older adults' decision-making and the law* (pp. 87–127). New York: Springer.

Willis, S. L., Blieszner, R., & Baltes, P. B. (1981). Intellectual training research in aging: Modification of performance on the fluid ability of figural relations. *Journal of Educational Psychology, 73*, 41–50.

Willis, S. L., & Nesselroade, C. S. (1990). Long-term effects of fluid ability training in old-old age. *Developmental Psychology, 26*, 905–910.

Wilson, R. S., Kaszniak, A. W., Bacon, L. D., Fox, J. H., & Kelly, M. P. (1982). Facial recognition in dementia. *Cortex, 18*, 329–336.

Wisocki, P. A. (Ed.). (1991). *Handbook of clinical behavior therapy with the elderly client.* New York: Plenum Press.

Witte, K. L., Freund, J. S., & Brown-Whistler, S. (1993). Age differences in free recall and category clustering. *Experimental Aging Research, 19*, 15–28.

Woods, B. (1999). The person in dementia care. *Generations, 23*(3), 35–39.

Woods, R. T. (1996). Psychological "therapies" in dementia. In R. T. Woods (Ed.), *Handbook of the clinical psychology of ageing* (pp. 575–600). New York: Wiley.

Yale, R. (1991). *A guide to facilitating support groups for newly diagnosed Alzheimer's patients.* San Francisco: Alzheimer's Association.

Yale, R. (1999, Fall). Support groups and other services for individuals with early-stage Alzheimer's Disease. *Generations, 23,* 57–61.

Yesavage, J. A. (1983). Imagery pretraining and memory training in the elderly. *Gerontology, 29,* 271–275.

Yesavage, J. A., & Jacob, R. (1984). Effects of relaxation and mnemonics on memory, attention and anxiety in the elderly. *Experimental Aging Research, 10,* 211–214.

Young, J. E. (1994). *Cognitive therapy for personality disorders: A schema-focused approach* (Rev. ed.). Sarasota, FL: Professional Resource Exchange.

Zarit, J. M., & Zarit, S. H. (1996). Ethical considerations in the treatment of older adults. In S. H. Zarit & B. G. Knight (Eds.), *A guide to psychotherapy and aging* (pp. 269–284) Washington, DC: American Psychological Association.

Zarit, S. H. (1996). Clinical interventions for family caregiving. In S. H. Zarit & B. G. Knight (Eds.), *A guide to psychotherapy and aging* (pp. 139–162). Washington, DC: American Psychological Association.

Zarit, S. H., Dolan, M. M., & Leitsch, S. A. (1998). Interventions in nursing homes and other alternative living settings. In I. H. Nordhus, G. VandenBos, S. Berg, & P. Fromholt (Eds.), *Clinical geropsychology* (pp. 329–344). Washington, DC: American Psychological Association.

Zarit, S. H., Femia, E. E., Johansson, B., & Gatz, M. (1999). Prevalence and incidence of depression in 80- and 90-year-olds: The OCTO study. *Aging and Mental Health, 3,* 119–128.

Zarit, S. H., Femia, E. E., Watson, J., Rice-Oeschger, L., & Kakos, B. (2004). Memory Club: A group intervention for people with early-stage dementia and their care partners. *Gerontologist, 44,* 262–269.

Zarit, S. H., Johansson, B., & Malmberg, B. (1995). Changes in functional competency in the oldest old: A longitudinal study. *Journal of Aging and Health, 7,* 3–23.

Zarit, S. H., Orr, N. K., & Zarit, J. M. (1985). *The hidden victims of Alzheimer's disease: Families under stress.* New York: New York University Press.

Zarit, S. H., Stephens, M. A. P., Townsend, A., & Greene, R. (1998). Stress reduction for family caregivers: Effects of adult day care use. *Journals of Gerontology: Social Sciences, 53B,* S267–S277.

Zarit, S. H., Stephens, M. A. P., Townsend, A., Greene, R., & Leitsch, S. A. (1999). Patterns of adult day service use by family caregivers: A comparison of brief versus sustained use. *Family Relations, 48,* 355–361.

Zarit, S. H., Todd, P. A., & Zarit, J. M. (1986). Subjective burden of husbands and wives as caregivers: A longitudinal study. *Gerontologist, 26,* 260–270.

Zarit, S. H., & Whitlatch, C. J. (1992). Institutional placement: Phases of the transition. *Gerontologist, 32,* 665–672.

Zarit, S. H., & Zarit, J. M. (1982). Families under stress: Interventions for caregivers of senile dementia patients. *Psychotherapy: Theory, Research and Practice, 19,* 461–471.

Zarit, S. H., Zarit, J. M., & Reever, K. E. (1982). Memory training for severe memory loss: Effects on senile dementia patients and their families. *Gerontologist, 22,* 373–377.

Zarit, S. H., Zarit, J. M., & Rosenberg-Thompson, S. (1990). A special treatment unit for Alzheimer's disease: Medical, behavioral, and environmental features. *Clinical Gerontologist, 9,* 47–63.

Zeiss, A. M., Lewinsohn, P. M., Rohde, P., & Seeley, J. R. (1996). Relationship of physical disease and functional impairment to depression in older people. *Psychology of Aging, 11*(4), 572–581.

Zeiss, A. M., & Steffen, A. (1996). Behavioral and cognitive treatments: Social learning in older adults. In S. H. Zarit & R. Knight (Eds.), *A guide to psychotherapy and aging* (pp. 35–60). New York: American Psychological Association.

Zelinski, E. M., & Burnight, K. P. (1997). Sixteen-year longitudinal and time lag change in memory and cognition in older adults. *Psychology and Aging, 12,* 503–513.

Zelinski, E. M., Crimmins, E., Reynolds, S., & Seeman, T. (1998). Do medical conditions affect cognition in older adults? *Health Psychology, 17,* 504–512.

Zgola, J. M. (1987). *Doing things: A guide to programming activities for persons with Alzheimer's disease and related disorders.* Baltimore: Johns Hopkins University Press.

Zgola, J. M. (1999). *Care that works: A relationship approach to persons with dementia.* Baltimore: Johns Hopkins University Press.

Zimmerman, S., & Sloane, P. D. (1999). Optimum residential care for people with dementia. *Generations, 23*(3), 62–68.

Zimmerman, S., Sloane, P. D., Eckert, J. K., Gruber-Baldini, A. L., Morgan, L. A., Hebel, J. R., et al. (2005). How good is assisted living?: Findings and implications from an outcomes study. *Journals of Gerontology: Social Science, 60*(4), S195–S204.

Zimmerman, S., Sloane, P. D., Heck, E., Maslow, K., & Schulz, R. (2005). Introduction: Dementia care and quality of life in assisted living and nursing homes. *Gerontologist, 45*(1), 5–7.

Zisook, S., Shuchter, S. R., Sledge, P. A., Paulus, M., & Judd, L. L. (1994). The spectrum of depressive phenomena after spousal bereavement. *Journal of Clinical Psychiatry, 55*(Suppl.), 29–36.

Zweig, R. A., & Hillman, J. (1999). Personality disorders in adults: A review. In E. Rosowsky, R. C. Abrams, & R. A. Zweig (Eds.), *Personality disorders in older adults: Emerging issues in diagnosis and treatment* (pp. 31–53). Mahwah, NJ: Erlbaum.

Zweig, R. A., & Hinrichsen, G. A. (1993). Factors associated with suicide attempts by depressed older adults: A prospective study. *American Journal of Psychiatry, 150,* 1687–1692.

Index

Page numbers followed by *f* indicate figure, *t* indicate table.

451